Orthopaedics

PreTest®
Self-Assessment
and Review

• NOTICE •

Orthopaedics

PreTest®
Self-Assessment and Review

Frank C. Wilson, M.D.
Kenan Professor of Surgery
Chief, Division of Orthopaedics
University of North Carolina School of Medicine
Chapel Hill, North Carolina

Douglas R. Dirschl, M.D.
Assistant Professor of Surgery
Division of Orthopaedics
University of North Carolina School of Medicine
Chapel Hill, North Carolina

McGraw-Hill
Health Professions Division
PreTest® Series

New York St. Louis San Francisco Auckland
Bogotá Caracas Lisbon London Madrid
Mexico City Milan Montreal New Delhi
San Juan Singapore Sydney Tokyo Toronto

McGraw-Hill
A Division of The ***McGraw-Hill*** *Companies*

Orthopaedics: PreTest® Self-Assessment and Review

1 2 3 4 5 6 7 8 9 MALMAL 9 9 8 7 6 5

ISBN 0-07-052076-3

The editors were Gail Gavert and Bruce MacGregor.
The production supervisors were Clara B. Stanley and Anna Lieggi.
This book was set in Times Roman by Digitype.
Malloy Lithographers was printer and binder.
This book is printed on acid-free paper.

Library of Congress Cataloging-in-Publication Data

Orthopaedics : PreTest self-assessment and review / Frank C. Wilson, Douglas R. Dirschl.
p. cm.
Includes bibliographical references.
ISBN 0-07-052076-3 (alk. paper)
1. Orthopedics—Examinations, questions, etc. I. Wilson, Frank C. II. Dirschl, Douglas R.
[DNLM: 1. Orthopedics—examination questions. WE 18.2 O67 1996]
RD732.6.0778 1996
617.3′0076—dc20
DNLM/DLC
for Library of Congress 95–21405

Contents

Contributors

H. Robert Brashear, M.D.
Emeritus Professor of Surgery
Division of Orthopaedics
University of North Carolina School of Medicine
Chapel Hill, North Carolina

Donald K. Bynum, M.D.
Associate Professor of Surgery
Division of Orthopaedics
University of North Carolina School of Medicine
Chapel Hill, North Carolina

Joseph T. Minchew, M.D.
Assistant Professor of Surgery
Division of Orthopaedics
University of North Carolina School of Medicine
Chapel Hill, North Carolina

Acknowledgments

No work such as this can be produced without the assistance of many people, and as we see this text come to print, we must acknowledge those to whom we are most indebted. Gail Gavert was thoughtful enough to give us the opportunity to work on this project, patient enough to work within our timetable, and kind enough to allow an adequate number of figures to make this text useful. We owe much to the contributors, who took time from busy clinical and academic schedules to provide questions and illustrations of the highest quality.

Special thanks are due J. Vincent Brown, who was responsible for nearly all the medical photography for this work, and to Jennifer Wilson, who drew the line art. We would also like to thank Robin Clark and Rockell Landry for their diligence and patience in the transcription of dictation and preparation of the manuscript.

Frank C. Wilson, M.D.
Douglas R. Dirschl, M.D.

Introduction

Orthopaedics: PreTest® Self-Assessment and Review is intended to provide both resident and practicing orthopaedists with a convenient instrument for self-evaluation and review in the areas of general and subspecialty orthopaedic practice. We hope the text will be helpful to residents preparing for the Orthopaedic In-Training Examination and Part I of the American Board of Orthopaedic Surgery Certifying Examination, as well as to board-certified orthopaedists preparing for recertification. Study of this review text should help the reader assess his or her knowledge of general and subspecialty orthopaedics, identify areas that require further study, and provide information on the chosen subjects.

The questions in this text are formatted to resemble those on the Orthopaedic In-Training Examination, which is composed of one best answer and matching set types of multiple-choice questions. The orthopaedic conditions covered and the weighting of the various subspecialty areas also correspond roughly to those on recent In-Training Examinations. We have used figures where we felt them necessary to make important teaching points and where the radiographic appearance was crucial to answering the question correctly. Each question has a corresponding answer, explanation, and reference.

No single source, no matter how comprehensive, can thoroughly cover every aspect of a field as broad as orthopaedics. This text is no exception and is intended as a guide. Should the reader feel the need for a more extensive discussion of the subject matter, he or she should consult the references listed in the bibliography or other textbooks and journals of orthopaedics.

The editors as well as the McGraw-Hill/PreTest® staff would be happy to receive your comments and suggestions.

Orthopaedics

PreTest®
Self-Assessment
and Review

Anatomy and Biomechanics

Douglas R. Dirschl, M.D.

DIRECTIONS: Each question below contains five suggested responses. Select the **one best** response to each question.

1. In the anterior surgical approach to the cervical spine, the sympathetic chain and stellate ganglion lie

(A) adjacent to the carotid sheath
(B) posterior to the longus colli muscle
(C) anterior to the longus colli muscle
(D) anterior to the longus capitis muscle
(E) anterior to the sternohyoid muscle

2. The cricoid cartilage lies opposite which vertebral level?

(A) C3
(B) C4
(C) C5
(D) C6
(E) C7

3. The greater occipital nerve exits the spine at which of the following vertebral levels?

(A) Occiput-C1
(B) C1-C2
(C) C2-C3
(D) C3-C4
(E) C4-C5

4. Which of the following statements most accurately describes the innervation and function of the right sternocleidomastoid muscle?

(A) Innervated by the spinal accessory nerve and branches of the ansa cervicalis; rotates the head to the left
(B) Innervated by the spinal accessory nerve and branches of the ansa cervicalis; rotates the head to the right
(C) Innervated by the spinal accessory nerve; rotates the head to the left
(D) Innervated by the spinal accessory nerve; rotates the head to the right
(E) Innervated by branches of the ansa cervicalis; rotates the head to the left

5. Which of the following muscles is innervated by the superficial peroneal nerve?

(A) Tibialis anterior
(B) Extensor hallucis longus
(C) Peroneus longus
(D) Peroneus tertius
(E) Extensor digitorum longus

6. In a posterolateral approach to the femur for fixation of an intertrochanteric fracture, bleeding is encountered as the vastus lateralis muscle is dissected from the linea aspera. The bleeding vessels are most likely branches of which of the following arteries?

(A) Medial femoral circumflex
(B) Transverse branch of the lateral femoral circumflex
(C) Deep femoral
(D) Superficial femoral
(E) Descending branch of the lateral femoral circumflex

7. Which of the following muscles is innervated by the peroneal division of the sciatic nerve?

(A) Biceps femoris, long head
(B) Biceps femoris, short head
(C) Semimembranosus
(D) Semitendinosus
(E) Adductor magnus

8. All the following structures have attachment to the medial femoral condyle EXCEPT the

(A) adductor magnus
(B) gastrocnemius, medial head
(C) popliteus
(D) superficial medial collateral ligament
(E) patellofemoral ligament

9. Which of the following most accurately describes the innervation and action of the popliteus muscle?

(A) Innervation by the common peroneal nerve; flexion of the knee and medial rotation of the femur on the tibia
(B) Innervation by the tibial nerve; flexion of the knee and lateral rotation of the femur on the tibia
(C) Innervation by the common peroneal nerve; flexion of the knee, medial rotation of the femur on the tibia, and retraction of the lateral meniscus
(D) Innervation by the tibial nerve; flexion of the knee, lateral rotation of the femur on the tibia, and retraction of the lateral meniscus
(E) Innervation by the tibial nerve; flexion of the knee, medial rotation of the femur on the tibia, and retraction of the lateral meniscus

10. During an anterolateral (Watson-Jones) approach to the hip, bleeding when the reflected head of the rectus femoris is detached from the joint capsule most likely indicates injury to which of the following arteries?

(A) Profunda femoris
(B) Medial femoral circumflex
(C) Ascending branch of the lateral femoral circumflex
(D) Transverse branch of the lateral femoral circumflex
(E) Common femoral

11. All the following structures are supplied by a branch of the obturator artery EXCEPT the

(A) obturator internus muscle
(B) obturator externus muscle
(C) pectineus muscle
(D) transverse acetabular ligament
(E) ligamentum teres

Questions 12–13

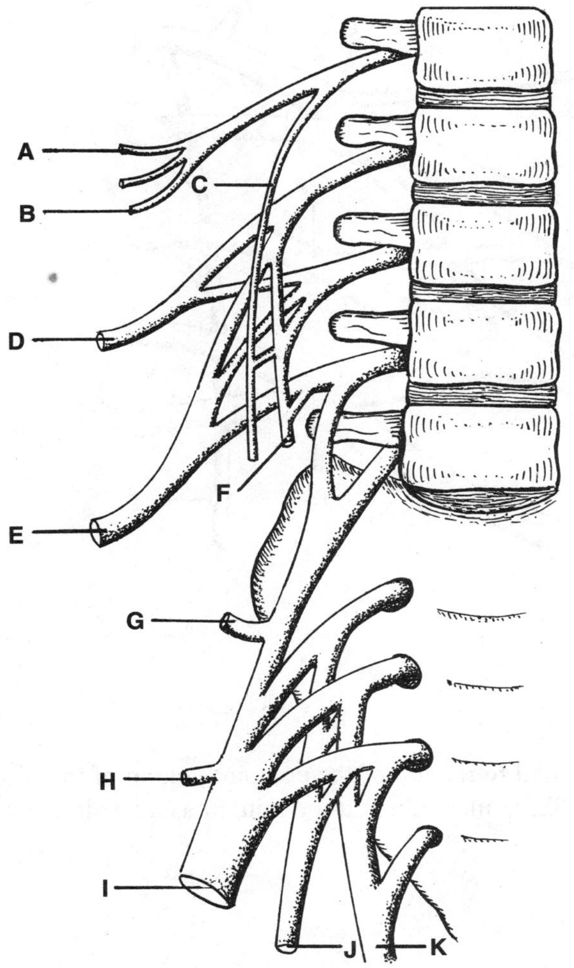

12. Following an anterior approach to the hip for joint replacement, a patient complains of numbness over the lateral thigh. The structure in the figure most likely to have been injured during the operative procedure is

(A) B
(B) C
(C) D
(D) E
(E) F

13. After undergoing intramedullary nailing for a fracture of the femur, a patient complains of numbness in the scrotum. The structure in the figure most likely to have been injured is

(A) G
(B) H
(C) I
(D) J
(E) K

14. In posterior approaches to the shoulder, the radial nerve is relatively well-protected from injury by the

(A) teres major
(B) teres minor
(C) latissimus dorsi
(D) trapezius
(E) subscapularis

15. The brachial plexus exits the neck between what muscles?

(A) Scalenus medius and scalenus posterior
(B) Scalenus medius and scalenus anterior
(C) Scalenus medius and pectoralis minor
(D) Serratus anterior and scalenus posterior
(E) Scalenus anterior and pectoralis minor

16. All the following are branches of the axillary artery EXCEPT the

(A) thoracoacromial artery
(B) subscapular artery
(C) supreme thoracic artery
(D) thyrocervical trunk
(E) lateral thoracic artery

17. In the posterior surgical approach to the humeral shaft, which of the following portions of the triceps muscle would be split?

(A) Long head
(B) Medial head
(C) Lateral head
(D) Long and medial heads
(E) Medial and lateral heads

Questions 18–20

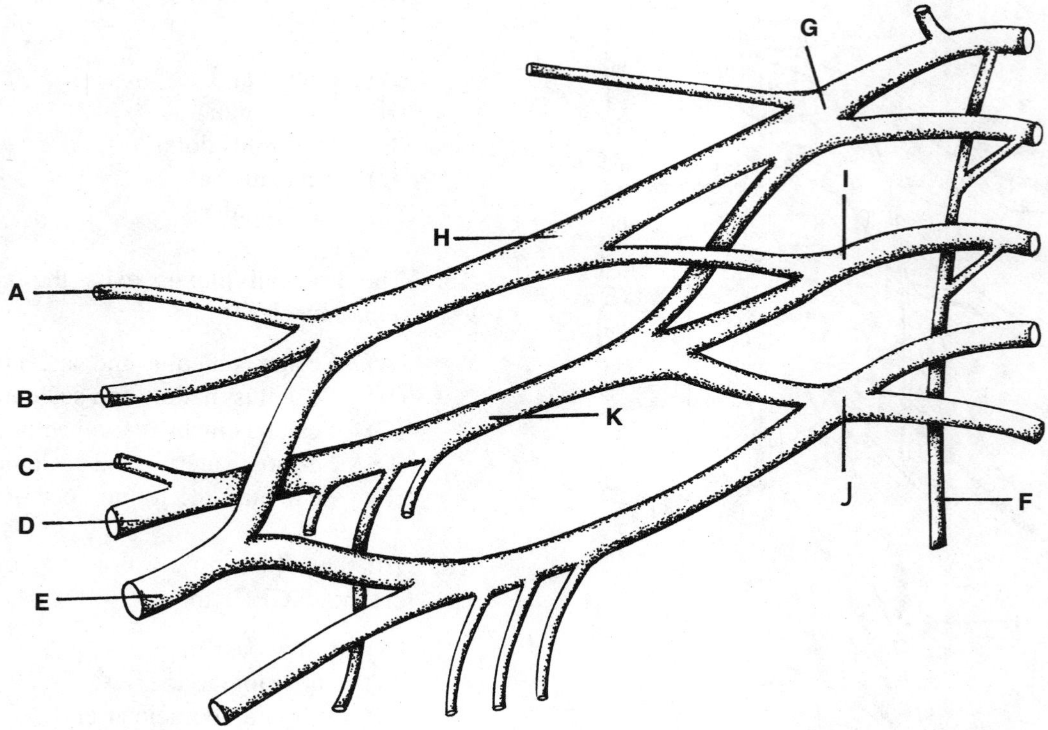

18. During an anterior surgical approach to the shoulder, medial retraction of the conjoint tendon of the biceps and coracobrachialis is carried out. The structure in the figure most likely to be injured as a result of forceful or prolonged retraction is

(A) A
(B) B
(C) C
(D) D
(E) E

19. The structure labeled *F* in the figure innervates what muscle?

(A) Serratus anterior
(B) Latissimus dorsi
(C) Rhomboid major
(D) Levator scapulae
(E) Teres major

20. Following an injury to the brachial plexus, a patient had weakness of shoulder abduction, no active external rotation of the shoulder or flexion of the elbow, and decreased sensation in the thumb and index fingers. There is no winging of the scapula. The most likely site of this patient's brachial plexus injury is

(A) G
(B) H
(C) I
(D) J
(E) K

21. The floor of the osteoligamentous sling that supports the head of the talus is formed by the

(A) bifurcate ligament
(B) interosseous ligament
(C) calcaneonavicular ligament
(D) anterior articular facet of the calcaneus
(E) navicular

22. Retraction of the scapula is brought about by the rhomboids and the

(A) latissimus dorsi
(B) trapezius
(C) levator scapulae
(D) levator scapulae and latissimus dorsi
(E) trapezius and latissimus dorsi

23. When performing a subtalar fusion, inadvertent posteromedial penetration of an osteotome is most likely to damage the

(A) tibialis posterior tendon
(B) flexor digitorum longus tendon
(C) flexor hallucis longus tendon
(D) posterior tibial artery
(E) calcaneal (Achilles) tendon

24. The most important stabilizer against valgus deformity in the flexed elbow is the

(A) radial head
(B) medial joint capsule
(C) anterior bundle of the medial collateral ligament
(D) posterior bundle of the medial collateral ligament
(E) transverse bundle of the medial collateral ligament

25. In the posterolateral approach to the radial head, the internervous plane lies between the

(A) radial and ulnar nerves
(B) radial and posterior interosseous nerves
(C) posterior interosseous and ulnar nerves
(D) radial and median nerves
(E) ulnar and median nerves

26. From lateral to medial, what is the normal anatomic arrangement of the following structures as they pass anterior to the elbow joint?

(A) Biceps tendon, brachial vein, brachial artery, median nerve
(B) Biceps tendon, median nerve, brachial vein, brachial artery
(C) Brachial vein, brachial artery, median nerve, biceps tendon
(D) Median nerve, brachial vein, brachial artery, biceps tendon
(E) Biceps tendon, brachial artery, brachial vein, median nerve

27. In the anterior approach to the proximal third of the radius, the deep muscle incised to gain access to the bone is innervated by which nerve?

(A) Radial
(B) Median
(C) Posterior interosseous
(D) Ulnar
(E) Musculocutaneous

28. The pronator quadratus has the same innervation as which of the following muscles?

(A) Flexor digitorum superficialis
(B) Flexor digitorum profundus
(C) Flexor carpi ulnaris
(D) Flexor pollicis longus
(E) Palmaris longus

29. The palmar cutaneous branch of the median nerve at the wrist is found most commonly between the

(A) flexor carpi radialis and radial artery
(B) flexor carpi radialis and flexor pollicis longus
(C) flexor carpi radialis and palmaris longus
(D) flexor pollicis longus and radial artery
(E) palmaris longus and flexor carpi ulnaris

Questions 30–31

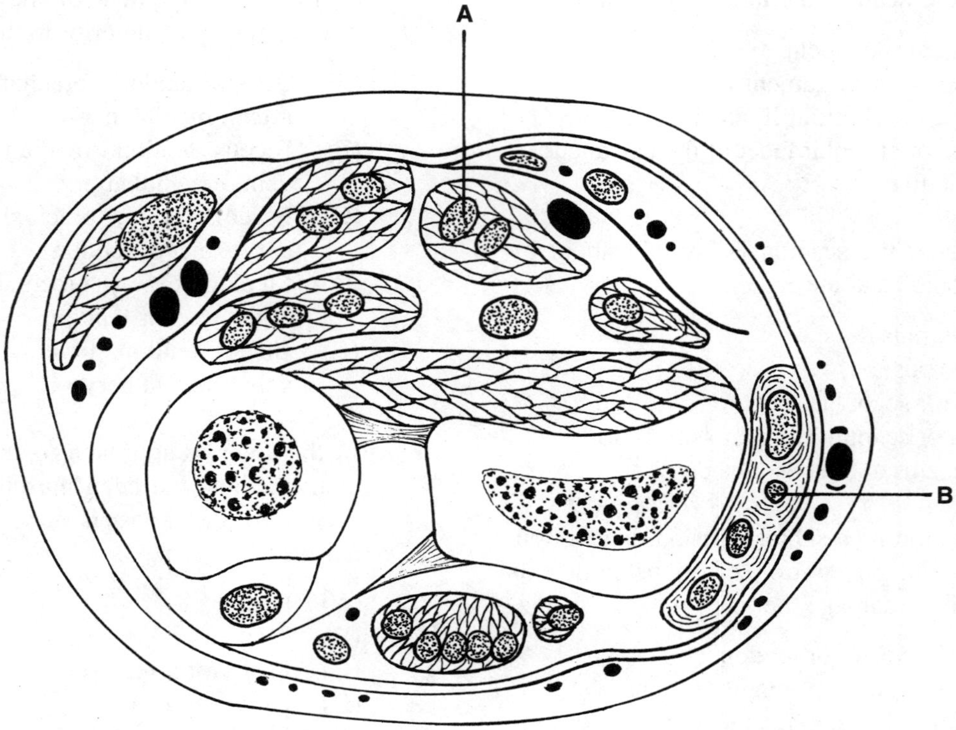

30. The figure is a cross section of the distal forearm just proximal to the wrist joint. The structure labeled *A* is the

(A) flexor digitorum superficialis to the index finger
(B) flexor digitorum superficialis to the long finger
(C) flexor digitorum profundus to the long finger
(D) median nerve
(E) flexor pollicis longus

31. The structure labeled *B* represents what musculotendinous unit?

(A) Abductor pollicis longus
(B) Abductor pollicis brevis
(C) Extensor pollicis longus
(D) Extensor pollicis brevis
(E) Extensor carpi radialis

Questions 32–33

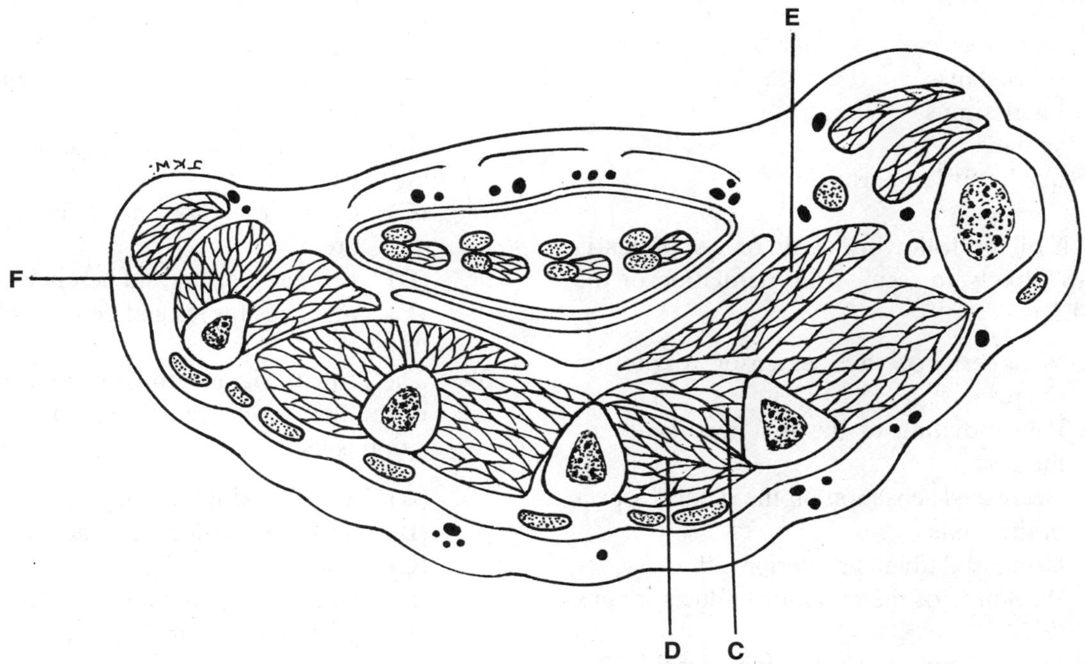

32. The figure is a cross section through the level of the mid-palm. The structure labeled *C* is the

(A) first dorsal interosseous
(B) second dorsal interosseous
(C) first palmar interosseous
(D) second palmar interosseous
(E) adductor pollicis (transverse head)

33. The structure labeled *F* is innervated by what nerve?

(A) Ulnar nerve, deep branch
(B) Ulnar nerve, superficial branch
(C) Median nerve, motor branch
(D) Ulnar nerve in the forearm
(E) Median nerve in the forearm

34. In the back, the most medial of the erector spinae muscles is the

(A) multifidus
(B) iliocostalis
(C) longissimus
(D) spinalis
(E) quadratus lumborum

35. Which of the following signs or symptoms is LEAST likely to result from herniation of the L4–L5 disk?

(A) Weakness of the extensor digitorum longus
(B) Pain radiating to the first web space of the foot
(C) Decreased sensation on the medial aspect of the ankle
(D) Decreased tibialis posterior reflex
(E) Weakness of the extensor hallucis longus

36. A 24-year-old man who sustained a spinal injury 3 days ago has slightly diminished strength in hip flexion but absent extension and adduction. Active motion of the knee and ankle is absent, as are the patellar and Achilles reflexes. Sensation is normal over the proximal thigh but absent below the middle third of the thigh. The patient's lowest functioning neurologic level is

(A) T12
(B) L1
(C) L2
(D) L3
(E) L4

37. When posterolateral bone grafting is performed for nonunion of the tibia, the structure at most risk for injury is the

(A) posterior tibial nerve
(B) sural nerve
(C) superficial peroneal nerve
(D) lesser saphenous vein
(E) peroneal artery

38. In the anterolateral approach to the ankle, dissection should proceed in the interval between the

(A) extensor digitorum longus and peroneus tertius
(B) extensor digitorum longus and tibialis anterior
(C) extensor digitorum longus and peroneus brevis
(D) peroneus tertius and peroneus brevis
(E) peroneus brevis and peroneus longus

39. The primary ligamentous restraint to inversion of the foot when the ankle is in the neutral position is the

(A) anterior talofibular ligament
(B) posterior talofibular ligament
(C) calcaneofibular ligament
(D) anterior tibiofibular ligament
(E) posterior tibiofibular ligament

40. Which of the following nerves supplies the extensor hallucis brevis muscle?

(A) Superficial peroneal
(B) Deep peroneal
(C) Posterior tibial
(D) Lateral plantar
(E) Medial plantar

41. The nerve that supplies the quadratus plantae muscle is the

(A) superficial peroneal
(B) deep peroneal
(C) posterior tibial
(D) lateral plantar
(E) medial plantar

42. The peroneus longus inserts on the same bone(s) as the

(A) long plantar ligament
(B) flexor hallucis brevis
(C) abductor hallucis
(D) oblique head of the adductor hallucis
(E) tibialis anterior

43. During insertion of an arthroscope into the ankle through the anterolateral portal, the structure at greatest risk for injury is

(A) the peroneus tertius tendon
(B) the dorsalis pedis artery
(C) a branch of the deep peroneal nerve
(D) a branch of the superficial peroneal nerve
(E) the saphenous nerve

44. While performing a total knee replacement, the surgeon determines that a lateral retinacular release is needed. What artery should the surgeon take particular care to preserve to prevent patellar ischemia?

(A) Middle genicular
(B) Superior lateral genicular
(C) Superior medial genicular
(D) Inferior lateral genicular
(E) Inferior medial genicular

45. The stress produced when a force is applied parallel to a surface is

(A) torque
(B) strain
(C) shear
(D) tension
(E) fatigue

46. A material that has the same mechanical properties in all directions is best described as

(A) elastic
(B) viscoelastic
(C) ductile
(D) anisotropic
(E) isotropic

47. When the thickness of a plate is increased by a factor of two, its bending stiffness increases by a factor of

(A) 2
(B) 4
(C) 6
(D) 8
(E) 16

48. The maximum tensile force that can be generated by a muscle is proportional to the

(A) physiologic cross-sectional area
(B) total muscle mass
(C) moment arm with respect to the joint it moves
(D) type of contraction (concentric or eccentric)
(E) applied external load

49. An increase in all the following will increase the rigidity of a unilateral external fixator EXCEPT the

(A) number of pins
(B) diameter of the pins
(C) separation of the pin groups
(D) number of side bars
(E) separation of the pins

50. Toughness is defined as the

(A) ratio of stress to corresponding strain
(B) strain energy at the point of ultimate stress
(C) resistance to indentation or scratching
(D) stress at the moment of failure
(E) stress beyond which plastic deformation occurs

Questions 51–52

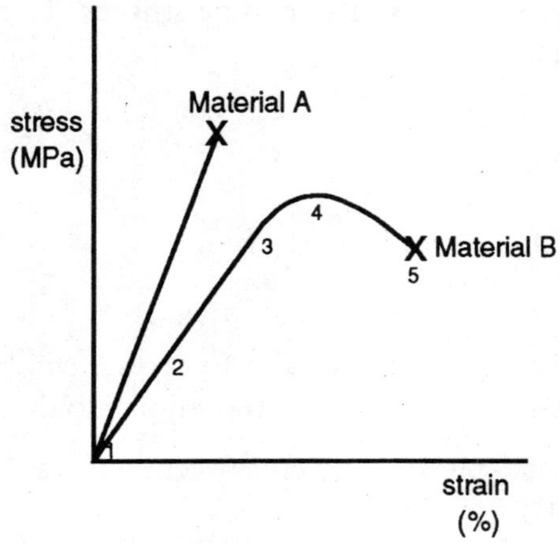

51. The figure shows the stress/strain diagram for two materials tested in tension. The yield point for material B is the point labeled

(A) 1
(B) 2
(C) 3
(D) 4
(E) 5

52. All the following are greater for A than B EXCEPT the

(A) elastic modulus
(B) ultimate load
(C) stiffness
(D) energy to failure
(E) load to failure

53. Which of the following items is a scalar quantity?

(A) Weight
(B) Velocity
(C) Force
(D) Moment
(E) Mass

54. The joint reaction force across the hip joint in unilateral stance is primarily due to the

(A) weight of the body above the hip
(B) lateral shift of the center of mass of the body
(C) contraction of the muscles crossing the hip
(D) weight of the contralateral leg
(E) inertial effect of the body above the hip

Questions 55–56

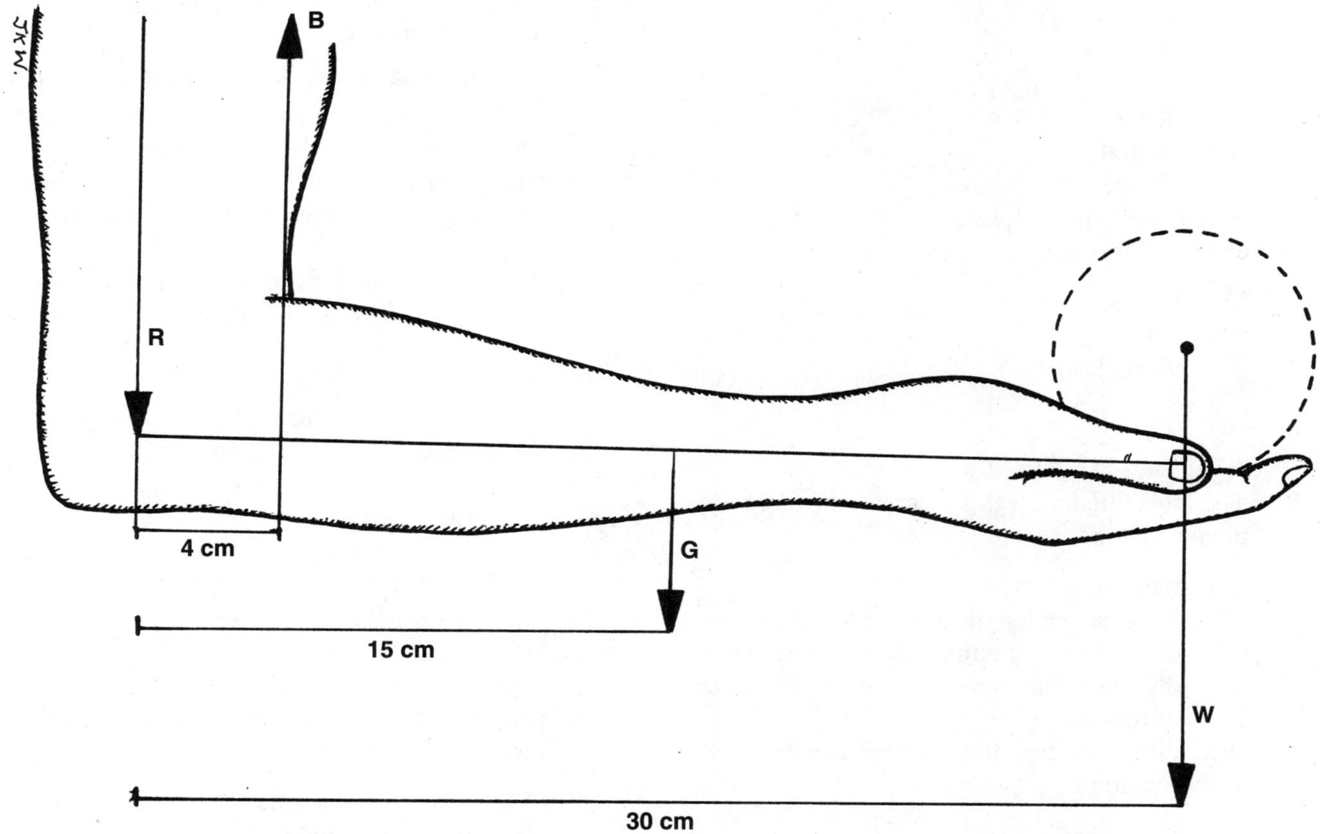

The figure represents a person holding a ball with the elbow flexed 90°. *W* represents the weight of the ball, *G* the weight of the forearm, *B* the force generated by the elbow flexors, and *R* the joint reaction force at the elbow.

55. The moment arm of force R is

(A) 0 cm
(B) 4 cm
(C) 15 cm
(D) 26 cm
(E) 30 cm

56. Which of the following statements about the magnitudes of the forces is true?

(A) B is equal to G + W
(B) B + R is equal to G + W
(C) B is more than 7 times W
(D) B is equal to W
(E) R is equal to W

57. Bone is weakest in resisting

(A) tension
(B) shear
(C) compression
(D) bending
(E) torsion

58. A material that deforms plastically to a great extent prior to failure is described as

(A) brittle
(B) elastic
(C) viscoelastic
(D) stiff
(E) ductile

59. The most efficient way to increase the area moment of inertia is to

(A) increase the area
(B) increase the length of the structure
(C) decrease the length of the structure
(D) distribute the mass away from the center of rotation
(E) distribute the mass nearer the center of rotation

60. All the following statements about the cubital tunnel are true EXCEPT that

(A) the proximal ulna forms one border
(B) the medial epicondyle of the humerus forms one border
(C) Osborne's fascia covers the tunnel
(D) the ulnar nerve enters the flexor carpi ulnaris in the tunnel
(E) it decreases in volume with elbow flexion

61. Which of the following muscles have their origin on the scapula and cross the elbow?

(A) Coracobrachialis and biceps
(B) Coracobrachialis and brachialis
(C) Brachialis and biceps
(D) Biceps and triceps
(E) Brachialis and triceps

62. Which of the following statements best describes the origin and insertion of the articularis genu muscle?

(A) It originates from the posterior fascia of the vastus intermedius and inserts into the tendon of the rectus femoris
(B) It originates from the anterior surface of the distal femur and inserts into the tendon of the rectus femoris
(C) It originates from the posterior fascia of the vastus intermedius and inserts into the upper part of the synovial membrane of the knee joint
(D) It originates from the anterior surface of the distal femur and inserts into the upper part of the synovial membrane of the knee joint
(E) It originates from the anterior surface of the distal femur and inserts into the superior aspect of the patella

63. The structure(s) LEAST likely to cause compression of the posterior interosseous nerve is (are) the

(A) fibrous bands anterior to the radial head
(B) recurrent radial vessels
(C) extensor carpi radialis longus
(D) arcade of Frohse
(E) distal border of the supinator

64. In the finger, the digital nerve is

(A) dorsal to the digital artery
(B) volar to the digital artery
(C) ulnar to the digital artery
(D) radial to the digital artery
(E) radiovolar in the proximal portion of the finger and ulnodorsal in the distal portion of the finger to the digital vessels

65. The structure nearest the nerve root as it exits the intervertebral foramen in the lumbar spine is the

(A) transverse process
(B) superior articular facet
(C) inferior articular facet
(D) vertebral body
(E) pars interarticularis

66. All the following statements about surgical wire are correct EXCEPT

(A) the strength of surgical wire in tension increases directly with its diameter
(B) twisted multistrand wire is less likely to slip than single-strand wire
(C) twisted wire is more flexible than a single-strand wire of equivalent maximum diameter
(D) the tensile strength of twisted wire is maximal at between four and eight turns per inch
(E) twisted multistrand wire is stronger in tension than a single-strand wire of equivalent maximum diameter

67. All the following decrease the joint reaction force in the hip during the stance phase of normal gait EXCEPT

(A) lateral shift of the center of mass of the body
(B) use of a cane in the ipsilateral hand
(C) use of a cane in the contralateral hand
(D) valgus-producing proximal femoral osteotomy
(E) varus-producing proximal femoral osteotomy

68. Clinically described sites of ulnar nerve compression include all the following EXCEPT the

(A) arcade of Struthers
(B) medial intermuscular septum
(C) ulnar recurrent arteries
(D) flexor carpi ulnaris
(E) Guyon's canal

Anatomy and Biomechanics

Answers

1. **The answer is D.** *(Hoppenfeld, deBoer, p 264.)* The stellate ganglion and cervical sympathetic chain lie anterior to the longus capitis muscle and lateral to the longus colli muscle. They are vulnerable to injury by overly zealous lateral retraction of the longus colli and longus capitis muscles during the anterior approach to the cervical spine.

2. **The answer is D.** *(Hoppenfeld, deBoer, p 258.)* The cricoid cartilage, a palpable anatomic reference point, is at the level of the sixth cervical vertebra. The hyoid bone is at the level of the third cervical vertebra, and the upper border of the thyroid cartilage is at the level of the fourth cervical vertebra. These landmarks are helpful in planning surgical approaches to the anterior cervical spine.

3. **The answer is B.** *(Hoppenfeld, deBoer, p 250.)* The greater occipital nerve is formed by the medial branch of the dorsal ramus of C2. This sensory nerve exits the spine at C1-C2, turns superiorly around the obliquus capitis inferior muscle, and pierces the trapezius to supply sensation to the posterior scalp as high as the vertex. This nerve should be protected in the posterior approach to the occiput and C1.

4. **The answer is A.** *(Jenkins, 6/e, p 80.)* The sternocleidomastoid muscle bends the head laterally to the ipsilateral side and rotates it to the contralateral side. It is innervated by the spinal accessory nerve (cranial nerve XI), as well as by branches of the ansa cervicalis (C2 and C3).

5. **The answer is C.** *(Jenkins, 6/e, pp 293–295.)* The superficial peroneal nerve branches from the common peroneal nerve as it passes between the two heads of the peroneus longus muscle. The nerve descends between the extensor digitorum longus and peroneal muscles and gives branches to the peroneus longus and brevis muscles. It also supplies sensation to the lateral leg and dorsum of the foot. The subcutaneous segment of this nerve may be injured during decompressive fasciotomy of the anterior and lateral compartments of the leg.

6. **The answer is C.** *(Hoppenfeld, deBoer, pp 362–363.)* The perforating arteries are usually three in number and arise from the posterior surface of the deep femoral artery. They pierce the linea aspera to supply the vastus lateralis muscle, where they are vulnerable to injury during the posterolateral approach to the femur.

7. **The answer is B.** *(Jenkins, 6/e, pp 262–267.)* The long head of the biceps femoris arises from a common origin with the semitendinosus and is innervated by the tibial division of the sciatic nerve. The sciatic contribution to the innervation of the adductor magnus muscle is from the tibial division of the sciatic nerve. The short head of the biceps femoris arises from the lateral lip of the linea aspera and is innervated by a branch of the peroneal division of the sciatic nerve. To avoid injury to this motor branch in the posterior ap-

proach to the middle third of the femur, the origin of the short head of the biceps femoris should be elevated from the femur in a lateral to medial direction and retracted medially.

8. The answer is C. *(Warren, J Bone Joint Surg 61-A:56–62, 1979.)* A number of structures are attached to the medial femoral condyle: the adductor magnus superiorly, the superficial medial collateral ligament inferiorly, and the medial head of the gastrocnemius inferiorly. The patellofemoral ligament courses anteriorly from the medial femoral condyle to the medial side of the patella, deep to the vastus medialis. The popliteus attaches to the posterior aspect of the *lateral* femoral condyle.

9. The answer is D. *(Hoppenfeld, deBoer, p 435.)* The popliteus originates from the medial surface of the proximal tibia, passes between the lateral meniscus and the capsule of the knee joint, and inserts into the lateral epicondyle of the femur and posterior aspect of the lateral meniscus. It is innervated by the tibial nerve. It is a weak flexor of the knee, rotates the femur laterally on the tibia, and retracts the lateral meniscus during knee flexion. Care must be taken to avoid injury to the popliteus during lateral approaches to the knee joint.

10. The answer is C. *(Hoppenfeld, deBoer, p 380.)* The lateral femoral circumflex artery usually originates from the profunda femoris artery and courses anteriorly and laterally from its site of origin. The ascending branch courses superiorly between the tensor fascia lata, sartorius, and rectus femoris muscles. It lies very near the hip joint capsule at the origin of the reflected head of the rectus femoris and is vulnerable to injury during surgical exposures that entail detachment of this muscle.

11. The answer is C. *(Hollinshead, p 389.)* The obturator artery arises in the pelvis from the internal iliac artery and supplies the obturator internus muscle prior to exiting the pelvis through the obturator foramen. It divides into anterior and posterior branches, the anterior branch supplying the obturator externus muscle and the posterior branch the transverse acetabular ligament and ligamentum teres. The pectineus muscle is supplied by branches of the femoral artery. Inadvertent division of branches of the obturator artery will not compromise the vascular supply to the femoral head.

12. The answer is C. *(Hoppenfeld, deBoer, p 312. Jenkins, p 239.)* The lateral femoral cutaneous nerve is formed from the posterior portions of the ventral rami of L2 and L3. It usually pierces the fascia lata slightly below the anterior superior iliac spine, although its course and location in this area are variable. Since the anterior approach to the hip is developed between the sartorius and tensor fascia lata muscles near their origins, the lateral femoral cutaneous nerve is vulnerable to injury near the anterior superior iliac spine.

13. The answer is E. *(Hollinshead, pp 810–811.)* The pudendal nerve usually arises from the ventral rami of S2–S4. Near the urogenital diaphragm, the pudendal nerve gives off the perineal nerve, which further divides into posterior scrotal branches that provide sensation to the scrotum. The pudendal nerve can be compressed as it courses around the ischial ramus by the central post of the fracture table during femoral nailing procedures.

14. The answer is A. *(Hoppenfeld, deBoer, pp 42–44.)* The radial nerve enters the arm through a triangular space bounded superiorly by the lower border of the teres major, medially by the long head of the triceps, and laterally by the lateral head of the triceps. The lower border of the teres minor is the superior border of the quadrangular space, which transmits the axillary nerve. In the posterior approach to the shoulder, the radial nerve is relatively well-protected from injury by the teres major, but the axillary nerve is vulnerable to injury by excessive inferior retraction of the teres minor.

15. The answer is B. *(Jenkins, p 345. Rockwood, Matsen, pp 250–254.)* The roots of the brachial plexus, accompanied by the subclavian artery, usually exit the neck between the scalenus anterior and medius muscles. This interval is used to locate the site for injection in interscalene block anesthesia for surgery on the upper limb. Anatomic variations of the scalene musculature may cause a thoracic outlet syndrome.

16. The answer is D. *(Jenkins, pp 77–78.)* The thyrocervical trunk is a branch of the subclavian artery. Because of extensive arterial anastomoses about the shoulder, ligation of the subclavian artery distal to the thyrocervical trunk may be carried out without devascularizing the upper limb. The supreme thoracic artery is the first branch of the axillary artery and supplies the upper thoracic wall. Awareness of the branches of the axillary artery is important when performing operative procedures around the shoulder.

17. The answer is B. *(Hoppenfeld, deBoer, pp 62–63.)* The long and lateral heads of the triceps muscle lie superficial to the medial, or deep, head. The posterior approach to the humerus uses the interval between the long and lateral heads of the triceps and splits the medial head to gain access to the shaft of the bone. Since the radial nerve lies just proximal to the medial head of the triceps in the spiral groove, it is avoided in this approach.

18. The answer is A. *(Hoppenfeld, deBoer, p 11.)* Excessive medial retraction on the conjoint tendon during an anterior approach to the shoulder may result in injury to the musculocutaneous nerve, which pierces the coracobrachialis 5 to 8 cm distal to the coracoid process. Stretch injury at this site causes weakness in elbow flexion and loss of sensation over the lateral forearm.

19. The answer is A. *(Jenkins, p 84.)* The long thoracic nerve is derived from the fifth, sixth, and seventh cervical nerve roots before they enter the brachial plexus. The chief contribution is usually from C6; contributions from either C5 or C7 may be lacking. The nerve runs posterior to the other elements of the brachial plexus on the outer surface of the serratus anterior, which it innervates. Absence of function in the serratus anterior, along with other signs of brachial plexus injury, indicates injury at the level of the nerve roots.

20. The answer is A. *(Jenkins, pp 84–86.)* The patient most likely sustained an injury to the upper trunk of the brachial plexus. Absence of scapular winging indicates the serratus anterior muscle is functioning, so the injury is not at the nerve root level. Weakness of abduction and loss of active external rotation follow loss of function of the suprascapular nerve. The deltoid is also weakened, since the upper trunk provides fibers to the posterior cord and axillary nerve. The sensory deficit and loss of active elbow flexion are due to loss of input from the C5 and C6 nerve roots to the brachial plexus.

21. The answer is C. *(Anderson, fig. 4-113.)* The calcaneonavicular ligament is a fibrocartilaginous structure coursing from the sustentaculum tali to the plantar surface of the navicular. One of the few ligaments containing fibers of elastin, it provides an elastic support for the head of the talus, which gives it an alternate name, the "spring" ligament. Elastic support of the talor head is necessary for normal biomechanics of the midfoot during walking.

22. The answer is E. *(Jenkins, pp 88–89.)* Retraction of the scapula is brought about primarily by the rhomboids and the middle fibers of the trapezius, but the latissimus dorsi also contributes via downward and posterior pull on the proximal humerus. The levator scapulae raises the medial border of the scapula but does not play a role in scapular retraction.

23. The answer is C. *(Anderson, fig. 4-88.)* The flexor hallucis longus tendon lies midway between the malleoli at the subtalar joint and grooves the talus as it passes inferiorly to go beneath the sustentaculum tali. It is directly apposed to the posterior facet of the subtalar joint and is easily damaged by penetration of an osteotome when one decorticates this facet. The vascular structures are medial to the flexor hallucis longus tendon at this level, and the posterior tibial and flexor digitorum tendons are anterior.

24. The answer is C. *(Hotchkiss, J Orthop Res 5:372–377, 1987.)* The medial collateral ligament of the elbow consists of anterior, posterior, and transverse bundles. The anterior bundle originates from the medial epicondyle of the humerus slightly posterior to the axis of elbow flexion and becomes taut with flexion of the elbow. This structure provides most of the resistance to valgus stress with the elbow flexed beyond 45°. The radial head and anterior bundle contribute equally to stability with the elbow in full extension. Preservation of a taut, functioning anterior bundle is essential to stability of the elbow in the throwing athlete or following total elbow replacement.

25. The answer is B. *(Hoppenfeld, deBoer, p 98.)* The posterolateral approach to the radial head exposes the interval between the anconeus, supplied by the radial nerve, and the extensor carpi ulnaris, supplied by the posterior interosseous nerve. Extension of the approach distally beyond the annular ligament may endanger the posterior interosseous nerve.

26. The answer is A. *(Hoppenfeld, deBoer, p 106.)* At the level of the elbow joint, the neurovascular structures lie medial to the biceps tendon as they pass beneath the lacertus fibrosus. From lateral to medial, they are the brachial vein, brachial artery, and median nerve. Understanding the relationship of these structures and identifying them are keys to operating successfully in the cubital fossa via either the anterolateral or anterior approach.

27. The answer is C. *(Hoppenfeld, deBoer, pp 114–115.)* The supinator muscle covers the proximal third of the radius and must be incised to gain access to the bone. It is innervated by the posterior interosseous nerve, which courses between the two heads of the muscle to enter the forearm. This nerve should be identified and retracted gently in approaches to the proximal forearm.

28. The answer is D. *(Hoppenfeld, deBoer, p 122.)* The pronator quadratus is innervated by the anterior interosseous nerve, which also innervates the flexor pollicis longus muscle. The flexor digitorum superficialis and palmaris longus are innervated by the median nerve, while the flexor digitorum profundus has both median and ulnar innervations. The flexor carpi ulnaris is innervated by the ulnar nerve. Isolated weakness of interphalangeal flexion of the thumb is highly suggestive of compression of the anterior interosseous nerve.

29. The answer is C. *(Anderson, fig. 6-74.)* The palmar cutaneous branch of the median nerve arises from the radial side of the median nerve proximal to the transverse carpal ligament. It lies between the flexor carpi radialis and the palmaris longus. The flexor pollicis longus is deeper in the distal forearm. Injury to the nerve during carpal tunnel release can be avoided by placing the skin incision in line with the long axis of the ring finger and incising the transverse carpal ligament on its ulnar border. The nerve is also at risk for injury during the volar approach to the scaphoid if the dissection extends ulnar to the flexor carpi radialis tendon.

30. The answer is B. *(Anderson, fig. 6-72.)* The flexor digitorum superficialis tendons lie beneath the transverse carpal ligament at the level of the wrist, ulnar to the median nerve and superficial to the flexor digitorum profundus tendons. The superficialis tendons to the long and ring fingers are volar to those to the index and small fingers. This relationship is important in the identification of tendons for transfer or repair.

31. The answer is D. *(Hoppenfeld, deBoer, p 150.)* The extensor pollicis brevis crosses the dorsal aspect of the forearm to reach the lateral side of the distal radius, where, along with the abductor pollicis longus, it enters a fibro-osseous tunnel that occupies the most radial aspect of the wrist. The fibro-osseous nature of this tunnel contributes to the development of stenosing tenosynovitis (de Quervain's disease).

32. The answer is C. *(Anderson, fig. 6-73.)* The three palmar interossei arise from the palmar aspects of the second, fourth, and fifth metacarpals. The first palmar interosseous lies between the second and third metacarpals and volar to the second dorsal interosseous (*D*). The transverse head of the adductor pollicis (*E*) lies palmar to the interossei.

33. The answer is A. *(Jenkins, p 166.)* The opponens digiti minimi arises from the flexor retinaculum and the hook of the hamate and inserts into the ulnar border of the entire fifth metacarpal. It aids opposition of the small finger to the thumb and is innervated by the deep branch of the ulnar nerve. Visible atrophy of this muscle may result from injury to the ulnar nerve.

34. The answer is D. *(Anderson, figs. 5-27 and 5-28.)* The erector spinae group of muscles (also known as the *sacrospinalis*) is composed, from medial to lateral, of the spinalis, longissimus, and iliocostalis muscles. The multifidus and quadratus lumborum lie deeper in the back and are not part of the erector spinae group.

35. The answer is C. *(Hoppenfeld, p 69.)* Herniation of the L4–L5 disk usually compresses the L5 nerve root, resulting in weakness of the extensor hallucis longus and extensor digitorum longus muscles and pain radiating to the first web space, a portion of the L5 dermatome. The tibialis posterior reflex, though often not elicited, is an L5 reflex and could be diminished in this case. The medial border of the ankle corresponds to the L4 dermatome; sensation here should be normal after herniation of the L4–L5 disk.

36. The answer is C. *(Hoppenfeld, p 94.)* There is only slight loss of strength in hip flexion because the iliopsoas (T12–L3) has almost complete innervation. Although the quadriceps and adductors (L2–4) receive partial innervation from L2, there is no clinically significant function. No other muscles in the lower limb have L2 innervation. The L2 dermatome ends approximately two-thirds of the way down the thigh. The patellar reflex is primarily an L4 reflex and would be absent.

37. The answer is E. *(Hoppenfeld, deBoer, pp 448–450.)* In the posterolateral approach to the tibia, dissection proceeds between the soleus, flexor hallucis longus, and peroneus longus muscles to reach the posterior surface of the fibula and interosseous membrane. The peroneal artery is at risk when dissecting along the interosseous membrane to reach the tibia.

38. The answer is D. *(Hoppenfeld, deBoer, pp 495–498.)* The anterolateral approach to the ankle exploits the internervous plane between the superficial peroneal and deep peroneal nerves. The peroneus tertius and extensor digitorum longus (deep peroneal nerve) are retracted medially and the peroneus brevis (superficial peroneal nerve) laterally.

39. The answer is C. *(Jenkins, pp 311–312.)* The calcaneofibular ligament assumes a nearly vertical orientation when the ankle is in the neutral position and is the primary ligamentous restraint against inversion of the foot in this position. The anterior talofibular ligament is the primary restraint when the ankle is in the plantarflexed position. Most sprains begin with the ankle in plantar flexion, injuring the anterior talofibular ligament initially. As the ankle moves toward neutral, stress is transferred to the calcaneofibular ligament, which may then be injured as well.

40. The answer is B. *(Jenkins, p 327.)* The extensor hallucis brevis muscle originates from the dorsal surface of the calcaneus and inserts into the base of the proximal phalanx of the great toe. It aids in extension of the great toe and is innervated by a branch of the deep peroneal nerve. It is vulnerable to denervation in approaches to the sinus tarsi that involve distal retraction of the muscle.

41. The answer is D. *(Jenkins, p 326.)* The quadratus plantae muscle, part of the second layer of muscles on the plantar aspect of the foot, extends from the calcaneus to the tendon slips of the flexor digitorum longus. The lateral plantar nerve innervates this muscle as it crosses its plantar surface in passing to the lateral side of the foot. The nerve may become entrapped following displaced fractures of the calcaneus or may be injured in surgical approaches to the plantar aspect of the hindfoot.

42. The answer is E. *(Jenkins, pp 303, 315–319.)* Both the peroneus longus and the tibialis anterior insert on the medial cuneiform and the base of the first metatarsal. Imbalance of these muscles may result in pronation or supination of the foot and disturbances of gait. The long plantar ligament inserts into the cuboid and lateral cuneiform. The plantar muscles to the great toe insert more distally than the peroneus longus.

43. The answer is D. *(Vota, Arthroscopy 5:41–52, 1989.)* The dorsal lateral cutaneous branch of the superficial peroneal nerve is at greatest risk for injury when the anterolateral portal is used for ankle arthroscopy. It is best avoided by remaining lateral to the peroneus tertius tendon.

44. The answer is B. *(Woodburne, pp 89–91.)* The blood supply to the patella is via the medial and lateral genicular arteries; however, the inferior lateral genicular artery usually has only a very small branch to the patella. After a medial parapatellar approach to the knee, the only important articular branch to the patella still intact is the superior lateral genicular artery, which should be preserved to prevent patellar ischemia.

45. The answer is C. *(Tencer, Instr Course Lect 42:46–47, 1993.)* A shear force is a force applied parallel to a defined face or surface. The resultant stress is a shear stress. Its magnitude is equal to the shear force divided by the cross-sectional area over which the force acts.

46. The answer is E. *(Tencer, Instr Course Lect 42:46–47, 1993.)* An isotropic material, such as rubber or a metal alloy, has mechanical properties that are independent of the orientation of the material in the testing apparatus. An anisotropic material, such as bone or ligament, has mechanical properties that differ with the orientation of the material in the testing apparatus. All biologic materials are anisotropic.

47. The answer is D. *(Tencer, Instr Course Lect 42:49–50, 1993.)* The stiffness of an object is directly related to its area moment of inertia. For a plate or any other object with a rectangular cross section, the area moment of inertia is proportional to the cube of the height, or thickness, of the object. Doubling the thickness of a plate would thus increase its bending stiffness by a factor of 8.

48. The answer is A. *(Mow, p 36.)* The maximum tensile force that can be actively generated by a muscle is an intrinsic property of the muscle and is unrelated to the moment arm, applied external load, or type of contraction. The physiologic cross-sectional area of the muscle is a measure of the number of muscle fibers per unit volume, the muscle fiber being the basic element of muscle that generates tension. The physiologic cross-sectional area is calculated by dividing the muscle volume by the average fiber length.

49. The answer is E. *(Mow, pp 314–315.)* Increasing pin separation, which entails placing pins farther from the fracture site, will decrease the rigidity of an external fixator. Rigidity is increased by placing pins closer to the fracture site, increasing pin number and diameter, increasing separation of pin groups, and adding additional side bars.

50. The answer is B. *(Mow, pp 332–333.)* Toughness is simply the strain energy in a material at the point of ultimate stress. The ratio of stress to strain is the modulus of elasticity, resistance to indentation is hardness, stress at the moment of failure is the ultimate stress, and the stress beyond which plastic deformation occurs is defined as the yield point.

51. The answer is C. *(Mow, pp 99–102. Tencer, Instr Course Lect 42:46–47, 1993.)* The yield point is the point at which the stress/strain behavior of a material changes from purely elastic to a combination of elastic and plastic deformation. The portion of the curve from 1 to 3 represents the elastic portion, and the portion from 3 to 5 represents a combination of elastic and plastic deformation. Material A undergoes only elastic deformation before failure; it has no yield point.

52. The answer is D. *(Tencer, Instr Course Lect 42:46–47, 1993.)* The energy to failure of a material is represented by the area under the stress/strain curve for that material, which is greater for material B than for material A. Elastic modulus and stiffness are measures of the same property and are represented by the slope of the elastic portion of the curve; they are both greater for material A than for material B. The ultimate load is the maximum stress the material can withstand, and the load to failure is the magnitude of the stress at the time of failure; both are greater for material A than for material B.

53. The answer is E. *(Tencer, Instr Course Lect 42:46–47, 1993.)* A scalar is a quantity having magnitude only, such as time, distance, or mass. A vector is a quantity that has both magnitude and direction, such as force, velocity, or acceleration. Weight is the force of gravity acting on an object, and moment is a force acting on a body at a distance that tends to cause rotation.

54. The answer is C. *(Norkin, pp 324–326.)* The muscles crossing the hip joint, particularly the abductors, are active in unilateral stance and have a very small moment arm. They must therefore generate a large amount of force to counteract the weight of the body, which acts at a greater distance from the joint. The abductors contribute the largest component of the joint reaction force.

55. The answer is A. *(Mow, pp 18–19.)* A joint reaction force, by definition, acts through the center of rotation of the joint and has a moment arm of zero. Force R acts through the center of rotation of the elbow joint and has a moment arm of 0 cm.

56. The answer is C. *(Mow, pp 18–19.)* For a system at equilibrium, the sum of the moments must be zero. Force R exerts no moment on the system; forces G and W will extend the elbow, while force B will flex the elbow. Thus, the equilibrium equation is (4 cm)B = (15 cm)G + (30 cm)W. Solving for B reveals that B = (3.75)G + (7.5)W, or B is at least 7 times W.

57. The answer is B. *(Tencer, Instr Course Lect 42:21–22, 1993.)* Bone is weakest in shear, followed by tension and then compression. Pure shear is not often applied to bone in clinical situations. Failure of bone with bending or torsion is the result of tension in a portion of the bone.

58. The answer is E. *(Tencer, Instr Course Lect 42:47–48, 1993.)* A ductile material is one that can undergo a large amount of plastic deformation prior to failure. Examples include polyethylene, rubber, and aluminum. Brittle materials deform very little prior to failure, and elastic materials do not undergo plastic deformation. Viscoelastic materials have properties that change with the rate of loading.

59. The answer is D. *(Mow, pp 104–109.)* The area moment of inertia is highly sensitive to the distribution of mass around the axis of rotation. Mass that is further from the axis of rotation is much more efficient in resisting bending with respect to that axis. This fact explains why a meterstick turned on edge is much more efficient at resisting bending than a meterstick turned horizontally.

60. The answer is D. *(Gelberman, J Bone Joint Surg 75-A:1854–1878, 1993.)* The cubital tunnel is a fibro-osseous tunnel through which the ulnar nerve passes at the level of the elbow joint. Its borders are the medial epicondyle of the humerus and the medial surface of the proximal ulna. These borders are bridged by a fascial roof, described in 1957 by Osborne. Because of the eccentric origin of the fascial roof, the cubital tunnel decreases in contour and volume with elbow flexion. The ulnar nerve enters the forearm by passing between the two heads of the flexor carpi ulnaris muscle distal to the lower border of the cubital tunnel. Osborne's fascia must be incised in transposition of the ulnar nerve.

61. The answer is D. *(Anderson, figs. 6–35 and 6–36.)* The long head of the biceps arises from the supraglenoid tubercle of the scapula and inserts on the bicipital tuberosity of the radius. The long head of the triceps arises from the infraglenoid tubercle of the scapula and inserts on the olecranon process of the ulna. The brachialis originates from the humerus; the coracobrachialis arises from the scapula but does not cross the elbow.

62. The answer is D. *(Jenkins, p 244.)* The articularis genu consists of a number of small muscular bundles that arise from the lower fourth of the anterior aspect of the femur. Lying deep to the vastus intermedius muscle, these bundles insert into the upper part of the synovial membrane of the knee joint.

63. The answer is C. *(Gelberman, J Bone Joint Surg 75-A:1854–1878, 1993.)* Compression of the posterior interosseous nerve by fibrous bands anterior to the radial head at the entrance to the radial tunnel is uncommon but does occur. The fan-shaped leash of recurrent radial vessels (leash of Henry) crosses the nerve and may cause compression. The extensor carpi radialis brevis has a thin proximal tendinous margin that may also compress the nerve. The arcade of Frohse, the free, fibrous proximal border of the supinator and the fibrous distal border of the supinator are also sites of compression. The extensor carpi radialis longus is more superficial and is not a source of compression.

64. The answer is B. *(Anderson, fig. 6–77.)* The digital nerves are volar to the digital vessels in the fingers but dorsal to the digital vessels in the palm. The digital nerve remains volar to the vessels throughout the length of the finger. Knowledge of this relationship is important in identification and repair of lacerations of the digital artery and nerve.

65. The answer is B. *(Hoppenfeld, deBoer, p 291.)* The superior articular process is the structure nearest the exiting nerve root in the intervertebral foramen in the lumbar spine. Hypertrophy of this structure can cause neurologic compression. The inferior articular facet is posterior and the transverse process and vertebral body anterior to the nerve root as it exits the foramen.

66. The answer is E. *(Tencer, Instr Course Lect 42:28, 1993.)* Twisted multistrand wire is more flexible and less likely to slip, but it is weaker in resisting tensile force than a single-strand wire of equivalent diameter. The tensile strength of wire increases directly with its diameter.

67. The answer is D. *(Norkin, pp 326–331. Fortune, pp 2796–2797.)* Valgus osteotomy of the proximal femur decreases the moment arm of the hip abductors, thereby causing increased abductor and joint reaction forces. Varus osteotomy of the proximal femur decreases the magnitude of the abductor pull and the joint reaction force by producing a longer moment arm for the abductors. Lateral tilt of the trunk moves the center of mass of the body closer to the hip joint and decreases joint reaction force. Use of a cane in either hand decreases the joint reaction force, but a cane is more effective in the contralateral hand because it acts through a longer moment arm.

68. The answer is C. *(Gelberman, J Bone Joint Surg 75-A:1854–1878, 1993.)* The most often mentioned but least often involved site of compression is the arcade of Struthers, which lies 8 cm proximal to the epicondyle and transmits the ulnar nerve from the anterior to the posterior compartments of the arm. The medial intermuscular septum fills the superior concavity formed by the medial epicondyle; the ulnar nerve may be compressed here if it subluxates anteriorly or if the septum is not adequately excised at the time of transposition of the ulnar nerve. Ulnar nerve compression between the two heads of the flexor carpi ulnaris and within Guyon's canal has been described. The anterior and posterior ulnar recurrent arteries do not cross or compress the ulnar nerve.

Physiology, Biochemistry, Pharmacology, and Microbiology

Douglas R. Dirschl, M.D.

DIRECTIONS: Each question below contains five suggested responses. Select the **one best** response to each question.

69. Each of the following substances is involved in the regulation of bone resorption. The only one for which osteoclasts have specific receptors is

(A) parathyroid hormone
(B) calcitonin
(C) thyroxine
(D) 1,25-dihydroxyvitamin D
(E) transforming growth factor beta

70. All the following are physiologic effects of parathormone EXCEPT

(A) increased hydroxylation of vitamin D in the renal tubule
(B) decreased resorption of calcium in the proximal renal tubule
(C) increased resorption of calcium in the distal renal tubule
(D) increased release of phosphate from bone
(E) increased serum levels of phosphate

71. Which of the following features is most consistently seen in osteoporosis?

(A) Increased serum alkaline phosphatase
(B) Decreased serum calcium
(C) Increased serum parathyroid hormone
(D) Impaired mineralization of osteoid
(E) Increased susceptibility to fractures

72. All the following bones are formed primarily by endochondral ossification EXCEPT the

(A) vertebra
(B) scapula
(C) clavicle
(D) patella
(E) scaphoid

73. Aging is associated with which of the following changes in cartilage proteoglycans?

(A) Increased keratan sulfate content
(B) Increased chondroitin sulfate content
(C) Increased aggregate size
(D) Increased length of glycosaminoglycan side chains
(E) Decreased rate of proteoglycan synthesis

74. A function of proteoglycan aggregates in articular cartilage is to

(A) regulate delivery of nutrients to components of the matrix
(B) regulate hydration of the matrix
(C) regulate hydration of the chondrocyte
(D) maintain alignment of the collagen fibers
(E) strengthen the attachment between articular cartilage and subchondral bone

75. The primary effect of bone morphogenetic proteins (BMPs) is to

(A) increase formation of osteoid by mature osteoblasts
(B) increase mineralization of osteoid
(C) induce migration of osteoblasts to the repair site
(D) induce differentiation of progenitor cells into chondrocytes
(E) induce migration of monocytes to the repair site

76. All the following are characteristics of demineralized bone implants EXCEPT that

(A) rapid osteoinduction occurs
(B) graft resorption occurs
(C) no immediate strength is provided
(D) the grafts are easily shaped
(E) the grafts are radiolucent

77. Osteomalacia resulting from liver disease is caused by impaired synthesis of which of the following metabolites?

(A) Calciferol
(B) Cholecalciferol
(C) 7-Dehydroxycholesterol
(D) 25-Hydroxycholecalciferol
(E) 1,25-Dihydroxycholecalciferol

78. The disease that results in deficient hydroxylation of the pro-alpha chains of collagen is known as

(A) scurvy
(B) rickets
(C) Ehlers-Danlos syndrome
(D) Marfan's syndrome
(E) lathyrism

79. All the following may be components of a proteoglycan subunit EXCEPT

(A) keratan sulfate
(B) chondroitin sulfate
(C) hyaluronic acid
(D) core protein
(E) dermatan sulfate

80. In the biology of bone grafts, osteoconduction is best defined as

(A) synthesis of new bone by the cells of the graft or the cells of host origin
(B) growth of capillaries and osteoprogenitor cells into the area of the graft
(C) recruitment of pleuripontential cells that differentiate into osteoblasts in the area of the graft
(D) resorption of graft bone and replacement with new host bone
(E) migration of monocytes into the area of the graft

81. Muscular strains occur typically

(A) in the muscle fiber
(B) at the Z line between fibers
(C) at the myotendinous junction
(D) in the tendon at the muscle's insertion
(E) in the fibrous portion of the muscle's origin

82. Endurance training increases all the following in muscle EXCEPT the

(A) number of mitochondria
(B) number of glycogen-synthesizing enzymes
(C) mass of protective connective tissue
(D) size of type I fibers
(E) strength

83. The gastrocnemius muscle in an animal is immobilized in a shortened position; the same muscle in another animal is immobilized in a lengthened position. After four weeks of immobilization, the two muscles will be equal in the

(A) degree of muscle atrophy
(B) maximum tension generated in a tetanic contraction
(C) loss of muscle weight
(D) loss of sarcoplasmic protein
(E) loss of myofibrillar protein

84. Which of the following statements is most likely to be true regarding the effects of immobilization on ligaments?

(A) Energy absorption to failure increases; normal insertional site
(B) Load to failure increases; osteoclastic activity at the insertional site
(C) Load to failure decreases; osteoclastic activity at the insertional site
(D) Load to failure increases; normal insertional site
(E) Load to failure decreases; normal insertional site

85. In a patient with a complete, unrepaired transection of the radial nerve at the level of the mid-humerus, an electromyogram of the brachioradialis muscle performed four weeks after injury will most likely demonstrate

(A) electrical silence
(B) positive waves
(C) reduced motor potentials
(D) fasciculations
(E) triphasic motor potentials

86. The collagen fibers in articular cartilage are best oriented to resist shear stress parallel to the motion of the joint in the

(A) gliding zone, superficial layer
(B) gliding zone, tangential layer
(C) transitional layer
(D) radial zone
(E) tidemark

87. Repeated impact loading of articular cartilage produces all the following changes EXCEPT

(A) surface fibrillation
(B) decreased tensile strength
(C) chondrocyte cloning
(D) osteophyte formation
(E) decreased synthesis of matrix

88. A 6-month-old infant with a history of poor weight gain, frequent vomiting, hypotonia, a rachitic "rosary," and a bulging anterior cranial fontanel has normal serum calcium and phosphate levels, normal serum vitamin D levels, and decreased serum alkaline phosphatase levels. The most likely diagnosis is

(A) vitamin D–deficient rickets
(B) vitamin D–resistant rickets
(C) hypophosphatemic rickets
(D) hypophosphatasia
(E) osteomalacia

89. Donation of autologous blood prior to spinal instrumentation and fusion for idiopathic scoliosis most significantly reduces the risk of transmission of

(A) bacterial infection
(B) hepatitis A
(C) hepatitis B
(D) hepatitis C (non-A, non-B hepatitis)
(E) AIDS

90. In an otherwise healthy 8-year-old child with acute osteomyelitis of the proximal tibia who is allergic to penicillin and cephalosporins, the most appropriate antibiotic treatment prior to identification of the causative organism is

(A) ciprofloxacin
(B) gentamicin
(C) clindamycin
(D) tetracycline
(E) amikacin

91. Patients with sickle cell disease are especially predisposed to bone and joint infections caused by

(A) *Pseudomonas aeruginosa*
(B) *Salmonella multilocida*
(C) *Escherichia coli*
(D) *Enterococcus faecalis*
(E) *Haemophilus influenzae*

92. In a patient receiving a general anesthetic for surgery, the earliest sign of developing malignant hyperthermia is

(A) muscle rigidity
(B) elevated temperature
(C) hypertension
(D) myoglobinuria
(E) hypercarbia

93. After transfusion of the first of 2 units of banked, packed red blood cells, a patient complains of pruritus, shaking chills, and urticaria. The patient's temperature is 38.5° C (101.3° F). The most appropriate course of action is to

(A) transfuse the second unit of blood
(B) administer diphenhydramine and acetaminophen; transfuse the second unit of blood
(C) stop the transfusion; administer diphenhydramine and acetaminophen
(D) stop the transfusion; send blood and urine samples for laboratory analysis
(E) stop the transfusion; send blood and urine samples for laboratory analysis; administer intravenous fluids

94. A 35-year-old farmworker sustained a grade II open tibial fracture when he was struck by a tractor. His last tetanus booster was given when he was 16. Appropriate tetanus prophylaxis for this patient is

(A) 0.5 mL of tetanus toxoid
(B) 0.5 mL of tetanus toxoid and 500 units of tetanus human immune globulin
(C) 0.5 mL of tetanus toxoid and 2.0 million units of penicillin
(D) 1.0 mL of tetanus toxoid
(E) 1.0 mL of tetanus toxoid and 500 units of tetanus human immune globulin

95. Heparin prevents thrombosis by the molecular action of

(A) inhibiting activation of factor X
(B) inhibiting activation of factor VIII
(C) inhibiting activation of factors VIII and X
(D) enhancing the action of antithrombin III
(E) inhibiting platelet aggregation

96. The earliest change in nerve conduction studies (NCS) following neural compression is

(A) decreased distal sensory amplitude
(B) increased distal sensory latency
(C) increased distal motor latency
(D) decreased distal motor amplitude
(E) the appearance of fibrillation potentials

97. All the following are neural responses to an acute, compressive episode EXCEPT

(A) blood supply is decreased
(B) axoplasmic transport is reduced
(C) Wallerian degeneration of the distal axons occurs
(D) recovery is seldom complete
(E) recovery may take months

98. The predominant cell type seen at sites of active osteolysis following arthroplasty of the hip is the

(A) lymphocyte
(B) polymorphonuclear leukocyte
(C) macrophage
(D) atypical fibroblast
(E) osteoclast

99. All the following factors that modulate the coagulation system require vitamin K as a cofactor EXCEPT

(A) factor VII
(B) factor VIII
(C) factor IX
(D) factor X
(E) protein C

100. The anticoagulant effects of warfarin are most rapidly reversed by which of the following agents?

(A) Vitamin K
(B) Protamine
(C) Whole blood
(D) Fresh frozen plasma
(E) Thrombin

101. The function of the groove of Ranvier is to provide

(A) mechanical support to the growth plate
(B) cells for growth in width of the growth plate
(C) vascular supply to the growth plate
(D) attachment for the joint capsule
(E) attachment for articular cartilage

102. Colchicine exerts an anti-inflammatory effect in the treatment of acute gouty arthritis by

(A) increasing excretion of uric acid
(B) promoting dissolution of urate crystals
(C) preventing phagocytosis of urate crystals
(D) inhibiting migration of granulocytes
(E) inhibiting the enzyme xanthine oxidase

103. For a 3-year-old girl with an acute pyarthrosis of the knee, antibiotic therapy prior to identification of the organism should be directed against *Staphylococcus aureus, Streptococcus pyogenes*, and

(A) *Escherichia coli*
(B) *Haemophilus influenzae*
(C) *Neisseria gonorrhoeae*
(D) *Pseudomonas aeruginosa*
(E) *Serratia marcescens*

104. Which of the following statements most correctly defines metastatic calcification?

(A) The presence of bone in a nonphysiologic location
(B) Calcium deposits and bone formation in a matrix produced by malignant cells
(C) Calcium deposits in damaged tissues, with normal extracellular calcium and phosphate concentrations
(D) Calcium deposits in tissues, with local elevation of extracellular calcium and phosphate concentrations
(E) The deposition of inorganic ions in tissues as a result of a metabolic abnormality

105. Surgical repair of a clean, complete, transverse mid-belly laceration of the biceps brachii muscle is most likely to result in

(A) scar formation at the laceration site, minimal regeneration of muscle fibers, and mild loss of muscle strength
(B) scar formation at the laceration site, minimal regeneration of muscle fibers, and progressive loss of muscle strength
(C) scar formation at the laceration site and progressive fibrosis of muscle fibers on both sides of the laceration
(D) regeneration of muscle fibers at the laceration site and atrophy of the muscle fibers distal to the laceration
(E) regeneration of muscle fibers at the laceration site and full strength

DIRECTIONS: Each group of questions below consists of lettered headings followed by a set of numbered items. For each numbered item, select the **one** lettered heading with which it is most closely associated. Each lettered heading may be used **once, more than once, or not at all**.

Questions 106–111

For each numbered item below, select the mediator of inflammation with which it is most closely associated.

(A) Prostaglandins
(B) Thromboxane A_2
(C) Histamine
(D) Leukotrienes
(E) Platelet activating factor

106. Impaired synthesis after administration of aspirin with a resulting decrease in platelet aggregation

107. Inhibition of gastric acid secretion and promotion of formation of cytoprotective mucus in the intestine

108. Synthesis by a small number of cell types, including platelets, endothelial cells, and leukocytes

109. Possible increase in synthesis following administration of aspirin or other nonsteroidal anti-inflammatory drugs (NSAIDs)

110. Intrinsically potent vasoconstrictor

111. Ability to directly increase vascular permeability

Questions 112–116

For each numbered item below, select the region of the fully developed growth plate with which it is most closely associated.

(A) Reserve zone
(B) Proliferative zone
(C) Hypertrophic zone
(D) Primary spongiosa
(E) Secondary spongiosa

112. Highest oxygen tension

113. Absence of vascular supply

114. Formation of bone

115. Lowest cell density

116. Chondrocyte cell division

Physiology, Biochemistry, Pharmacology, and Microbiology

Answers

69. The answer is B. *(Favus, pp 43–58.)* Parathyroid hormone stimulates both differentiation of osteoclastic progenitor cells and bone resorption by mature osteoclasts. These effects, however, are indirect, being mediated through cells of osteoblastic lineage. Vitamin D is a potent stimulator of osteoclastic bone resorption, but this effect is also mediated through osteoblastic cells. Thyroxine stimulates bone resorption but will not do so in the presence of osteoclasts alone because there are no thyroxine receptors on the osteoclast. Transforming growth factor beta appears to act through stimulation of cells of osteoblastic lineage and not directly on the osteoclast. Since calcitonin receptors are present on the osteoclast, calcitonin causes shrinkage of the osteoclast within minutes of administration.

70. The answer is E. *(Favus, p 45.)* Parathyroid hormone stimulates increased release of phosphate from bone, but serum phosphate falls because of the rapid phosphaturia induced by parathormone stimulation of phosphate excretion in the distal tubule. Although the net effect of parathormone administration is to increase calcium resorption by the kidney, this effect results from a decrease in calcium resorption in the proximal tubule coupled with a much larger increase in calcium resorption in the distal tubule. Parathormone also stimulates 1-hydroxylation of vitamin D in the kidney.

71. The answer is E. *(Favus, p 151.)* Osteoporosis is a metabolic bone disorder in which the loss of mineralized bone increases the risk of fractures after minimal trauma. The mineralization of osteoid is normal, but the amount of osteoid produced is decreased. Serum markers such as alkaline phosphatase, calcium, and parathormone are generally normal.

72. The answer is C. *(Albright, pp 52–55.)* Membranous bone formation is responsible for the cranial bones, facial bones, mandible, and clavicle. Secondary endochondral ossification of the clavicle occurs at one or both ends of the bone, but the substance of the bone is intramembranous in origin. The remainder of the axial and appendicular skeleton is formed by endochondral ossification, although growth in the width of these bones by periosteal bone formation is a form of membranous ossification.

73. The answer is A. *(Albright, pp 362–363.)* Aging is associated with a shift in gylcosaminoglycan side chains from predominantly chondroitin sulfate to an increasing content of keratan sulfate. The length of the glycosaminoglycan side chains decreases with aging; the size of the proteoglycan aggregates also decreases with aging. The rate of synthesis of proteoglycans is constant throughout adult life, but the size and composition of the proteoglycans synthesized changes with aging.

74. The answer is B. *(Albright, pp 356–358.)* The negative charges on the glycosaminoglycan side chains of the proteoglycan molecules repel one another and force the aggregate to occupy the largest possible space. These negative charges also attract and hold positively charged water molecules, allowing the proteoglycan molecules to regulate hydration of the cartilage matrix. The proteoglycan concentration is directly related to the stiffness and shear strength of the cartilage. Proteoglycan molecules have no effect on the hydration of chondrocytes, the delivery of nutrients, or the alignment of collagen fibers.

75. The answer is D. *(Friedlaender, pp 75–83.)* The bone morphogenetic proteins act on local mesodermal progenitor cells to induce differentiation into chondrocytes. These chondrocytes form cartilage, which subsequently undergoes endochondral ossification to bone. BMPs appear to have no direct effect on mature osteocytes to synthesize or mineralize osteoid. Being local agents, BMPs do not cause such remote effects as migration of osteoblasts or monocytes to the area of bone repair.

76. The answer is B. *(Friedlaender, pp 60–62.)* Most allograft bone materials and bone substitutes undergo resorption as part of the incorporation process, which is not the case with demineralized materials. Demineralized bone grafts are soft and easily shaped at the time of surgery. Because of removal of the mineral elements of bone in processing, these grafts have no inherent strength at the time of implantation and are radiolucent.

77. The answer is D. *(Albright, pp 312–314.)* Vitamin D_3 (cholecalciferol) is the most important form in man and is formed in the skin by the ultraviolet irradiation of 7-dehydroxycholesterol. Vitamin D_3 is hydroxylated in the liver to 25-hydroxycholecalciferol, synthesis of which is impaired in liver disease. Hydroxylation to the active form, 1,25-dihydroxycholecalciferol, occurs in the kidney. Calciferol, or vitamin D_2, is relatively unimportant in humans and is produced by irradiation of ergosterol.

78. The answer is A. *(Gamble, pp 64–67.)* Proline hydroxylase and lysine hydroxylase are responsible for hydroxylation of the pro-alpha chains of collagen in the endoplasmic reticulum. These enzymes require ferrous iron, molecular oxygen, and ascorbic acid (vitamin C) as cofactors. Scurvy, or vitamin C deficiency, impairs the function of these enzymes. Patients with Ehlers-Danlos syndrome have defects in the cross-linking of mature collagen fibers. Marfan's syndrome has many variants, most of which exhibit extra amino acids on the procollagen chains. Lathyrism is a disease of animals caused by eating the seeds of sweet peas, which contain a substance that inhibits cross-linking of mature collagen fibers.

79. The answer is C. *(Gamble, pp 68–72.)* A proteoglycan subunit is composed of a core protein with numerous attached glycosaminoglycan side chains. In skeletal tissue, these side chains are most commonly chondroitin sulfate and keratan sulfate, but dermatan sulfate and heparan sulfate are also found. Hyaluronic acid is the central organizing molecule of a proteoglycan aggregate; 100 to 500 proteoglycan subunits form noncovalent associations with the hyaluronic acid molecule to form an aggregate.

80. The answer is B. *(Friedlaender, pp 3–5, 55–60.)* Osteogenesis is the synthesis of new bone at the graft site, and graft remodeling is the process of resorbing the graft material and replacing it with newly formed host bone. Osteoinduction refers to the recruitment of mesenchymal progenitor cells to the area of the graft, and the induction of their differentiation into bone-forming cells. The migration of mononuclear cells into an area of bone injury occurs normally in the inflammatory phase of fracture healing. Osteoconduction is the three-dimensional process whereby vascular and perivascular tissues, accompanied by osteoprogenitor cells, grow into the area of the graft.

81. The answer is C. *(Poss, p 98.)* Animal and clinical studies support the assertion that the site of injury in muscular strains is the myotendinous junction. Even "mid-belly" tears actually occur at central myotendinous attachments. At the myotendinous junction, the muscle cells are extensively involuted to afford a greater surface area for attachment to the tendon fibers.

82. The answer is D. *(Albright, pp 420–421.)* Endurance training of muscles results in more efficient use of glycogen and an increased capacity for aerobic metabolism. This leads to increases in the number of mitochondria, the number of glycogen-synthesizing and oxidative enzymes, the mass of contractile protein and protective connective tissue, and strength. Type 1, or fast-twitch muscle fibers, undergo hypertrophy with high-resistance training but not with endurance training.

83. The answer is D. *(Jokl, Clin Orthop 174:222–229, 1983.)* Investigations done in animals have shown clear differences in function and protein composition between muscles immobilized in a shortened versus a lengthened position. The loss of muscle weight, a measure of muscle atrophy, was significantly greater in shortened muscles than in lengthened muscles. The maximum tension generated in a tetanic contraction, as well as muscle endurance, were decreased in shortened muscles. Myofibrillar protein loss was greater in shortened muscles than in lengthened muscles, but sarcoplasmic protein loss was similar in the two groups. Muscles immobilized in a lengthened position retain better physiologic function than those immobilized in a shortened position.

84. The answer is C. *(Poss, p 100.)* Immobilization significantly decreases the strength, load to failure, and the energy-absorbing capacity of ligaments. These effects are most pronounced at the bone-ligament junction, which shows increased osteoclastic activity and bone resorption. When tested in tension, immobilized ligaments commonly fail at the bone-ligament interface, while normal ligaments fail more often in midsubstance.

85. The answer is B. *(Albright, pp 440–441.)* In this situation, the brachioradialis muscle has been completely denervated. Electrical signs of denervation may be seen as early as 2 days or as late as 2 weeks after injury and consist of fibrillation potentials and positive waves. Fasciculations and reduced motor potentials are seen in injured muscles with intact innervation or in primary diseases of muscle or motor nerves. Triphasic motor potentials are characteristic of the normal state.

86. The answer is B. *(Albright, pp 348–351.)* The superficial layer of the gliding zone is a thin layer consisting of a flat sheet of randomly oriented collagen fibers. The tangential layer of the gliding zone has collagen fibers arranged parallel to one another in the direction of joint motion. This layer resists shear stress in the direction of joint motion but not in the direction perpendicular to joint motion. The collagen fibers of the transitional and radial layers are primarily perpendicular to the joint surface to resist compression. The tidemark resists shear in all directions, anchoring the articular cartilage to the underlying zone of calcified cartilage.

87. The answer is E. *(Brandt, pp 36–38.)* Models of impact loading of articular cartilage have produced changes very similar to those seen in human osteoarthritis. These include fibrillation, decreased tensile strength, altered proteoglycan content, chondrocyte cloning, increased hydration, and osteophyte formation. Biosynthesis of matrix increases with repeated impact loading of cartilage in an attempt to repair the injury.

88. The answer is D. *(Favus, pp 171–190.)* Hypophosphatasia is a rare, heritable type of rickets characterized by a reduction of activity in the tissue-nonspecific isoenzyme of alkaline phosphatase. Its clinical appearance may be identical to that of nutritional rickets, although affected children may become extremely ill and die. Unlike other types of rickets, serum levels of calcium, phosphate, vitamin D, and parathormone are normal. Alkaline phosphatase levels in the serum are, however, quite low, which is important in the diagnosis.

89. The answer is D. *(Poss, pp 159–162.)* Prior to transfusion, donated blood is screened for the presence of bacterial infection, antibodies to the hepatitis A and hepatitis B antigens, and human immunodeficiency virus (HIV). A screening test for hepatitis C (non-A, non-B hepatitis) is currently not in widespread commercial use. Although transfusion of autologous blood reduces the risk of transmission of all of these conditions, it most significantly reduces the risk of transmission of the condition for which donated blood is not screened.

90. The answer is C. *(Morrissy, pp 539–561.)* The most likely causative organism for osteomyelitis in this child is *Staphylococcus aureus*. The recommended initial treatment is a semisynthetic penicillin or, for patients allergic to penicillin, a cephalosporin. Patients allergic to both penicillins and cephalosporins should be given clindamycin or vancomycin as empiric treatment. Ciprofloxacin is not currently approved for use in children. Gentamicin and amikacin have spectra of activity primarily against gram-negative organisms.

91. The answer is B. *(Dirschl, Orthop Rev 23:305–312, 1994.)* Osteomyelitis in patients with sickle cell disease is most commonly caused by staphylococci, but salmonellae also cause a large percentage of cases. It is postulated that microinfarcts in the bowel wall cause salmonellal bacteremia, which may result in osteomyelitis. Osteomyelitis in patients with sickle disease often occurs in the diaphysis, in contrast to the metaphyseal location of most other osseous infections.

92. The answer is E. *(Poss, pp 240–242.)* Malignant hyperthermia is a hypermetabolic disorder of skeletal muscle and may be a heritable condition. It can be triggered intraoperatively by certain anesthetic agents or may occur during the early postoperative period. Hypermetabolism causes hypercarbia (the earliest detectable change), which causes tachycardia and tachypnea via sympathetic stimulation. Arrhythmias, muscle rigidity, oxygen desaturation, hypertension, and elevation of body temperature often follow. Hyperkalemia, hypercalcemia, and myoglobinuria may also be present.

93. The answer is B. *(Poss, pp 158–159.)* Febrile and allergic reactions to transfusion of banked blood are common and self-limiting. They generally occur after transfusion of more than 300 mL of blood and are characterized by shaking chills, pruritus, urticaria, and fever. Treatment is supportive, and pretreatment with diphenhydramine and acetaminophen prior to subsequent blood transfusions diminishes such reactions. Hemolytic transfusion reactions occur after very small volumes (30 to 40 mL) of blood are transfused. In addition to the signs and symptoms noted above, these reactions can cause dyspnea, nausea, hemoglobinuria, and shock.

94. The answer is B. *(Browner, p 324.)* Tetanus is caused by *Clostridium tetani,* an anaerobe that produces a neurotoxin. Active immunization with tetanus toxoid is the most effective way to prevent the disease. Any patient who has not completed a series of three toxoid immunizations or has not received a booster dose in the 10 years prior to being injured should receive 0.5 mL of tetanus toxoid. Patients with severe wounds, such as open fractures, should receive 250 to 500 units of tetanus human immune globulin in addition to tetanus toxoid. Although this patient should receive antibiotics to reduce the risk of infection from other organisms, antibiotics are not required for effective tetanus prophylaxis.

95. The answer is D. *(Poss, pp 107–108.)* Antithrombin III is a naturally occurring inhibitor of the activation of factor X and thrombin. Heparin combines with antithrombin III to increase markedly its antithrombotic activity. It appears to have no direct effects on any of the clotting factors or on platelet aggregation. Because the clotting mechanism is truly a cascade, less heparin and antithrombin III are required to neutralize factor X than are required to neutralize the thrombin produced once the thrombotic process is under way, which is the rationale for the prophylactic administration of heparin in low doses.

96. The answer is A. *(Gelberman, J Bone Joint Surg 75–A:1854–1878, 1993.)* Abnormal distal sensory conduction values are the most specific findings in neural compression. The earliest of these changes is a decrease in the distal sensory amplitude, followed by an increase in distal sensory latency. Changes in distal motor conduction values lag well behind changes in sensory values. Fibrillation potentials seen on electromyograms (EMGs) are indicative of muscle denervation. In clinical use, the distal sensory latency has the greatest diagnostic value, since it is the most consistent finding from one patient to another.

97. The answer is D. *(Albright, pp 438–439.)* Acute compression of a nerve interferes with the nerve's blood supply and axoplasmic transport. Ischemia results in degeneration of the compressed axon's distal segments, followed by Wallerian degeneration, which results in a recovery period measured in months. Unlike findings after transection, the endoneural tubules remain in continuity throughout the process, guiding the regrowth of axons and ensuring contact with the structure each originally innervated. Thus, recovery is generally complete after this type of injury but is seldom complete after transection of the nerve.

98. The answer is C. *(Schmalzried, J Bone Joint Surg 74–A:849–863, 1992.)* In histologic studies, all sites of active bone resorption around the prosthetic components were populated predominantly by macrophages. These cells were often seen in Howship's lacunae in the absence of osteoclasts, which suggests direct resorption of bone by macrophages. The macrophages and the extracellular matrix were, in all cases, filled with particulate debris; polyethylene particles were present and were combined, in some cases, with polymethylmethacrylate or metal particles. Small numbers of lymphocytes and osteoclasts were also seen at these sites. Fibroblasts were present in small numbers at sites of active bone resorption, but they were the predominant cell type at sites where bone resorption was not taking place.

99. The answer is B. *(Gilman, pp 1317–1320.)* Some clotting factors remain biologically inactive unless carboxylated by an enzyme that requires vitamin K as a cofactor. These so-called vitamin K–dependent clotting factors include factors VII, IX, X, and prothrombin (factor II). Two anticoagulant proteins, protein C and protein S, which are synthesized in the liver, are also vitamin K–dependent. The oral anticoagulants, such as warfarin, prevent the activation of vitamin K and thereby indirectly inhibit the formation of the vitamin K–dependent modulators.

100. The answer is D. *(Gilman, pp 1317–1320.)* Administration of vitamin K reverses the anticoagulant effects of warfarin, but the response may take 24 h or longer, since carboxylation of new coagulation factors must first occur. Fresh frozen plasma, which contains high concentrations of already carboxylated clotting factors, provides immediate hemostatic action. Whole blood contains very low concentrations of clotting factors and is ineffective in this setting. Thrombin is indicated for topical use only, since high parenteral concentrations are required to gain hemostatic effects. Protamine sulfate, which binds to and inactivates heparin, is used for rapid reversal of bleeding complications following heparin therapy.

101. The answer is B. *(Brighton, Instr Course Lect 33:3–25, 1984.)* Encircling the growth plate of a long bone is a wedge-shaped groove of cells called the *ossification groove* and a ring of fibrous tissue and bone called the *perichondrial ring*. The ossification groove is named after Ranvier, who first described these structures in 1873. LaCroix studied the perichondrial ring, which now bears his name. The groove of Ranvier contains cells that flow into the cartilage at the beginning of the reserve zone of the growth plate to provide chondrocytes for growth in width of the growth plate. The perichondrial ring of LaCroix acts as a limiting membrane that provides mechanical support for the growth plate. The perichondrial artery supplies both of these structures but does not penetrate the growth plate.

102. The answer is D. *(Gilman, pp 674–680.)* The anti-inflammatory effect of colchicine is relatively selective for acute gouty arthritis; it is generally not effective for other forms of arthritis. Colchicine interferes with the function of the fibrillar microtubules in granulocytes, inhibiting their migration to the inflamed area. Colchicine also prevents elaboration of a leukocytic glycoprotein that causes joint pain and inflammation in gouty arthritis. Colchicine does not alter phagocytosis of urate crystals. Allopurinol inhibits the enzyme xanthine oxidase, which is necessary for the synthesis of uric acid in man, and thereby lowers serum levels of uric acid. Probenecid increases urinary excretion of uric acid.

103. The answer is B. *(Dirschl, Orthop Rev 23:305–312, 1994.)* In otherwise healthy children between the ages of 1 and 16 years, acute suppurative arthritis is caused by *Staphylococcus aureus* in up to 90 percent of cases. *Streptococcus pyogenes* and *Haemophilus influenzae* are responsible for nearly all the remaining cases. *Escherichia coli* infection is seen in neonates, especially those requiring intensive care. *Pseudomonas aeruginosa* and *Neisseria gonorrhoeae* arthritides are usually not seen in children but are much more common in adults.

104. The answer is D. *(Gamble, pp 77–78.)* The hallmark of metastatic calcification is the presence of elevated concentrations of calcium and phosphate in the extracellular fluid at the site of calcification. Calcification in a matrix produced by malignant cells is referred to as *tumoral calcification*. Dystrophic calcification occurs in damaged tissues in the presence of normal concentrations of extracellular ions (e.g., calcific tendonitis). Metabolic abnormalities, such as gout, result in crystalline deposition disease. The presence of bone in soft tissues is heterotopic ossification.

105. The answer is A. *(Poss, pp 94–95.)* Although myoblasts have the potential to regenerate muscle fibers after laceration of a muscle, this capacity exists only in muscles with very small cross-sectional areas. In large muscles, such as the biceps, dense scar accumulates at the repair site, allowing only minimal fiber regeneration. The innervation of the distal segment of the muscle is disrupted, and this portion of the muscle becomes fibrotic, resulting in a minimal, static loss of muscle strength. The proximal portion of the muscle functions normally, with no apparent loss of muscle strength.

106–111. The answers are 106–B, 107–A, 108–E, 109–D, 110–B, 111–C. *(Gilman, pp 600–614, 638–644.)* Thromboxane A_2 is a potent stimulator of platelet aggregation and is synthesized, as are prostaglandins, by the cyclooxygenase pathway of arachidonic acid metabolism. Aspirin and other NSAIDs inhibit cyclooxygenase and prevent synthesis of thromboxane A_2, which causes decreased platelet aggregation and increased bleeding time. In addition to its role in platelet aggregation, thromboxane A_2 is also a potent vasoconstrictor by direct stimulation of smooth muscle cells in vascular walls.

Prostaglandin E and prostacyclin inhibit gastric acid secretion by a direct action on the cells of the gastric mucosa. These prostaglandins also are responsible for increasing secretion of mucus in the stomach and small intestine.

Most mediators of inflammation, with the exception of platelet activating factor, are synthesized in a wide variety of tissues. Platelet activating factor is synthesized in the vascular endothelium, polymorphonuclear leukocytes, and platelets. It is a potent stimulator of platelet aggregation, vasodilatation, and leukocyte migration and activation. It is not a metabolite of arachidonic acid, and its synthesis is not inhibited by NSAIDs.

Aspirin and other NSAIDs inhibit the enzyme cyclooxygenase, which allows increased accumulation of its substrate, arachidonic acid. This action may increase activity in the lipooxygenase pathway of arachidonic acid metabolism, leading to increased synthesis of leukotrienes, which also are potent mediators of inflammation.

Both prostaglandins and leukotrienes cause increased blood flow in the area of inflammation but do not increase vascular permeability directly. Histamine and bradykinin have this ability and allow serum and other proteinaceous fluid to collect in the extravascular space.

112–116. The answers are 112–B, 113–C, 114–E, 115–A, 116–B. *(Brighton, Instr Course Lect 33:3–25, 1984.)* Epiphyseal arteries pass through the reserve zone and arborize extensively atop the proliferative zone, which results in the highest oxygen tension of any region of the growth plate in the proliferative zone. The reserve zone is not actually supplied by the epiphyseal artery and has a relatively low oxygen tension.

The epiphyseal arteries end in the proliferative zone and do not pass downward into the hypertrophic zone. The metaphyseal arteries do not pass any higher than the last intact transverse septum of calcified cartilage and thus do not pass upward into the hypertrophic zone. This zone, then, is entirely avascular and has the lowest oxygen tension of any region of the growth plate.

Beneath the last intact transverse septum lies a region of vascularized calcified cartilage, the primary spongiosa, in which little or no bone formation occurs, even though plump osteoblasts line the calcified columns. A short distance down these calcified longitudinal bars, the osteoblasts begin to lay down bone. This area of bone formation on the calcified cartilage bars is the secondary spongiosa.

The reserve zone lies immediately next to the bony epiphysis and contains a few small cells separated by large amounts of extracellular matrix. No active cell division is demonstrable in this zone. For all practical purposes, the proliferative zone is the only region of the growth plate where mitosis of chondrocytes occurs.

Pathology

H. Robert Brashear, M.D. and Frank C. Wilson, M.D.

DIRECTIONS: Each question below contains five suggested responses. Select the **one best** response to each question.

117. If, on microscopic examination of the metaphysis of a long bone, all the trabeculae of cancellous bone—even well away from the epiphyseal plate—contained cores of cartilage matrix, the most likely diagnosis would be

(A) osteopetrosis
(B) osteomalacia
(C) achondroplasia
(D) Ollier's disease
(E) spondyloepiphyseal dysplasia

118. If a biopsy of the distal femoral metaphysis of an 8-month-old infant showed that all the cancellous trabeculae consisted of very immature woven bone, the two most likely diagnoses would be

(A) osteogenesis imperfecta and rickets
(B) rickets and osteopetrosis
(C) rickets and scurvy
(D) scurvy and osteopetrosis
(E) scurvy and osteogenesis imperfecta

119. Osteogenesis imperfecta is associated with a defect in the synthesis of

(A) type I collagen
(B) type II collagen
(C) type IV collagen
(D) chondroitin sulfate
(E) keratan sulfate

120. All the following are complications of type I Gaucher's disease EXCEPT

(A) osteonecrosis of the femoral head
(B) pathologic fracture
(C) sarcomatous degeneration
(D) hematogenous osteomyelitis
(E) failure of remodeling of the distal femoral metaphysis

121. In patients with chronic inflammatory arthritis, which of the following accounts for the majority of acute phase effects?

(A) Interleukin 1
(B) Hageman factor
(C) Complement proteins
(D) Circulating immune complexes
(E) Antinuclear antibodies

122. Proliferation of synovial endothelial cells in rheumatoid arthritis is stimulated by

(A) abnormal gamma globulins
(B) transforming growth factor beta
(C) B lymphocytes
(D) parvoviruses
(E) macrophages

123. The earliest observed pathologic feature in the development of gouty arthritis is the

(A) deposition of monosodium urate crystals in synovium and periarticular tissues
(B) appearance of monosodium urate crystals in the renal collecting ducts
(C) appearance of monosodium urate crystals in synovial fluid
(D) appearance of monosodium urate crystals in polymorphonuclear leukocytes
(E) formation of microtophi in the articular cartilage of axial joints

Questions 124–125

An adult patient with osteoarthritis of the hip underwent total hip arthroplasty. A histologic section of the patient's femoral head is shown in the figure.

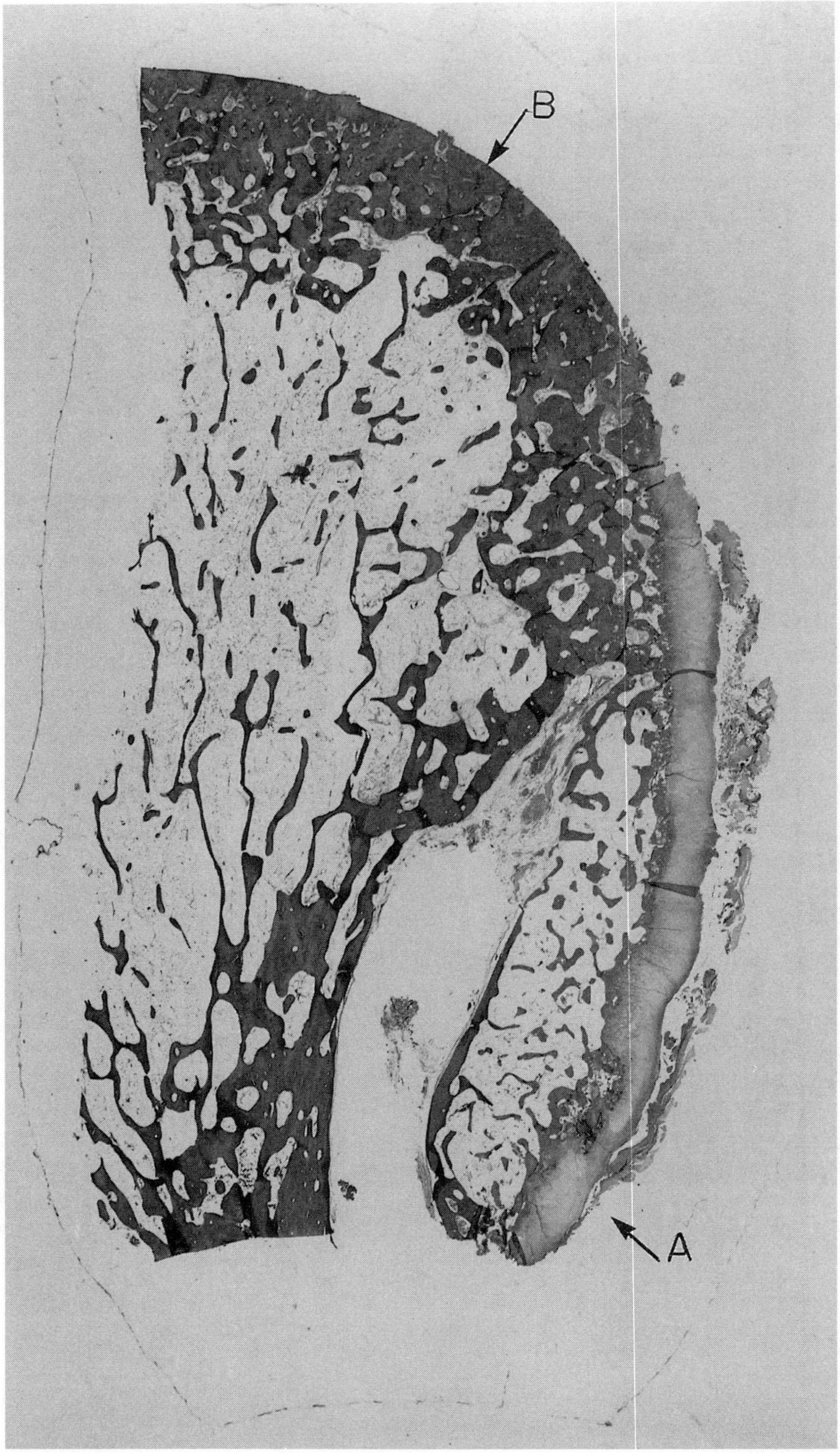

124. The cartilage covering the surface of the large osteophyte (*A*) in the figure

(A) has all the microscopic features of articular cartilage
(B) is supported by subchondral bone of endochondral origin
(C) is joined to the subchondral bone by a tide mark
(D) is likely to be necrotic because of its precarious circulation
(E) has a small but significant incidence of later sarcomatous change

125. At the tip of the arrow labeled *B* in the figure, high-power magnification would most likely reveal

(A) a thin layer of articular cartilage with flattened cells aligned parallel to the surface
(B) degenerated articular cartilage with marked fibrillation
(C) immature woven bone
(D) dense lamellar bone
(E) numerous osteoclasts and resorption canals

---

126. The microscopic structure of a subcutaneous nodule in a patient with rheumatoid arthritis most closely resembles that of a

(A) granulamatous lesion of tuberculosis
(B) lymphoma
(C) focus of pigmented villonodular synovitis
(D) giant cell tumor of bone
(E) ganglion of tendon sheath

127. In acute hematogenous osteomyelitis of childhood, the earliest microscopic changes in bone are in the

(A) epiphysis
(B) metaphyseal-physeal junction
(C) subperiosteal portion of the metaphysis
(D) subperiosteal portion of the diaphysis
(E) metaphyseal-diaphyseal junction

128. An involucrum seen 3 weeks after the onset of acute hematogenous osteomyelitis would consist principally of

(A) lamellar bone with hematopoietic marrow
(B) woven or fiber bone
(C) a mixture of cartilage and immature bone
(D) lamellar bone with a fibrous marrow
(E) endochondral bone

129. A synovial biopsy of the ankle pictured in the figure would most likely show

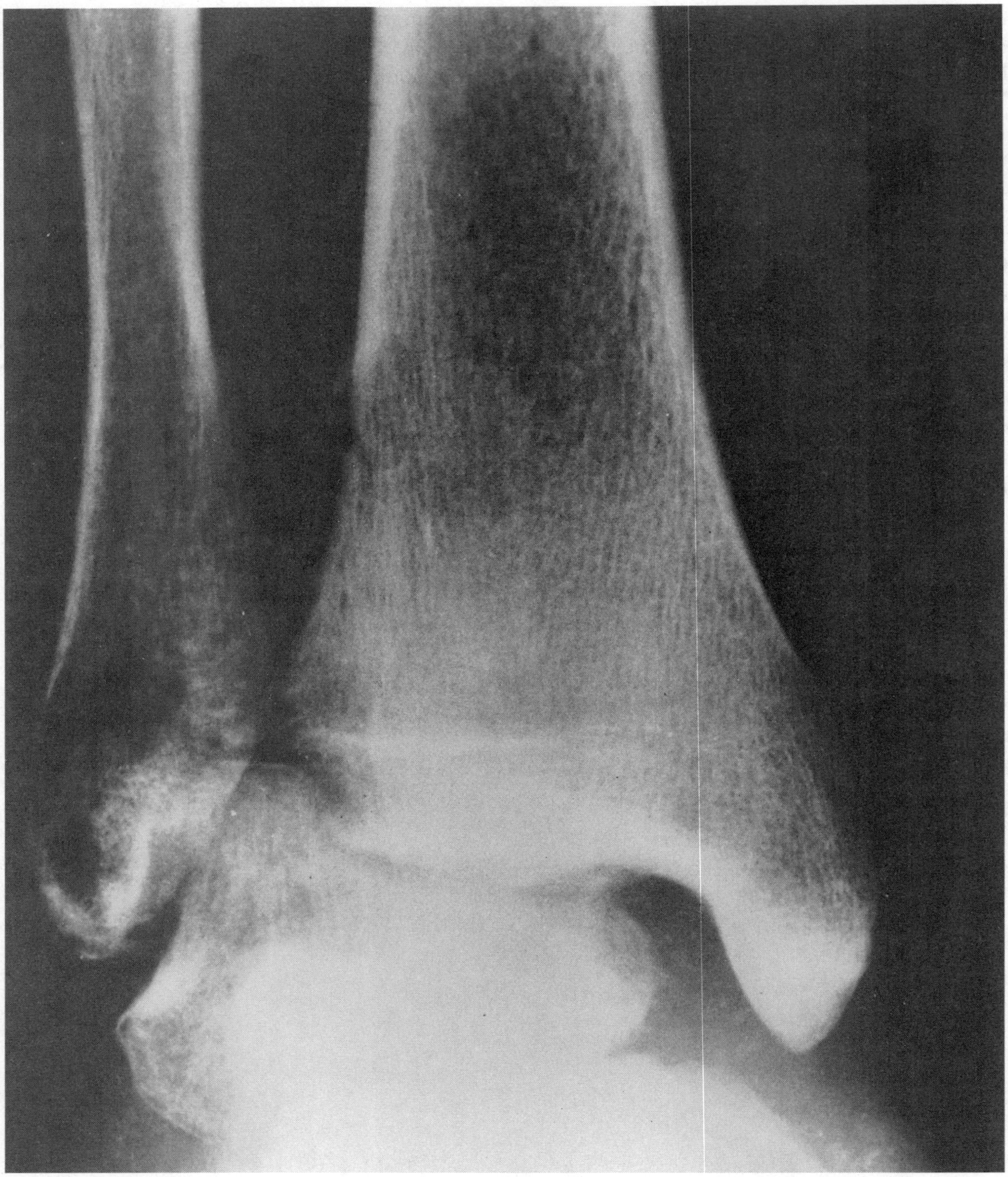

(A) numerous monosodium urate crystals
(B) Charcot-Leyden crystals
(C) numerous polymorphonuclear leukocytes
(D) minimal inflammatory changes
(E) granulomatous changes with caseation

Questions 130–131

A 45-year-old man has had 2 years of chronic, draining osteomyelitis of the femur. An anteroposterior (AP) radiograph and sinogram of the femur are shown in the figure. (*Questions follow on next page.*)

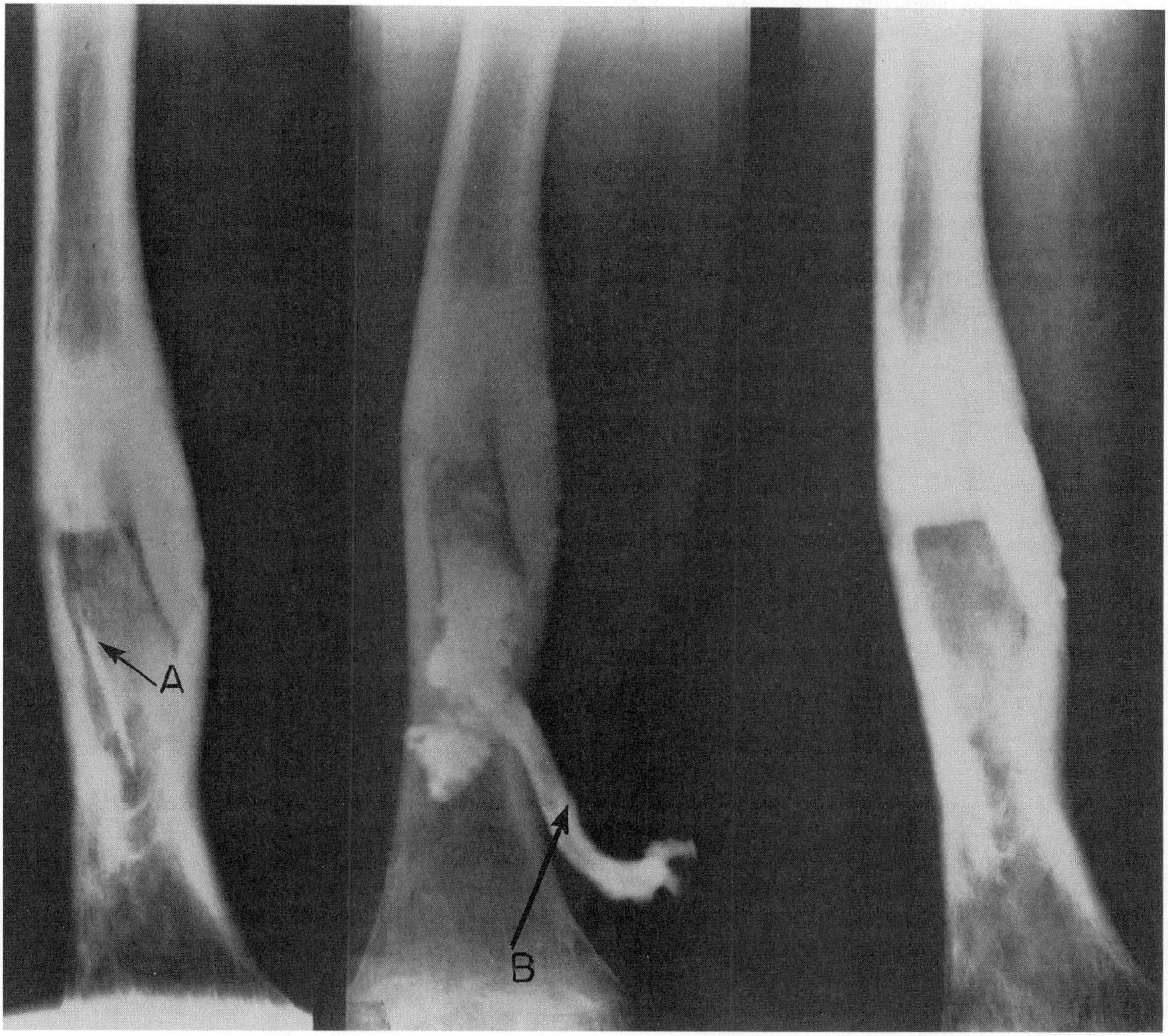

130. Histologic examination of the bone at the tip of arrow *A* would most likely show

(A) trabeculae lined with osteoblasts
(B) immature woven bone
(C) mature cortical bone with osteoclasts covering the surface
(D) surfaces devoid of osteoclasts and osteoblasts
(E) surrounding granulomatous tissue undergoing caseating necrosis and containing Langerhans giant cells

131. Arrow *B* points to a channel leading from the skin surface to the medullary cavity. The channel, outlined by radiopaque dye, would most probably be lined by

(A) squamous epithelium
(B) columnar epithelium with mucous cells
(C) ciliated columnar epithelium
(D) cuboidal transitional epithelium
(E) endothelium

Questions 132–133

A 7-year-old boy had sustained a fracture of the tibia and fibula 3 weeks ago. An AP radiograph of the leg is shown in the figure.

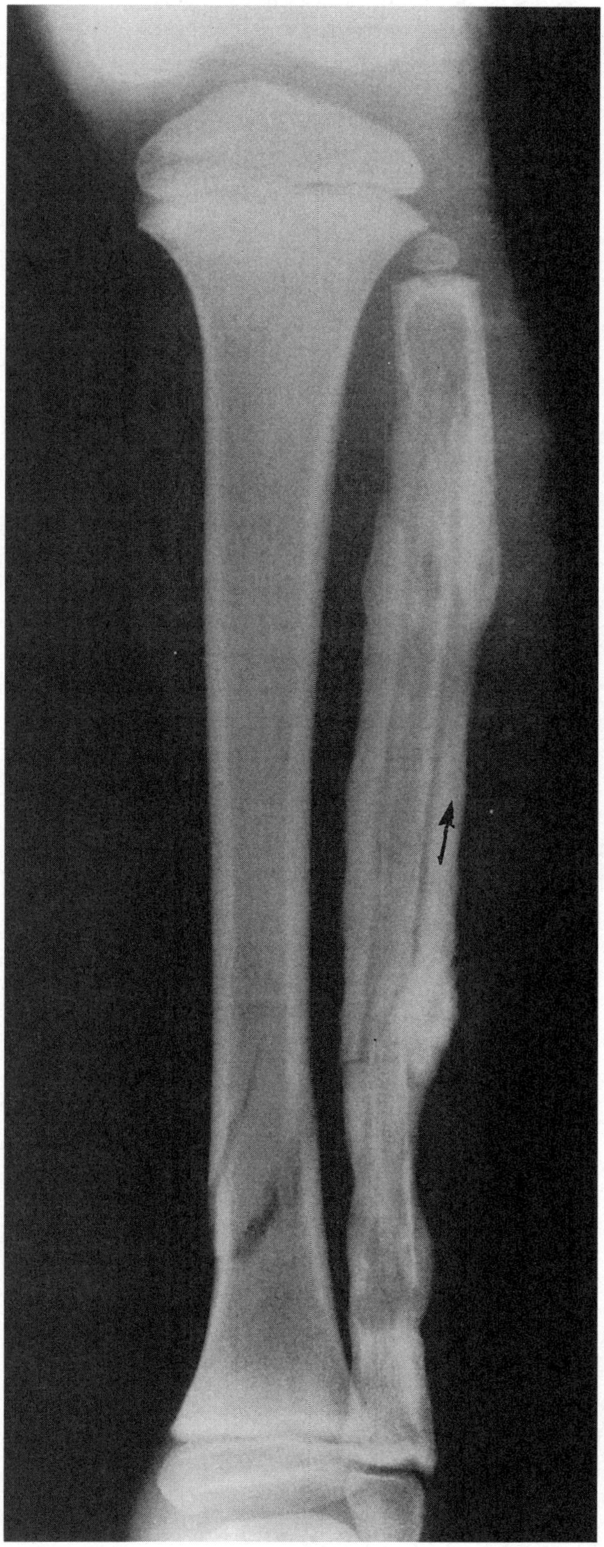

132. The changes in the fibula in the figure are most likely caused by

(A) parosteal osteosarcoma
(B) Ewing's sarcoma
(C) osteogenesis imperfecta
(D) tuberculous osteomyelitis
(E) hematogenous osteomyelitis

133. The bone at the tip of the arrow in the figure is most likely

(A) tumor bone
(B) fracture callus
(C) an involucrum
(D) a sequestrum
(E) viable endochondral bone

134. Histologic examination of cancellous bone from the vertebra of a 90-year-old woman with osteoporosis would most likely reveal

(A) thin trabeculae whose surfaces contain numerous Howship's lacunae
(B) normal trabeculae whose surfaces are lined by osteoid
(C) trabeculae of immature bone
(D) thin trabeculae with neither formation nor resorption surfaces
(E) thin trabeculae with numerous resorption surfaces

135. The biochemical change that reflects increased osteoclastic activity in patients with Paget's disease is elevation of the

(A) serum calcium
(B) serum phosphorus
(C) serum alkaline phosphatase
(D) urinary hydroxyproline
(E) urinary chondroitin sulfate

Questions 136–137

A 4-year-old boy had progressive genu valgum since he began walking at the age of 16 months. The child had a serum calcium of 8.6 mg/dL and phosphorus of 2.2 mg/dL. An AP radiograph of the knee is shown in the figure. (*Questions follow on next page*.)

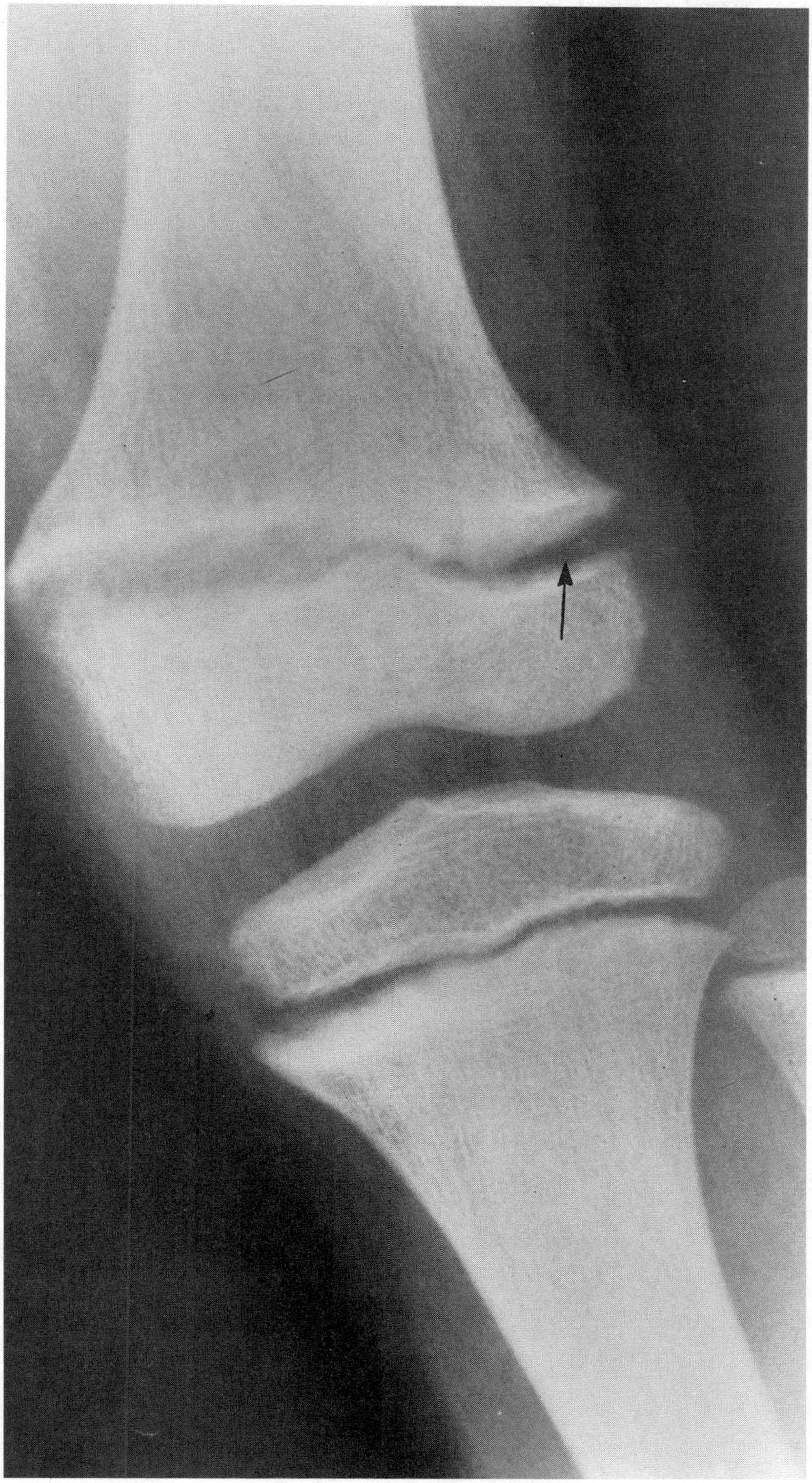

136. A biopsy of the physis at the site indicated by the arrow in the figure would most likely show a marked increase in the number of cells in the

(A) resting zone
(B) zone of cell columns
(C) hypertrophic zone
(D) zone of provisional calcification
(E) zone of endochondral ossification

137. When this child grows up and marries, which, if any, of his children will be likely to have the same disorder?

(A) All of his sons and none of his daughters
(B) All of his daughters and none of his sons
(C) Half of his sons and half of his daughters
(D) All of his children
(E) None of his children

138. Biopsy of a 10-day-old lesion of myositis ossificans traumatica could most easily be misinterpreted as

(A) fibrous dysplasia
(B) chondrosarcoma
(C) Paget's disease
(D) osteogenic sarcoma
(E) Ewing's sarcoma

139. Two days after a sudden interruption of the blood supply to the femoral head in a child (e.g., following fracture or dislocation), the most striking microscopic changes would most likely occur in the

(A) osteocytes
(B) red marrow
(C) synovium
(D) overlying cartilage
(E) woven (immature) bone

140. A 36-year-old man has had osteonecrosis of the femoral head for 1 year. Histologic examination of the marrow in the part of the femoral head that had undergone creeping substitution would reveal

(A) necrosis
(B) regeneration to normal marrow
(C) loose fibrous tissue with numerous vessels
(D) dense scarring with few blood vessels
(E) replacement by cartilage

141. Two months following avascular necrosis of the entire femoral head in a 32-year-old man, histologic examination of the center of the necrotic area would most often reveal

(A) viable fatty marrow
(B) osteoclastic activity along the necrotic trabeculae
(C) osteoblasts lining the necrotic trabeculae
(D) no evidence of cellular activity
(E) fibrous tissue within the marrow spaces

Questions 142–143

The figure is a histologic section of a fractured rib 2 weeks following the fracture in a 22-year-old man who expired due to complications of multiple trauma.

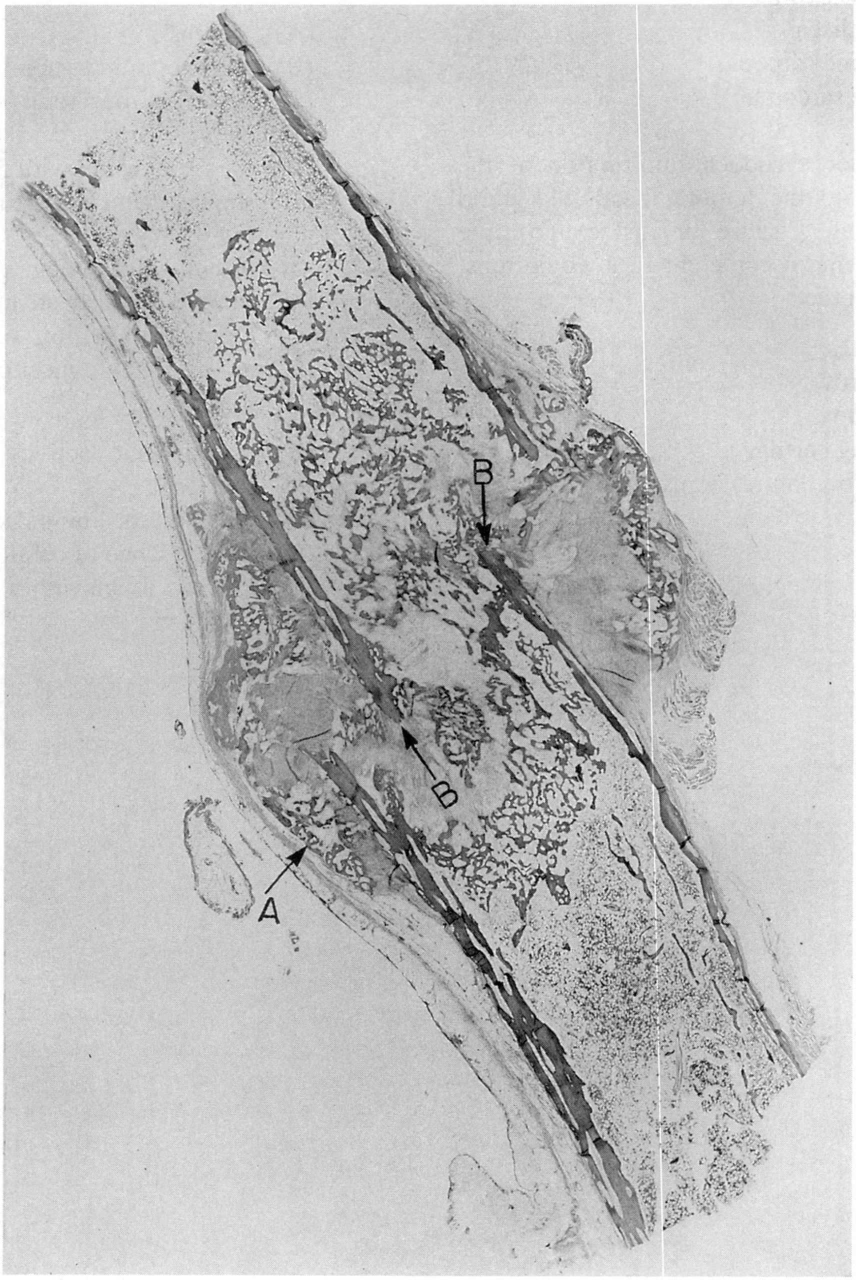

142. The tissue at the tip of arrow *A* is

(A) viable lamellar bone
(B) necrotic lamellar bone
(C) woven bone
(D) haversian bone
(E) unmineralized osteoid

143. The bone at the tip of arrow *B* is most likely

(A) necrotic woven bone
(B) viable lamellar bone
(C) necrotic lamellar bone
(D) unmineralized osteoid
(E) bone of endochondral origin

144. A biopsy taken from the site of implantation of an autogenous tibial cortical bone graft 2 months after surgery would most likely show

(A) the original viable osteocytes within the original bone lacunae
(B) new osteocytes within the original lacunae of the graft
(C) original lacunae containing a mixture of new and old osteocytes
(D) empty original and new lacunae
(E) empty original lacunae and new osteocytes within the new lacunae

145. Following a fracture of the femoral shaft, the most abundant external callus would be most likely to form in

(A) an adult treated with intramedullary fixation
(B) an adult treated with plate fixation
(C) an adult with a closed head injury treated in skeletal traction
(D) a child treated in a spica cast
(E) a child treated with an external skeletal fixator

146. Which of the following lesions is most likely to be confused histologically with a giant cell tumor of bone?

(A) Chondroblastoma
(B) Osteoblastoma
(C) Brown tumor of hyperparathyroidism
(D) Nonossifying fibroma
(E) Osteogenic sarcoma

147. Functionally defective osteoclasts are most likely to be found in

(A) an osteoid osteoma
(B) a chondrosarcoma
(C) hyperparathyroidism
(D) an osteoblastoma
(E) osteopetrosis

148. In patients with metastases to bone, the bony lesion will be symptomatic in

(A) less than 5 percent
(B) 15 to 20 percent
(C) 25 to 30 percent
(D) 35 to 40 percent
(E) Over 50 percent

149. Paget's disease is most likely caused by

(A) an inherited factor
(B) a "slow virus" infection
(C) a hormonal imbalance
(D) a metabolic disease
(E) an immunologic disorder

150. In Paget's disease, progressive osteolysis is most likely to be encountered in the

(A) vertebrae
(B) pelvis
(C) skull
(D) tibiae
(E) metatarsals

151. The clinical feature of an atypical enchondroma that distinguishes it from a typical enchondroma is

(A) location in the bones of the hands and feet
(B) the size of the lesion
(C) occurrence in patients over 50 years of age
(D) an associated history of pain
(E) the appearance of other cartilaginous lesions

152. The likelihood that an enchondroma will develop into a secondary chondrosarcoma is most closely related to the

(A) size of the lesion
(B) extent of calcification within the lesion
(C) presence of binucleated chondrocytes within the lesion
(D) finding of increased uptake on bone scanning
(E) epiphyseal location of the enchondroma

153. Chondrosarcomas are thought to arise from precursory enchondromas in what percentage of cases?

(A) 5 percent
(B) 20 percent
(C) 50 percent
(D) 75 percent
(E) 90 percent

154. In patients over 60 years of age, secondary osteosarcoma occurs most often in association with

(A) prior radiation of a benign lesion
(B) Paget's disease
(C) retinoblastoma
(D) chondrosarcoma
(E) osteochondroma

155. A Codman's triangle is LEAST likely to be seen in association with

(A) an aneurysmal bone cyst
(B) osteomyelitis
(C) a fracture
(D) hemophilic pseudotumor
(E) nonossifying fibroma

156. Which of the following radiographic features is LEAST common in osteogenic sarcoma?

(A) Metaphyseal location
(B) Fluffy, or cloudlike, radiopacities
(C) Periosteal reaction
(D) A soft tissue mass
(E) A complete periosteal collar of bone

157. On histologic examination, an aneurysmal bone cyst can most easily be confused with

(A) an osteogenic sarcoma
(B) a nonossifying fibroma
(C) a chondroblastoma
(D) a hemangioendothelioma
(E) a giant cell tumor

158. The most likely cause of a firm, 9-cm mass in the mid-thigh of a 63-year-old man is

(A) aggressive fibromatosis
(B) malignant fibrous histiocytoma
(C) rhabdomyosarcoma
(D) fibrosarcoma
(E) hemangioma

159. A 15-year-old boy has a 3-cm synovial sarcoma in the midlateral thigh and no palpable lymph nodes. The most appropriate treatment is wide

(A) local excision
(B) local excision and resection of inguinal nodes
(C) local excision and chemotherapy
(D) local excision, with resection of inguinal nodes and chemotherapy
(E) local excision and radiation

160. In contrast to neurilemomas, neurofibromas occur in

(A) younger patients, contain a homogeneous cell population, commonly affect viscera, and have a lower risk of malignant degeneration
(B) older patients, contain a mixture of cell types, rarely affect viscera, and have a higher risk of malignant degeneration
(C) older patients, contain a homogeneous cell population, commonly affect viscera, and have a lower risk of malignant degeneration
(D) younger patients, contain a mixture of cell types, commonly affect viscera, and have a higher risk of malignant degeneration
(E) older patients, have a homogeneous cell population, rarely affect viscera, and have a higher rate of malignant degeneration

161. Cavernous hemangiomas usually require

(A) treatment with sclerosing agents
(B) radiation
(C) surgery
(D) a combination of surgery and radiation
(E) observation only

Pathology

Answers

117. The answer is A. *(Rubin, p 1286.)* The characteristic feature of osteopetrosis (marble bones) is the persistence (failure of resorption) of the primary trabeculae of endochondral bone, i.e., bone that was formed on cartilage cores. The primary spongiosa with its cartilage cores does not persist in any of the other listed conditions.

118. The answer is E. *(Rubin, p 1287.)* Defective formation of bone resulting in the accumulation of trabeculae of very immature, woven bone is characteristic of infantile scurvy and osteogenesis imperfecta. Both of these disorders are associated with defective formation of collagen. In rickets, the formation of collagen is normal but mineralization is impaired. In osteopetrosis, the resorption of the primary trabeculae of endochondral bone is impaired.

119. The answer is A. *(Cotran, p 1218.)* Type I collagen is the main collagenous component of bone and its synthesis is impaired in osteogenesis imperfecta. Type II collagen is found in cartilage, as are chondroitin and keratan sulfates, while type IV collagen occurs in basement membranes. Formation of type II and type IV collagen is normal in osteogenesis imperfecta.

120. The answer is C. *(Rubin, p 1313.)* Gaucher's disease is characterized by failure of remodeling of the distal femur, resulting in a widened, misshapen metaphysis on radiographs. Osteonecrosis of the femoral head and pathologic fracture may occur as a result of Gaucher's disease, and hematogenous osteomyelitis occurs more frequently in patients with Gaucher's disease than in the general population. Sarcomatous transformation has not been reported in bone affected by Gaucher's disease.

121. The answer is A. *(Kelley, pp 288–289.)* Increased levels of interleukin 1, by inducing release of prostaglandins, cause multiple metabolic, hematologic, physiologic, and immunologic effects. The Hageman factor is a protein that contributes to host defense mechanisms. Complement and immune complexes mediate local inflammatory effects, such as attraction of leukocytes. Antinuclear antibodies are antibodies to nuclear antigens found in the sera of patients with a variety of rheumatic diseases, and the detection of these antibodies may serve as a screening test for rheumatic diseases.

122. The answer is E. *(Kelley, p 915.)* Proliferation of endothelial cells is responsible for the angiogenesis critical to the development of synovitis in patients with rheumatoid arthritis. Macrophages in rheumatoid synovium have the capability to induce neovascularization through production of endothelial growth cell factors and interleukin 1. Transforming growth factor beta inhibits formation of endothelial cells. B lymphocytes play no role in the inflammatory process.

123. The answer is A. *(Wilson, p 246.)* Most investigators agree that deposition of monosodium urate crystals in synovium and periarticular tissues is the earliest pathologic change in gouty arthritis. These crystals later appear in synovial fluid, where they are phagocytized by polymorphonuclear leukocytes. Nephrolithiasis is the major extra-articular manifestation of gout, but it occurs later in the course of the disease. The formation of microtophi also occurs later and favors peripheral rather than axial joints.

124. The answer is B. *(Rubin, p 1327.)* The bone of osteophytes is generally derived from cartilage overgrowth and is thus of endochondral origin. The cartilage of the osteophyte in the figure does not have the fine, organized structure of articular cartilage and has no well-defined tide mark. Osteophytes associated with osteoarthritis are intrasynovial, are not necrotic, and have no tendency toward malignant degeneration.

125. The answer is D. *(Cotran, p 1247.)* Advanced osteoarthritis is characterized by loss of articular cartilage and thickening of the subchondral bone (eburnation). This is a slow process, and the bone formed is mature lamellar rather than woven bone. The cartilage is entirely absent in this area, and the remaining eburnated bone would likely harbor few osteoclasts.

126. The answer is A. *(Rubin, p 1333.)* A rheumatoid nodule resembles a granuloma, with a central core of fibrinoid necrosis surrounded by macrophages. It is not cystic, and giant cells of the osteoclastic type are not present.

127. The answer is B. *(Wilson, p 146.)* Hematogenous osteomyelitis of childhood begins as a focus of infection in the metaphysis adjacent to the epiphyseal plate; it is there that the earliest microscopic changes would be found. Only later does the infection extend to the diaphysis or subperiosteal area, and the infection involves the epiphysis only if concurrent septic arthritis is present.

128. The answer is B. *(Wilson, p 147.)* The early subperiosteal bone (involucrum) formed as a result of pus extending beneath the periosteum in hematogenous osteomyelitis is immature and is referred to as fiber or woven bone. This bone is formed directly by pluripotential osteoprogenitor cells residing in the periosteum; thus, no cartilaginous phase is seen.

129. The answer is C. *(Wilson, p 153.)* The marked destruction of the joint seen in the figure is characteristic of infectious (pyogenic) arthritis, and the synovium would be filled with polymorphonuclear leukocytes. This radiographic appearance is not characteristic of gout, and Charcot-Leyden crystals are seen in asthma. Tuberculosis is quite rare in the ankle and would be associated with marked osteoporosis.

130. The answer is D. *(Wilson, p 147.)* The structure labeled *A* is a sequestrum, surrounded by pus, which is generally devoid of cellular elements. A sequestrum has no blood supply; osteoblasts and osteoclasts require a good vascular supply to remain viable. Langerhans giant cells and caseating necrosis are characteristic of tuberculosis, which rarely affects the shafts of long bones.

131. The answer is A. *(Wilson, p 148.)* The sinuses of chronic osteomyelitis are generally lined by squamous epithelium derived from the overlying skin. Specialized columnar or cuboidal epithelium would be unlikely, and endothelial linings occupy the heart and vessels. Metaplasia of the squamous epithelium lining these sinuses can result in squamous cell carcinoma.

132. The answer is E. *(Wilson, p 147.)* The radiographic changes are typical of hematogenous osteomyelitis that has involved the entire shaft of the fibula. Tumors are unlikely to involve the entire bone, tuberculosis rarely affects the shafts of long bones, and osteogenesis imperfecta would involve both the tibia and fibula.

133. The answer is C. *(Wilson, p 148.)* The radiographic appearance is typical for an involucrum of hematogenous osteomyelitis. Tumors are unlikely to involve the entire length of the bone or to leave the cortex of the old shaft as a sequestrum. This is reactive, viable bone and thus is not necrotic. Periosteal bone, such as that of an involucrum, is of membranous rather than cartilaginous origin.

134. The answer is D. *(Rubin, p 1303.)* In senile osteoporosis, the trabeculae are generally thin but show little evidence of resorption or formation of bone on their surfaces. The trabeculae are composed of mature, lamellar bone. Unmineralized osteoid would be present only with osteomalacia.

135. The answer is D. *(Poss, p 41.)* Even in the most active stages of Paget's disease, the serum calcium and phosphorus remain in the normal range. The serum alkaline phosphatase may be very high in active Paget's disease, but this reflects increased osteoblastic rather than osteoclastic activity. Hydroxyproline is a major breakdown product of the collagen in bone, and its increased excretion in the urine is indicative of increased osteoclastic activity.

136. The answer is C. *(Cotran, p 417.)* The clinical history and the radiograph are characteristic of hypophosphatemic (vitamin D–resistant) rickets. The diagnosis is substantiated by the low normal serum calcium and the low phosphorus. In rickets the cells of the growth plate mature normally but, because of failure of calcification, cells in the hypertrophic layer accumulate in great numbers.

137. The answer is B. *(Wilson, p 26.)* Hypophosphatemic rickets is inherited as an X-linked dominant disorder. Because the father will contribute an X chromosome to each of his daughters and a Y chromosome to each of his sons, only the daughters will inherit the disorder.

138. The answer is D. *(Cotran, p 1264.)* The rapid formation of very immature bone and osteoid in the early stages of myositis ossificans can easily be mistaken for osteogenic sarcoma. The absence of active osteoblasts and the benign fibrous stroma seen in fibrous dysplasia would not pose a diagnostic problem. Although cartilage may be present in myositis ossificans, it is not as prominent a feature as new bone. The lesion does not resemble Paget's disease or Ewing's sarcoma, which are round cell tumors.

139. The answer is B. *(Wilson, p 133.)* The marrow elements are extremely sensitive to ischemia and would be the first to show obvious changes. Loss of osteocytes from lacunae within the bone, the hallmark of osteonecrosis, would not be present for several days following the ischemic event. Although there may be minimal hyperemia of the synovium, changes in it and in articular cartilage would not be striking.

140. The answer is C. *(Rubin, p 1291.)* In the repair of osteonecrosis, revascularization is accompanied by the formation of a loose fibrovascular marrow. The former necrotic marrow (red or fatty) rarely regenerates, but the necrotic debris is removed by macrophages and does not persist. Heavy, dense, hypovascular scarring within the marrow spaces is not usually seen.

141. The answer is D. *(Rubin, p 1291.)* Two months following necrosis of the entire femoral head in an adult, the center of the necrotic area would not have revascularized, and only necrotic, acellular debris would be present. Neither bone formation nor resorption would be apparent.

142. The answer is C. *(Albright, pp 328–333.)* The bone indicated by arrow *A* is the woven or fiber bone characteristic of early callus formation. It is well supplied with blood vessels but has no lamellae or haversian systems. In the absence of metabolic disease, this early callus would be ossified almost as quickly as it was formed, and significant amounts of osteoid would not be present.

143. The answer is C. *(Albright, pp 328–333.)* Arrow *B* indicates the cortical margin of the rib at the fracture site. Cortical bone is of periosteal, not endochondral, origin and is mature lamellar bone. The cortical bone at the site of a fracture is deprived of its blood supply by disruption of the periosteum at the time of injury and is necrotic for at least a few millimeters from the fracture site.

144. The answer is E. *(Poss, p 167.)* Two months following implantation, the original lacunae of an autogenous cortical bone graft would be empty. New osteocytes do not enter these old lacunae; rather, new bone is formed on the surfaces of the graft, and all osteocytes present are within the newly formed bone.

145. The answer is C. *(Wilson, p 268.)* Rigid stabilization of a fracture tends to diminish the amount of external callus, and excessive motion, especially early in the healing process, tends to increase it. A child treated by spica immobilization may develop considerable callus, but this is not nearly as great as that produced in a patient with a closed head injury treated in skeletal traction. The formation of massive amounts of heterotopic bone is not uncommon in patients with severe closed head injuries.

146. The answer is C. *(Mirra, p 982.)* The histologic appearance of a brown tumor of hyperparathyroidism may be identical to that of a giant cell tumor of bone. Ten to 20 percent of chondroblastomas have prominent giant cells with little chondroid or "chicken wire" calcification, but closer analysis of biopsy material will reveal the chondroid. Only giant cell tumors rich in reactive osteoid resemble osteoblastomas histologically. Nonossifying fibromas have fewer and less prominent nuclei than all but low-grade giant cell tumors. Osteosarcomas rich in giant cells and relatively deficient in osteoid production may be confused with giant cell tumors, but closer examination of the stroma in osteosarcomas always reveals osteoid production by the malignant cells.

147. The answer is E. *(Mirra, p 992.)* Osteoclasts resorb bone and in this manner participate in calcium homeostasis. Normally, osteoclasts lie adjacent to the spicules of bone they are resorbing, but once resorption is complete, there may be no osteoclasts in contact with bone spicules. In osteopetrosis, a genetic defect impairs the ability of the osteoclast to resorb bone. Osteoclastic function is normal in the other conditions listed.

148. The answer is B. *(Mirra, p 1498.)* Skeletal metastases outnumber primary bone tumors by a ratio of approximately 25 to 1. Fifteen to 20 percent of patients with bony metastases have clinical symptoms (pain or a mass). More than 80 percent of bone metastases are from carcinomas of the breast, prostate, lung, kidney, and thyroid.

149. The answer is B. *(Mirra, p 899.)* The first clinically recognizable event in Paget's disease is lysis of bone; therefore, the etiology is most likely to be a factor that stimulates osteoclastic hyperactivity. For the past 20 years, viruslike inclusions have been found consistently in the nuclei of osteoclasts in patients with Paget's disease. Proof of their etiologic role, however, awaits isolation of the virus and satisfaction of Koch's postulates. The focal nature of osteoclastic proliferation in Paget's disease makes it unlikely to be the result of generalized or systemic factors, i.e., hormonal, metabolic, or immunologic disorders.

150. The answer is A. *(Mirra, p 917.)* Osteolysis of the vertebrae is progressive in patients with Paget's disease. As the vertebral bodies collapse and become more compacted, they also become increasingly osteolytic. Whether these changes result from resorption following insufficiency fractures, disuse, or some other factor is unknown.

151. The answer is D. *(Mirra, p 479.)* Atypical enchondromas are those associated with a complaint of pain, whereas typical enchondromas are incidental radiographic findings. Their association with pain makes atypical lesions more ominous, and, since a small percentage of these lesions have undetectable low-grade malignant changes at the time of discovery, they must be followed more closely for growth or spread. Patients with atypical lesions are, as a group, slightly younger than patients with typical enchondromas, but the clinical pictures are similar in other respects.

152. The answer is A. *(Mirra, p 480.)* As a general principle, the potential for malignant change in hamartomatous tissue is in direct proportion to the volume of tissue present. For that reason, the smallest enchondromas, i.e., those of the hands and feet, have the least propensity for malignant change. In contrast, patients with large or multiple enchondromas are at considerably greater risk for sarcomatous degeneration. Chondrocytes with double nuclei occur in almost every enchondroma, and most enchondromas are "hot" on bone scanning. The rare epiphyseal enchondroma carries no increased risk of malignant transformation.

153. The answer is C. *(Mirra, p 493.)* In Mirra's studies, approximately 50 percent of chondrosarcomas showed evidence of a preexisting enchondroma. This incidence is higher among large, centrally located lesions, such as those in the pelvis or femur, and lower for enchondromas of the feet and hands.

154. The answer is B. *(Mirra, p 351.)* In patients over 60 years of age, 56 percent of osteosarcomas occur in association with Paget's disease. Osteosarcoma occasionally develops in patients with retinoblastoma who have not had radiation or chemotherapy. Ten percent of chondrosarcomas dedifferentiate into fibrosarcoma, malignant fibrocystiocytoma, or osteosarcoma. Solitary osteochondromas rarely undergo malignant change; when they do, it is usually to chondrosarcoma.

155. The answer is E. *(Mirra, p 271.)* A Codman's triangle is a triangle of reactive, subperiosteal new bone seen at the edge of a benign or malignant process that has rapidly elevated the periosteum. While most common in malignancies, especially osteosarcomas, it may be seen in rapidly expanding aneurysmal bone cysts, hemophilic pseudotumors, fractures in which blood elevates the periosteum, and in acute osteomyelitis, in which pus elevates the periosteum. It is rarely encountered in benign tumors such as nonossifying fibromas.

156. The answer is E. *(Mirra, p 263.)* Ninety percent of osteosarcomas occur in the metaphysis, although the tumor may cross the epiphyseal plate or expand into the diaphysis. Fluffy, or cloudlike, radiodensities that are eccentric in location are almost pathognomonic for osteosarcoma. In about 80 percent of osteosarcomas, some type of periosteal reaction is seen, with a Codman's triangle being the most frequent. Although soft tissue masses are not always visible on standard radiographs, almost 90 percent of osteosarcomas have a mass that can be demonstrated with computed tomography (CT) or magnetic resonance imaging (MRI) scans. A complete periosteal collar of new bone around the lesion is not characteristic of osteosarcoma.

157. The answer is E. *(Rubin, p 1315.)* The septa of an aneurysmal bone cyst contain numerous multinucleated giant cells and in areas appear quite like a giant cell tumor of bone. Giant cells associated with giant cell tumors of bone generally contain more nuclei (greater than 15 per cell) than do those associated with aneurysmal bone cysts.

158. The answer is B. *(Miller, p 173.)* Soft-tissue masses greater than 5 cm in diameter are likely to be malignant. Malignant fibrous histiocytoma is the most common sarcoma of late adulthood. Aggressive fibromatosis, rhabdomyosarcoma, and hemangiomas are more common in children. Fibrosarcoma is an uncommon soft-tissue malignancy.

159. The answer is E. *(Enzinger, p 172.)* While there is no clear agreement on the optimal treatment of synovial sarcoma, excision and radiotherapy are particularly effective for small, accessible tumors. There is no evidence that chemotherapy suppresses metastases, and inguinal nodes are radiated (in preference to excision) only when they are clearly enlarged.

160. The answer is D. *(Enzinger, p 821.)* Neurofibromas tend to occur in a younger age group, usually with neurofibromatosis. Visceral involvement and malignant degeneration are much more common than with neurilemomas. Whereas the cell population of neurilemomas is relatively homogeneous, that of neurofibromas is a mixture of cell types.

161. The answer is C. *(Enzinger, p 587.)* Cavernous hemangiomas, most common during childhood and in the upper limb, differ from capillary hemangiomas in several important areas: they are larger and less circumscribed, rarely regress, and may erode adjacent structures. For these reasons, most cavernous hemangiomas require surgery; their capillary counterparts often regress spontaneously.

Musculoskeletal Imaging

Douglas R. Dirschl, M.D.

DIRECTIONS: Each question below contains five suggested responses. Select the **one best** response to each question.

162. The best method to assess congruity of the hip joint following closed reduction of a traumatic dislocation of the hip is

(A) AP radiography of the pelvis
(B) AP radiography of the hip
(C) CT of the pelvis
(D) MRI of the pelvis
(E) polytomography of the pelvis

163. The radiographic view most useful for identifying superior displacement of the posterior hemipelvis is the

(A) AP pelvic
(B) pelvic inlet
(C) pelvic outlet
(D) obturator oblique
(E) iliac oblique

164. The muscle identified by the arrow on the MRI scan in the figure exerts what action on the humerus?

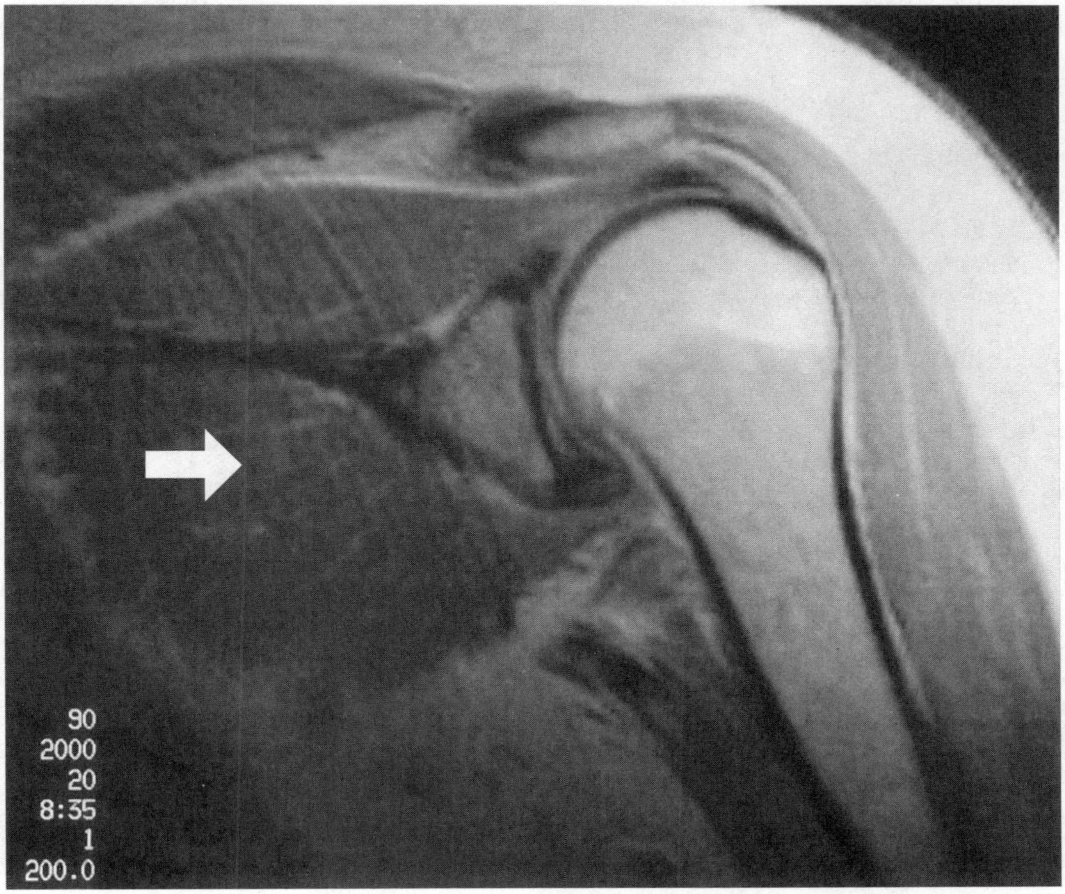

(A) Flexion
(B) Extension
(C) Abduction
(D) Internal rotation
(E) External rotation

---

165. The minimum amount of bone mineral that must be lost from the skeleton before the loss can be detected on plain radiographs is

(A) 10 percent
(B) 30 percent
(C) 50 percent
(D) 70 percent
(E) 90 percent

166. The anatomic structure that is well delineated in a CT scan of the pelvis but not in iliac or obturator oblique radiographic views is the

(A) pubic symphysis
(B) anterior rim of the acetabulum
(C) posterior rim of the acetabulum
(D) sciatic notch
(E) sacroiliac joint

167. The figure shows a T1-weighted MRI image of the shoulder region. The area identified by the arrow contains a significant amount of

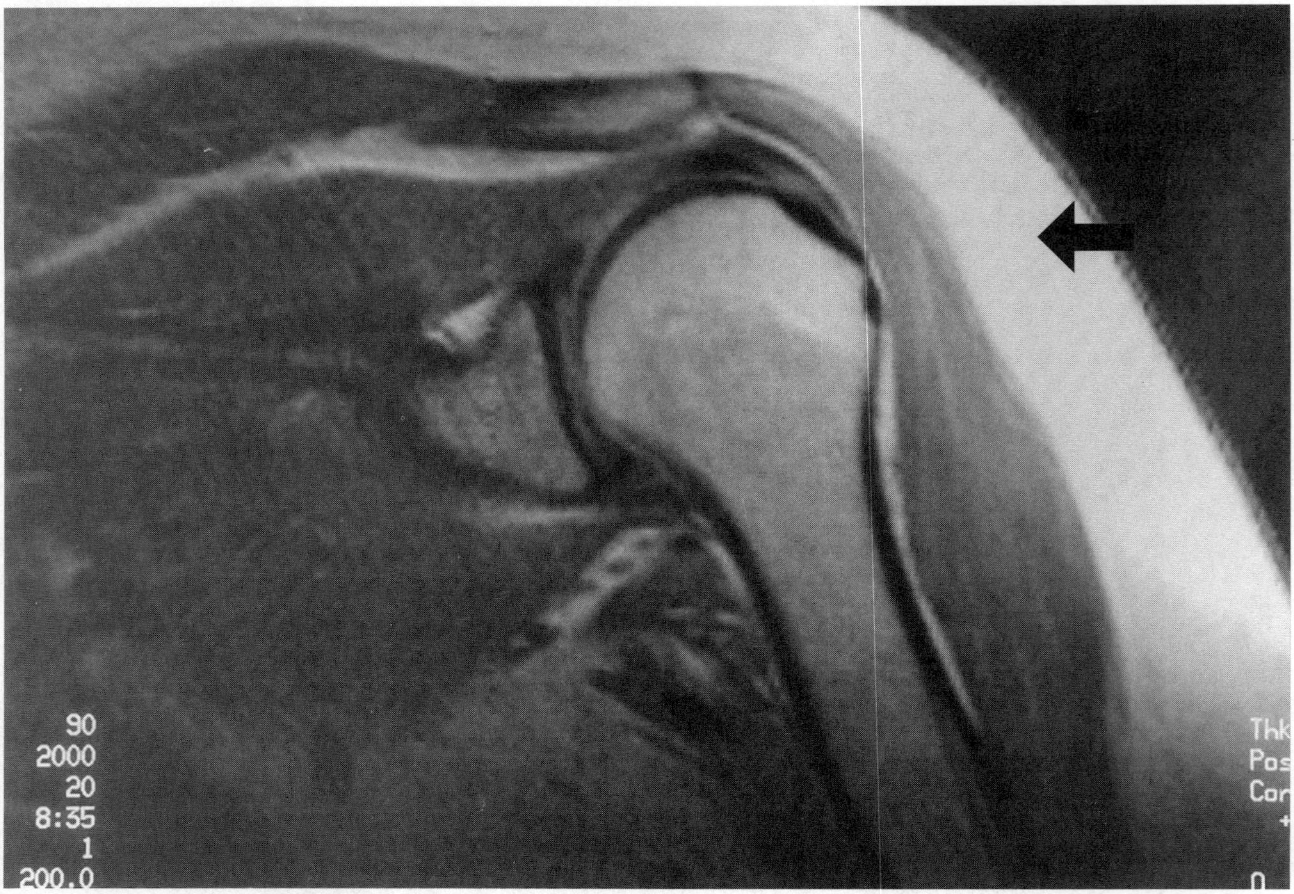

(A) cartilage
(B) calcium
(C) water
(D) fat
(E) necrotic tissue

168. The study with the highest specificity for identifying a talocalcaneal coalition is the

(A) oblique radiograph of the foot
(B) Harris radiographic view of the foot
(C) lateral radiograph of the foot
(D) radionuclide bone scan
(E) CT scan

169. The figure is a T1-weighted MRI scan of the knee. The structure identified by the arrow is the

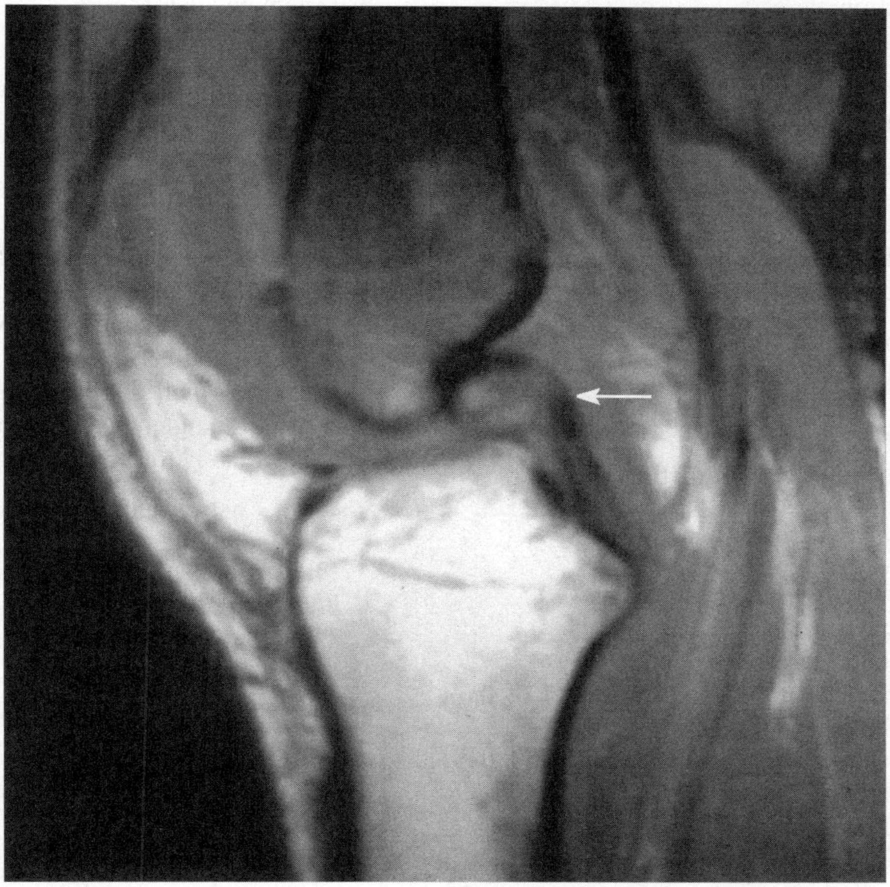

(A) popliteus tendon
(B) posterior cruciate ligament
(C) anterior cruciate ligament
(D) Wrisberg's ligament
(E) Humphry's ligament

---

170. The technique for measuring bone mineral density that exposes the patient to the LEAST amount of radiation is

(A) single-photon absorptiometry
(B) dual-photon absorptiometry
(C) quantitative computed tomography
(D) quantitative digital radiography
(E) neutron activation

171. A 12-year-old girl injured her knee while playing soccer. Examination revealed tenderness over the distal femur and instability to valgus stress. Plain radiographs were normal. The most appropriate next step in evaluation is

(A) a stress radiograph
(B) a CT scan
(C) an MRI scan
(D) an arthrogram
(E) an angiogram

172. In a patient with sickle cell hemoglobinopathy, acute osteomyelitis is best distinguished from bone infarction by

(A) plain radiographs of the tibia
(B) a technetium-99 bone scan
(C) a gallium scan
(D) a CT scan
(E) aspiration of bone

173. All the following may be sequelae of Paget's disease of bone EXCEPT

(A) bowing of the tibia
(B) osteoporosis circumscripta
(C) neurologic impairment
(D) "codfish" vertebrae
(E) sarcomatous transformation

174. The iliac oblique radiograph of the pelvis is most useful for demonstrating the

(A) pubic rami
(B) acetabular teardrop
(C) anterior column and posterior lip of the acetabulum
(D) posterior column and anterior lip of the acetabulum
(E) sacral foramina

175. The radiographic view that best delineates anteroposterior displacement of the posterior hemipelvis is the

(A) AP pelvic
(B) pelvic inlet
(C) pelvic outlet
(D) obturator oblique
(E) iliac oblique

176. An 18-year-old man has had a history of two traumatic anterior shoulder dislocations and now has signs and symptoms suggestive of anterior shoulder instability. You suspect he may have a small avulsion fracture of the anterior rim of the glenoid. The plain radiographic view most likely to show this finding is

(A) a true anteroposterior radiograph of the shoulder
(B) an axillary view of the shoulder
(C) a West Point axillary lateral
(D) a Stryker notch view
(E) a "serendipity" view

DIRECTIONS: Each group of questions below consists of lettered headings followed by a set of numbered items. For each numbered item, select the **one** lettered heading with which it is **most** closely associated. Each lettered heading may be used **once, more than once, or not at all.**

Questions 177–180

For each patient below, select the most likely bone tumor.

(A) Conventional osteosarcoma
(B) Periosteal osteosarcoma
(C) Telangiectatic osteosarcoma
(D) Secondary osteosarcoma
(E) Chondrosarcoma

177. An asymptomatic, 24-year-old man with a sclerotic, oval mass on the posterior surface of the distal femur

178. A 12-year-old boy with a purely lytic, permeative lesion involving the distal femoral metaphysis

179. A 62-year-old woman with an ill-defined, destructive lesion in the ischium and an associated soft-tissue mass containing osteoblastic tissue

180. A 46-year-old man with an expansile lesion in the center of the femoral metaphysis; endosteal scalloping and punctate calcifications are present

Questions 181–184

For each numbered radiographic feature below, select the type of inflammatory arthritis with which it is most closely associated.

(A) Rheumatoid arthritis
(B) Juvenile rheumatoid arthritis
(C) Psoriatic arthritis
(D) Erosive osteoarthritis
(E) Reiter's syndrome

181. Heberden's nodes

182. Ankylosis of the interphalangeal joints of the hand

183. Erosion of the tufts of the distal phalanges of the hand

184. Involvement of the metacarpophalangeal joints

Questions 185–188

For each numbered anatomic region of the shoulder below, select the radiographic view that best images that region.

(A) Stryker notch view
(B) Fisk view
(C) Scapular outlet view
(D) Zanca view
(E) Apical-oblique view

185. The bicipital groove

186. The anteroinferior rim of the glenoid

187. The undersurface of the acromion

188. The acromioclavicular joint

Musculoskeletal Imaging

Answers

162. The answer is C. *(Browner, pp 1344–1347.)* Computerized tomography (CT) of the pelvis should be routinely obtained following successful closed reduction of a dislocation of the hip. The value of CT lies in its ability to evaluate the femoral head, demonstrate small intraarticular fragments, and assess congruence of the femoral head and acetabulum. MRI scanning may prove useful as an adjunct to CT in the evaluation of the integrity of the labrum and vascularity of the femoral head. Radiographs are an important screening tool, but they may not reveal small intraarticular fragments.

163. The answer is C. *(Browner, pp 869–870.)* The pelvic outlet view is obtained with the patient supine and the x-ray beam directed 45° cephalad. This view is useful for identifying superior migration of the hemipelvis and fractures through the sacral foramina. The pelvic inlet radiograph is most useful for identifying anterior or posterior displacement of the posterior hemipelvis, and iliac and obturator oblique views are most appropriate for evaluating fractures of the acetabulum.

164. The answer is E. *(Chan, pp 10–17.)* The infraspinatus muscle lies posterior to the body of the scapula and inferior to the scapular spine. It attaches to the greater tuberosity of the humerus and participates in external rotation of the humerus relative to the scapula.

165. The answer is B. *(Greenspan, p 18.6.)* Although very small increases in bone mineral density can be detected on plain radiographs, decreases in overall bone mineral density are usually not detected until the reduction reaches at least 30 percent. Also, technical factors, such as improper settings for millivoltage and milliamperage, can lead to apparently decreased bone mineral density on radiographs of normal bones.

166. The answer is E. *(Browner, p 872.)* Plain radiographs of the pelvis aid in identification of fractures of the sacrum, iliac wing, acetabulum, and pubic rami. They can also show displacement of the posterior hemipelvis and injuries of the acetabular rims and anterior and posterior columns. A CT scan is necessary, however, to determine the congruity of and the exact nature of injury to the sacroiliac joints.

167. The answer is D. *(Chan, pp 58–68.)* The differences in relaxation characteristics between water and fat can be used in the interpretation of MRI scans. Fatty tissue is characteristically bright on T1-weighted MRI scans and much less so on T2-weighted scans. Water is extremely bright on T2-weighted MRI scans, but not on T1-weighted scans. Bone and calcified tissue have no signal on MRI scans. Cartilage has intermediate signal intensity on both T1- and T2-weighted scans.

168. The answer is E. *(Greenspan, pp 25.28–25.29.)* Although talocalcaneal coalitions may be demonstrated on the oblique and Harris radiographic views of the foot, polytomography and CT scanning are more sensitive and specific. The CT scan is the most specific test, followed by polyspiral tomography. A technetium-99m (^{99m}Tc) bone scan is extremely sensitive but nonspecific for tarsal coalition.

169. The answer is B. *(Chan, pp 30–35.)* The posterior cruciate ligament (PCL) extends between the anteromedial aspect of the intercondylar notch of the femur and the posterolateral surface of the proximal tibia. The course of the anterior cruciate ligament is just the reverse: posterolateral femur to anteromedial tibia. The image in the figure is through the center of the knee joint; the popliteus tendon is farther lateral and would be seen in images in which the fibular head also appeared. The meniscofemoral ligament of Wrisberg is a very thin structure occasionally seen end-on just posterior to the PCL in a sagittal image of the knee. Humphry's ligament is not visualized on an MRI scan of the knee.

170. The answer is D. *(Greenspan, pp 19.2–19.4.)* Quantitative digital radiography, also known as dual-energy x-ray absorptiometry, is a very sensitive and reliable means of measuring bone mineral density that exposes the patient to approximately 5 millirads (mrad) of radiation per scan. Single- and dual-photon absorptiometry and quantitative computed tomography expose the patient to 10 to 100 times the radiation of quantitative digital radiography. Neutron activation is not used to determine bone mineral density.

171. The answer is A. *(Rockwood, pp 1176–1177.)* Making the diagnosis of a fracture-separation of the distal femoral epiphysis can be difficult. Plain radiographs may reveal only a nondisplaced widening of the physis without fracture of the adjacent metaphysis. Stress radiographs are recommended if multiple routine views are negative in the presence of suggestive clinical findings. Although a CT or MRI scan would reveal the fracture-separation, a stress radiograph can be quickly and simply performed and is far more cost-effective.

172. The answer is E. *(Dirschl, Orthop Rev 23:305–312, 1994.)* Radiographs are poor tools for distinguishing bone crises from foci of osteomyelitis in patients with sickle cell hemoglobinopathy since infarcts and fissures in the bone will be present with both conditions. Similarly, technetium-99 and gallium scans may show increased uptake of radioisotope in both clinical conditions. Aspiration of bone and subsequent culture of the material obtained remains the best method for distinguishing bone infarction from osteomyelitis in patients with sickle cell disease.

173. The answer is D. *(Greenspan, pp 22.3–22.11.)* Osteoporosis circumscripta is a characteristic osteolytic lesion in the skull associated with the early phases of Paget's disease. Severe bowing of the long bones, especially the tibia, can occur and can lead to stress fractures. Bony overgrowth and collapse of vertebral bodies can lead to neurologic impairment and paraplegia. Secondary sarcomatous transformation is a major but rare sequela of Paget's disease. "Codfish" vertebrae are associated with osteoporosis, whereas Paget's disease often produces a bone-within-a-bone appearance, often referred to as a "picture-frame" vertebra.

174. The answer is D. *(Browner, pp 899–900.)* The iliac oblique view of the pelvis is taken with the injured side rotated 45° away from the x-ray tube. This view shows the iliac wing in its largest dimension and profiles the posterior column of the pelvis and anterior lip of the acetabulum. The obturator oblique view profiles the anterior column of the pelvis and posterior lip of the acetabulum.

175. The answer is B. *(Browner, pp 869–870.)* The pelvic inlet view is obtained with the patient supine and the x-ray beam directed 60° caudad. This view is useful for determining anteroposterior displacement of the sacroiliac joint, sacrum, and iliac wing. It is also useful for identifying internal rotation deformities of the ilium. The pelvic outlet view is best for identifying superior migration of the posterior hemipelvis.

176. The answer is C. *(Rockwood, Matsen, pp 184–196.)* Although the true anteroposterior radiograph may demonstrate large avulsion fractures of the inferior glenoid, the West Point axillary view and the apical-oblique view provide more information about small abnormalities of the anterior rim of the glenoid. The Stryker notch view is best for delineating a compression fracture of the humeral head associated with anterior dislocation of the shoulder, and a "serendipity" view is used for imaging the sternoclavicular joint.

177–180. The answers are 177-B, 178-C, 179-D, 180-E. *(Greenspan, pp 16.2–16.12.)* Periosteal osteosarcoma occurs largely in the third and fourth decades of life, with nearly all lesions occurring on the posterior aspect of the distal femur. Conventional radiography is adequate for making the diagnosis and reveals a dense, oval or spherical mass attached to the posterior surface of the distal femur, which is sharply demarcated from the surrounding soft tissue.

Telangiectatic osteosarcoma is twice as common in males as in females and occurs predominantly in the second and third decades of life. The typical radiographic appearance is of a poorly demarcated, destructive lesion that is almost entirely osteolytic. A soft tissue mass may also be present. These tumors are highly vascular and can be confused with aneurysmal bone cysts on histologic examination.

Secondary osteosarcoma, most often due to Paget's disease, occurs in the older population. The typical radiographic appearance is that of a destructive, osteoblastic lesion in an area of Pagetic bone. An associated soft-tissue mass containing tumor bone is often seen.

Conventional chondrosarcomas are slow-growing lesions, often discovered incidentally, that occur most frequently in the pelvis, distal femur, and proximal humerus. The typical radiographic appearance is that of a central, expansile lesion, with thickening and scalloping of the endosteal cortex. Speckled or popcornlike calcifications are often present.

181–184. The answers are 181-D, 182-B, 183-C, 184-A. *(Greenspan, pp 11.2–11.19.)* Erosive osteoarthritis combines certain clinical features of rheumatoid arthritis with certain radiographic signs of degenerative joint disease. Involvement is limited to the hands, with proximal and distal interphalangeal joints being most frequently affected. Heberden's nodes are characteristic of this condition.

Juvenile rheumatoid arthritis exhibits many of the features of adult rheumatoid arthritis. Additional features that are almost pathognomonic for this condition include ankylosis of the interphalangeal joints and cervical spine, and periosteal reactions along the shafts of the metacarpals and proximal phalanges.

Psoriatic arthritis involves predominantly the distal interphalangeal joints of the hands and feet. Characteristic radiographic changes include destruction of the distal interphalangeal joints in the hand and erosion of the terminal tufts of the distal phalanges. This condition may also be manifest as the so-called sausage digit or as arthritis mutilans.

Involvement of the metacarpophalangeal joints is nearly pathognomonic for rheumatoid arthritis. The most common pattern is ulnar subluxation of the metacarpophalangeal joints with ulnar deviation of the fingers. The swan neck and boutonnière deformities are seen more often with this form of arthritis than with other inflammatory arthritides.

185–188. The answers are 185-B, 186-E, 187-C, 188-D. *(Rockwood, Matsen, pp 187–200.)* Although bicipital tendinitis is rarely the primary cause of shoulder pain, the anatomy of the bicipital groove can be evaluated by the Fisk view. In this view, the x-ray machine is superior to the shoulder, and the patient leans forward over the x-ray table, holding the cassette on the supinated forearm. Flattening of the medial wall may predispose to subluxation of the biceps tendon.

Small avulsion fractures or calcifications of the anteroinferior rim of the glenoid are often seen in anterior shoulder instability and following traumatic anterior dislocation of the glenohumeral joint. This region is best imaged with the apical-oblique view or with the West Point axillary view.

Subacromial impingement is a frequent cause of pain and disability in the adult shoulder. A spur on the undersurface of the anteroinferior acromion, which may impinge on the subdeltoid bursa and rotator cuff, is best seen on scapular outlet or 30° caudal tilt views. These views also demonstrate shapes of the acromion that favor impingement.

Fractures of the distal clavicle or acromion, osteolysis of the distal clavicle, and degenerative arthritis of the acromioclavicular joint may not be identified on routine anteroposterior radiographs of that joint since the inferior portion of the distal clavicle is frequently obscured by the spine of the scapula. To obtain an unobstructed view of the acromioclavicular joint, Zanca has recommended that the x-ray beam be tilted 10° cephalad and aimed at the acromioclavicular joint.

Amputations, Prosthetics, Orthotics, and Rehabilitation

Douglas R. Dirschl, M.D.

DIRECTIONS: Each question below contains five suggested responses. Select the **one best** response to each question.

189. Each of the following statements regarding the energy expenditure by lower limb amputees during ambulation is correct EXCEPT that the

(A) use of a prosthesis results in a lower rate of energy expenditure than use of crutches
(B) oxygen demand increases progressively as the level of lower limb amputation moves proximally
(C) average rate of oxygen consumption increases as the level of lower limb amputation moves proximally
(D) chosen speed of walking decreases as the level of lower limb amputation moves proximally
(E) energy expenditure is greater in bilateral than in unilateral lower limb amputees

190. All the following criteria can be satisfied with a custom molded ankle-foot orthosis (AFO) EXCEPT

(A) immobilization of the subtalar joint
(B) selective limitation of plantar flexion of the ankle
(C) inhibition of tonic reflexes in spastic patients
(D) allowing weight-bearing on the patellar tendon
(E) controlling rotation of the distal leg

191. A significant problem associated with plastazote shoe inserts is

(A) their high cost
(B) inadequate support of the midfoot
(C) difficulty in molding the material
(D) inadequate durability for long-term wear
(E) the high incidence of decubiti in diabetic patients

192. Rigid foot orthoses have been associated with all the following problems EXCEPT

(A) poor patient compliance
(B) stress fractures
(C) plantar fibromatosis
(D) sesamoiditis
(E) irritation of a Morton's neuroma

193. The shortest functional level for a transtibial amputation is

(A) just proximal to the tibial tuberosity
(B) just distal to the tibial tuberosity
(C) 7 cm distal to the joint line
(D) 10 cm distal to the joint line
(E) 15 cm distal to the joint line

194. A conical shape of the residual limb following a transtibial amputation results from

(A) improper selection of the amputation level
(B) failure to bevel the anterior tibial surface
(C) an anterior flap that is excessively long
(D) an anterior flap that is excessively short
(E) leaving the fibula over 2 cm shorter than the tibia

195. In performing a transtibial amputation, myodesis is contraindicated in

(A) all patients
(B) amputations performed for trauma
(C) severely dysvascular limbs
(D) residual limbs shorter than 9 cm
(E) residual limbs longer than 15 cm

196. All the following can be associated with delayed skin healing following transtibial amputations EXCEPT

(A) grasping of the skin with forceps
(B) skin closure under tension
(C) use of a thigh tourniquet during the procedure
(D) separation of layers in the creation of myofasciocutaneous flaps
(E) inversion of the skin edges at closure

197. A rigid, plastic, patellar tendon–bearing (PTB) socket for a transtibial prosthesis is contraindicated for all the following residual limbs EXCEPT those with

(A) length greater than 12 cm
(B) thin skin
(C) scarring
(D) split-thickness skin grafts
(E) prior skin breakdown

198. Supracondylar cuff suspension, when combined with a patellar tendon–bearing (PTB) socket,

(A) is appropriate for use with short residual limbs
(B) can make the prosthesis difficult to don
(C) cannot completely eliminate pistoning of the socket
(D) is recommended for residual limbs with poor knee stability
(E) provides excellent control of knee extension

199. A 23-year-old man sustained a fracture of the throacic spine, with complete paralysis below the level of the 11th thoracic nerve root. To balance his weight over his feet using an above-knee orthosis, the patient's line of gravity must pass

(A) through the hip and knee joints
(B) anterior to the hip and knee joints
(C) posterior to the hip and knee joints
(D) anterior to the hip joint and posterior to the knee joint
(E) posterior to the hip joint and anterior to the knee joint

200. The multiaxial foot, when applied to a transtibial prosthesis, is NOT recommended for patients who

(A) are strong and athletic
(B) walk frequently on uneven ground
(C) need to reduce torque on the residual limb
(D) require added shock absorption
(E) have limited access to prosthetic follow-up

201. The proper alignment of the socket in a transtibial prosthesis will place the socket in slight

(A) flexion
(B) extension
(C) adduction
(D) abduction
(E) flexion and internal rotation

202. A patient who has a unilateral transtibial prosthesis complains of pain over the lateral aspect of the knee with prolonged weight-bearing. Examination reveals a wide-based gait, medial shoe wear, and evidence of increased pressure on the skin over the lateral aspect of the knee. The most likely cause of the problem is that the prosthetic

(A) socket is too flexed
(B) limb is too short
(C) foot is too inset
(D) foot is too outset
(E) heel is too firm

203. A patient with a unilateral transtibial prosthesis has knee extension that persists from heel strike to the mid-stance phase of gait. All the following may be causes of this gait pattern EXCEPT that the

(A) prosthetic foot is too anterior
(B) prosthetic socket is in insufficient flexion
(C) heel of the SACH (solid ankle cushion heel) foot is too soft
(D) foot is excessively dorsiflexed
(E) heel on the shoe is too low

204. Which of the following conditions poses the LEAST challenge to the design of orthotic devices?

(A) Hyperreflexia
(B) Spasticity
(C) Clonus
(D) Muscular weakness
(E) Abnormal motor integration

205. When compared with transfemoral amputation, knee disarticulation has all the following potential benefits EXCEPT

(A) increased weight-bearing on the end of the residual limb
(B) increased suspension requirement for the prosthetic socket
(C) decreased surgical blood loss
(D) better cosmetic appearance
(E) increased resistance to infection

206. When a transfemoral amputation is performed, the adductor magnus should be sutured to the

(A) quadriceps tendon with the thigh in adduction
(B) quadriceps tendon with the thigh in abduction
(C) the lateral aspect of the femur with the thigh in abduction
(D) the lateral aspect of the femur with the thigh in adduction
(E) the quadriceps and hamstring tendons with the thigh in neutral position

207. If the clinical situation permits, an elbow disarticulation is preferred over a transhumeral amputation in children because

(A) control of the terminal device will be easier for the patient
(B) a stronger, more functional elbow joint can be fabricated
(C) a more durable prosthesis can be fabricated
(D) fitting of the myoelectric prosthesis is easier
(E) humeral overgrowth is avoided

208. All the following would decrease flexibility at the ankle of a polypropylene ankle-foot orthosis (AFO) EXCEPT

(A) using a more rigid polypropylene
(B) increasing the thickness of the polypropylene
(C) adding graphite to the composite
(D) moving the trimline posteriorly
(E) increasing the width of the orthosis

209. For correct anteroposterior alignment of a transfemoral prosthesis in the mid-stance phase of gait, a plumb line from the greater trochanter should fall

(A) anterior to the axis of the knee
(B) through the axis of the knee
(C) posterior to the axis of the knee
(D) medial to the axis of the knee
(E) lateral to the axis of the knee

210. A patient with a transfemoral prosthesis who has a vaulting gait on the prosthetic side most likely has a prosthesis that is too

(A) short
(B) long
(C) adducted
(D) abducted
(E) loose

211. Which of the following patients who ambulates with a transfemoral prosthesis will obtain the greatest benefit from a hydraulically controlled knee?

(A) A 6-year-old with a congenitally short femur
(B) A 17-year-old with a traumatic amputation
(C) A 32-year-old secretary
(D) A 55-year-old executive
(E) A 65-year-old diabetic

212. In a 36-year-old man with hemiparesis, a footdrop, and spasticity of the ankle plantar flexors, ambulation using a rigid ankle-foot orthosis (AFO) will result in all the following EXCEPT

(A) greater clearance of the foot in the swing phase
(B) improved mediolateral stability of the ankle
(C) improved heel strike
(D) improved push off at the end of the stance phase
(E) an increased flexion moment at the knee

213. Overgrowth of amputation stumps in children occurs by

(A) physeal growth
(B) appositional bone growth
(C) epiphyseal hypertrophy
(D) heterotopic ossification
(E) soft tissue atrophy

214. When performing a transradial amputation, the optimal length for the residual forearm is

(A) 5 cm
(B) 10 cm
(C) 15 cm
(D) 20 cm
(E) as long as possible

215. The primary value in the treatment of flexible flatfeet in the young child with a scaphoid pad, a long medial counter, and a Thomas heel is to

(A) extend shoe life
(B) improve the height of the longitudinal arch
(C) relieve foot pain
(D) relieve leg pain
(E) prevent early arthritic changes in the tarsus

216. For a neonate with a unilateral congenital transradial amputation, the most appropriate terminal device and age for initial prosthetic fitting is a

(A) passive hand at 2 months
(B) passive hand at 4 months
(C) passive hand at 6 months
(D) voluntary opening hook at 6 months
(E) voluntary closing hook at 6 months

217. The use of wrist orthotics in the treatment of patients with hemiplegic hand deformities has all the following goals EXCEPT to

(A) reduce flexor tone at the wrist and fingers
(B) utilize pressure points at the forearm, wrist, and fingers
(C) provide direct contact between the splint and the palm of the hand
(D) prevent the development of edema
(E) maintain the wrist in a neutral position

218. For a neonate with fibular hemimelia and a congenital transtibial amputation, the initial prosthetic fitting would be best accomplished when the child is

(A) rolling prone to supine
(B) sitting independently
(C) crawling
(D) pulling to a stand
(E) standing unsupported

219. A 4-year-old boy sustains a transfemoral amputation in an automobile accident. The most appropriate knee unit for this child's initial prosthesis is

(A) manual locking
(B) constant friction
(C) variable friction
(D) hydraulic
(E) polycentric

220. The primary bodily control motion required for opening the terminal device of a standard transradial prosthesis is

(A) glenohumeral flexion
(B) glenohumeral extension
(C) glenohumeral abduction
(D) biscapular adduction
(E) glenohumeral flexion and biscapular adduction

221. Following repair of a complete laceration of the median nerve at the wrist flexion crease, the most important use for an orthotic is to

(A) protect the asensate index and long fingers
(B) block extension of the interphalangeal joint of the thumb
(C) block adduction of the thumb
(D) block extension of the metacarpophalangeal joints of the index and long fingers
(E) block flexion of the wrist

222. The bodily control motion required to lock or unlock the prosthetic elbow of a standard transhumeral prosthesis is

(A) shoulder depression, glenohumeral flexion and abduction
(B) shoulder depression, glenohumeral extension and abduction
(C) shoulder elevation, glenohumeral flexion and abduction
(D) shoulder elevation, glenohumeral extension and abduction
(E) biscapular abduction, shoulder depression and abduction

223. A spiral or hemispiral AFO design is most useful in patients with

(A) hemiparesis
(B) spastic cerebral palsy
(C) cervical myelopathy
(D) idiopathic toe-walking
(E) sciatic nerve lacerations

224. The use of an orthosis is contraindicated in a

(A) blind patient
(B) nonambulatory patient
(C) patient who cannot don and doff the device independently
(D) patient with a bleeding diathesis
(E) patient in whom energy consumption increases when using the device for functional tasks

225. For a transradial amputee, all the following are advantages of a myoelectric prosthesis over a mechanical prosthesis EXCEPT

(A) improved cosmetic appearance
(B) fewer harness straps
(C) superior grip strength
(D) greater ability to operate the terminal device close to the body and overhead
(E) decreased weight of the prosthetic unit

226. The most common reason for the use of orthotics in young children with cerebral palsy is to

(A) correct deformity
(B) prevent contractures
(C) control tone
(D) improve functional capability
(E) enhance the stability of lax joints

227. A 25-year-old man has a complete thoracic level paraplegia as a result of a motor vehicle accident. The maximum level of independent function he may be expected to achieve is

(A) use of a motorized wheel chair
(B) use of a manual wheel chair
(C) household ambulation with a knee-ankle-foot orthosis
(D) household ambulation with a hip-knee-ankle-foot orthosis
(E) household ambulation with a reciprocating walker

228. Forty-eight hours after sustaining a T12 burst fracture, a patient had a complete neurologic deficit below the L2 level. The chance for recovery of functional motor activity below this level is

(A) 0
(B) 5 percent
(C) 10 percent
(D) 25 percent
(E) 50 percent

229. On examination of a patient ambulating with a unilateral transtibial prosthesis, the foot can be seen to swing out laterally away from the sound leg during the initial swing phase of gait. The most likely cause for this gait abnormality is that the

(A) prosthetic foot is too inset
(B) prosthetic foot is too outset
(C) prosthetic socket is rotated medially with respect to the line of progression
(D) prosthetic socket is rotated laterally with respect to the line of progression
(E) prosthesis is too long

230. In performing a transfemoral amputation, the quadriceps should be sutured to the

(A) adductor magnus with the hip in flexion
(B) adductor magnus with the hip in extension
(C) posterior aspect of the residual femur with the hip held in flexion
(D) posterior aspect of the residual femur with the hip held in extension
(E) posterior aspect of the residual femur with the hip in neutral

231. The socket of a standard transfemoral prosthesis should be placed in a position of

(A) adduction
(B) abduction
(C) slight flexion and adduction
(D) slight flexion and abduction
(E) neutral flexion/extension and adduction/abduction

232. The energy required to ambulate with a hip disarticulation prosthesis is approximately what percentage of normal?

(A) 150 percent
(B) 175 percent
(C) 200 percent
(D) 250 percent
(E) 300 percent

233. The most common site of terminal bony overgrowth in children with acquired amputations is the

(A) humerus
(B) radius
(C) femur
(D) tibia
(E) fibula

234. For an 18-month-old child with a congenital unilateral transradial amputation, the most appropriate management is

(A) a passive hand prosthesis
(B) a voluntary opening hook prosthesis
(C) a voluntary closing hook prosthesis
(D) a myoelectric hand prosthesis
(E) no prosthesis

235. In a standard transradial prosthesis, when terminal device operation close to the midline of the body is required, as when buttoning a shirt, body motion necessary to operate the terminal device is

(A) shoulder depression
(B) shoulder elevation
(C) biscapular adduction
(D) biscapular abduction
(E) glenohumeral abduction

236. Operation of the terminal device in a standard shoulder disarticulation prosthesis is accomplished through

(A) shoulder elevation
(B) shoulder depression
(C) biscapular adduction
(D) biscapular abduction
(E) rotation of the chin away from the prosthetic side

237. The main effect of a step-up elbow hinge in a transradial prosthesis is to

(A) decrease the force required to flex the prosthetic forearm
(B) decrease the cable excursion required to activate the terminal device
(C) increase the arc of motion of the prosthetic forearm
(D) reduce the number of control cables
(E) decrease the weight of the prosthetic device

238. A 5-year-old boy who sustained a traumatic transtibial amputation complained, 3 years later, of pain and tenderness over the lateral aspect of his residual limb. Radiographs revealed terminal overgrowth of the fibula, and prosthetic modifications did not relieve his symptoms. The preferred management is

(A) shortening of the residual fibula
(B) shortening of the residual fibula and tibia with myodesis and closure
(C) proximal fibular epiphysiodesis
(D) resection of the entire fibula
(E) conversion to a knee disarticulation

239. All the following statements concerning the Krukenberg operation are correct EXCEPT that

(A) it is especially valuable for patients without access to prosthetic limbs
(B) it is not useful for the blind, bilateral amputee
(C) the power of pincer grip is greater with the elbow flexed than extended
(D) it is contraindicated in patients with burns of the forearm
(E) sensibility at the tip can approach the sensibility of a normal finger

Amputations, Prosthetics, Orthotics, and Rehabilitation

Answers

189. The answer is C. *(Bowker, pp 382–387.)* As the level of a lower limb amputation moves proximally, both energy expenditure and oxygen demand increase. Because the chosen walking speed decreases as the amputation moves proximally, the average rate of oxygen consumption with ambulation for lower limb amputees does not change with the level of amputation and is approximately the same as for normal subjects. Bilateral amputees expend greater energy during ambulation than do unilateral amputees.

190. The answer is E. *(Bunch, pp 194–210.)* The many variations of ankle-foot orthoses support the foot and ankle complex over a wide range of applications. They may control the subtalar joint, selectively limit dorsiflexion and plantar flexion, assist in dorsiflexion during the swing phase of gait, and inhibit tonic reflexes in patients with spasticity. A double upright AFO with a patellar tendon–bearing brim can partially unload the ankle joint by allowing weight-bearing through the patellar tendon region. AFOs do not control rotation of the distal leg.

191. The answer is D. *(Bordelon, p 37.)* Plastazote is an extremely useful material for custom orthoses. It is especially useful for patients with diabetes and rheumatoid arthritis who have bony prominences on the soles of their feet. The material is easy to mold and inexpensive. Its durability, however, is poor, and a new orthosis is usually required within 3 to 6 months.

192. The answer is C. *(Bordelon, p 43.)* Rigid orthoses are difficult to utilize and should be reserved for patients with flexible foot deformities. Patients frequently have a difficult time adjusting to the orthosis, making compliance a problem. The rigid nature of the orthosis can result in local irritation, leading to sesamoiditis or irritation of preexisting neuromas or nodules. Stress fractures can result from altered weight distribution. Plantar fibromatosis has not been associated with use of rigid foot orthoses.

193. The answer is B. *(Bowker, p 435.)* Although there is much disagreement as to the ideal length of a transtibial amputation stump for optimal prosthetic function, it is universally agreed that the shortest functional amputation level is just distal to the tibial tuberosity. This level allows preservation of knee extension by the quadriceps mechanism, while flexion is provided by the semimembranosus and biceps femoris. Control of flexion and extension of the knee is lost with amputations proximal to the tibial tuberosity.

194. The answer is E. *(Bowker, pp 436–437.)* A cylindrically shaped residual limb is desirable following a transtibial amputation to provide a better prosthetic fit. A cylindrical residual limb results from cutting the fibula only minimally shorter than the tibia. A conical shape results from cutting the fibula more than 2 cm shorter than the tibia, making the distal portion of the tibia unduly prominent.

195. The answer is C. *(Bowker, p 438.)* Wound closure following a transtibial amputation may be achieved using either a myodesis or myoplasty technique. Myodesis provides firm fixation of the posterior muscles to the tibia, preventing later retraction of muscle tissue. Since myodesis places the muscle under greater tension than does myoplasty, myodesis is contraindicated in patients with severely dysvascular limbs.

196. The answer is C. *(Bowker, p 445.)* To achieve successful healing of an amputation, the one tissue structure that *must* heal is the skin; therefore, it must be handled gently with gloved fingers or skin hooks rather than forceps. The skin must be precisely approximated without inverted edges or tension. There should be no separation of layers in the creation of myofasciocutaneous flaps, as this may interfere with the blood supply to the skin. Use of a thigh tourniquet during the procedure has not been associated with impaired skin healing following transtibial amputations.

197. The answer is A. *(Bowker, pp 454–455.)* The PTB hard socket is made of rigid plastic, is indicated primarily for residual limbs with good soft tissue coverage and no sharp bony prominences, has excellent durability, and can be fitted to residual limbs of any length. It is not recommended for residual limbs with thin skin coverage, scarring, skin grafts, or a predisposition to breakdown of the skin.

198. The answer is C. *(Bowker, pp 454–458.)* Supracondylar cuff suspension, when combined with a PTB socket, is appropriate for average length residual limbs with good knee stability. It is not recommended for short residual limbs, since control of rotation and of knee extension are poor with this type of suspension. Although adequate for most transtibial amputees, this mode of suspension cannot completely eliminate pistoning of the socket.

199. The answer is E. *(Bordelon, pp 89–91.)* In the absence of muscular control of the hip and knee joints, stability can still be achieved at these joints if an extension moment is applied to both joints, since both are more stable in full extension than in any amount of flexion. To this end, the brace must be fabricated so that the line of gravity of the patient passes posterior to the hip joint and anterior to the knee joint.

200. The answer is E. *(Bowker, pp 465–466.)* The multiaxial foot provides more ankle motion than any other prosthetic foot, and it is particularly suitable for patients who walk on uneven terrain. Shock absorption with this foot is excellent, and it decreases torque on the residual limb. The increased weight of this foot makes it unsuitable for weak or debilitated patients, and its increased maintenance needs make it unsuitable for those with limited access to prosthetic follow-up.

201. The answer is A. *(Bowker, pp 469–470.)* The socket of a transtibial prosthesis should be tilted slightly posteriorly, creating an initial knee flexion moment upon heel strike, which loads the areas of skin in the socket that are more tolerant of pressure. Proper flexion of the socket not only improves weight-bearing characteristics, but it also provides a smoother gait pattern by placing the quadriceps muscle on stretch, giving it a mechanical advantage for control of the prosthesis. Additionally, flexion of the socket limits recurvatum forces during the mid-stance and terminal phases of gait.

202. The answer is D. *(Bowker, pp 470–474.)* When the foot on a transtibial prosthesis is too outset, the pilon will lean medially, the gait will be wide-based, and excessive medial shoe wear will be apparent. The patient may also have excessive pressure over the lateral aspect of the knee and the medial side of the residual limb. Heel firmness, flexion of the socket, and shortness of the prosthetic limb should have no effect on the mediolateral alignment of the prosthesis.

203. The answer is D. *(Bowker, pp 470–474.)* A properly aligned transtibial prosthesis allows for a knee-flexion moment at the time of heel strike that persists through mid-stance. An increased extension moment on the knee can be caused by a socket that is insufficiently flexed, a prosthetic foot that is too anterior, a SACH heel that is too soft, or a heel on the shoe that is too low. This gait pattern can also be caused by a prosthetic foot that is excessively plantar flexed; excessive dorsiflexion of a prosthetic foot results in an *increased* knee flexion moment at heel strike.

204. The answer is D. *(Aisen, pp 1–2.)* Early orthotic devices were designed based solely on biomechanical principles. These orthoses were well suited for patients with muscular weakness but failed to take into consideration complex patterns of abnormal motor integration frequently seen in patients with "upper motor neuron syndrome." Orthotists have learned that spasticity, clonus, and abnormal reflexes pose a much greater challenge to orthotic design than does simple muscular weakness.

205. The answer is D. *(Bowker, pp 479–485.)* When compared with transfemoral amputation, knee disarticulation offers a durable weight-bearing residual limb, decreased surgical blood loss, and increased resistance to infection by preserving the articular cartilage as a barrier to infection. The resulting bulbous residual limb is less cosmetic than that following transfemoral amputation, yet this makes socket suspension much easier than with a transfemoral amputation.

206. The answer is D. *(Bowker, pp 504–506.)* Preservation of the adductor magnus muscle is desirable when performing a transfemoral amputation because it helps maintain balance between the abductor and adductor muscle forces. A residual limb with dynamically balanced function will allow the amputee to function better and use a prosthesis with greater ease. Therefore, the adductor magnus should be sutured securely to the lateral aspect of the residual femur with the thigh held in maximum adduction. This position provides the appropriate balance with the stronger hip abductors.

207. The answer is E. *(Bowker, pp 251–252.)* Elbow disarticulation remains controversial even though it provides improved suspension capabilities and rotational stability of the prosthesis. The elbow disarticulation amputee is limited to simple cable controls, a weak terminal device, and weak external elbow hinges. In addition, the full humeral length in an elbow disarticulation precludes the use of a myoelectric elbow. Disarticulation is clearly the level of choice, however, for child amputees. The high incidence of humeral overgrowth requiring stump revision following transhumeral amputation in children can be avoided with elbow disarticulation.

208. The answer is D. *(Aisen, p 6.)* The use of plastics provides great versatility in construction of AFOs. The flexibility at the ankle may be decreased by increasing the thickness of the polypropylene or by incorporating graphite into the composite, making the polypropylene more rigid. The width of the AFO also affects flexibility at the ankle; a wider AFO (anterior trimline) is less flexible than a narrower AFO (posterior trimline).

209. The answer is B. *(Bowker, pp 509–511.)* The goal in aligning a transfemoral prosthesis in the coronal plane is to achieve a balance between voluntary and involuntary knee control. Voluntary knee control is achieved through active use of the hip extensor muscles. Involuntary control occurs when the axis of the prosthetic knee is posterior to the biomechanical weight line, such that further weight-bearing forces the knee into greater extension and increased stability. The ideal balance between voluntary and involuntary knee control occurs when the plumb line from the greater trochanter falls directly through the axis of the knee in the mid-stance phase of gait.

210. The answer is B. *(Bowker, pp 509–515.)* A vaulting gait on the prosthetic side in a patient ambulating with a transfemoral prosthesis is usually due to a prosthesis that is too long. This gait pattern can also occur if the socket is too far anterior to the knee, which causes an extension moment at the knee throughout the stance phase of gait. A prosthesis that is too loose would cause a vaulting gait during stance phase on the normal limb.

211. The answer is B. *(Bowker, pp 528–529.)* By providing normal heel rise and extension in the swing phase independent of walking speed, hydraulic control offers nearly normal knee action over a very wide cadence range. The hydraulic knee mechanism is indicated for amputees who can take advantage of this cadence response function. Teenage and young adult males are the most common users of hydraulic knee joints. Young children, older adults, and sedentary persons are poor candidates for hydraulic knee control.

212. The answer is D. *(Aisen, p 13.)* Although the use of an orthosis may assist some functional movements, it will invariably limit or resist other desirable movements. In this patient, a rigid AFO will improve clearance of the foot in the swing phase, heel strike, and the mediolateral stability of the ankle. There is, however, a trade-off because elimination of normal plantar flexion results in decreased push off at the end of the stance phase and limits forward displacement of the tibia after heel strike, causing an increased flexion moment at the knee.

213. The answer is B. *(Bowker, pp 677–678.)* Following amputations in children, especially amputations performed for trauma, rapid growth of the residual limb may occur, even to the extent that the bone grows through the skin. This process occurs by appositional growth rather than physeal stimulation, even though the bony overgrowth usually ceases when physeal growth ceases. It is most commonly seen in the humerus, fibula, tibia, and femur, in that order of frequency.

214. The answer is E. *(Bowker, pp 238–239.)* In performing a transradial amputation, as much residual limb as possible should be preserved. A longer residual forearm will result in a stronger lever arm and more complete pronation and supination. Five centimeters of length is required to preserve elbow function, and at least 10 cm of length is needed for adequate pronation and supination.

215. The answer is A. *(Morrissy, p 992.)* There are no valid data to support the hypothesis that use of shoe modifications for flexible flatfeet improves the arch or influences the development of degenerative changes. Foot or leg pain in children is more likely to be related to causes other than flexible flatfeet. Medial breakdown of shoes in these patients can be delayed by appropriate modifications and inserts.

216. The answer is A. *(Bowker, pp 761–763.)* A child with a congenital forearm amputation may be provided with a passive hand within 60 to 90 days of birth. Theoretically, this affords the child more normal quadripedal development. Voluntary opening and voluntary closing hooks are very difficult for a child to manage before 1 year of age.

217. The answer is C. *(Aisen, pp 50–51.)* The orthotic treatment of the hemiplegic hand has five main goals: (1) to reduce flexor tone at the wrist and fingers; (2) to prevent flexion contractures; (3) to maintain the wrist in a neutral position; (4) to prevent edema of the hand and fingers, and (5) to apply pressure at points overlying the forearm, wrist, and fingers. Direct contact between the splint and the palm is avoided so as not to elicit a grasp reflex, resulting in increased flexor tone.

218. The answer is D. *(Bowker, p 835.)* A lower limb prosthesis is not recommended for children under 6 months of age because they are growing so rapidly at this age that they will quickly outgrow the prosthesis. Furthermore, the child must master sitting balance and other developmental tasks before standing and walking become realistic goals. Most authors recommend initial prosthetic fitting when the child is almost ready to pull to a stand.

219. The answer is A. *(Bowker, pp 836–837.)* A functional knee is generally not introduced for children with transfemoral amputations until the age of 3 to 6 years, at which time the knee usually features a manual locking mechanism. As the child masters the prosthesis, the knee can be unlocked, first at home and later at school. As the child grows and masters the prosthesis, a variable friction knee can be substituted, usually by the age of 6 years.

220. The answer is A. *(Bowker, pp 134–136.)* The control cable for opening the terminal device of a standard transradial prosthesis passes posterior to the elbow joint, along the posterior arm, and attaches to the posterior support strap of a figure-of-eight harness. This arrangement allows glenohumeral flexion to produce tension in the cable and open the terminal device. Glenohumeral extension and biscapular adduction decrease tension in the control cable.

221. The answer is C. *(Aisen, pp 74–76.)* In patients with lacerations of the median nerve at the wrist resulting in paralysis of thumb abduction and opposition, it is imperative to prevent a disabling adduction contracture of the thumb. The orthosis employed for this purpose must position the thumb in palmar abduction and opposition to both prevent contracture and promote function during the reinnervation period. Extension contractures of the index and long fingers do not occur unless the ulnar nerve is lacerated as well.

222. The answer is A. *(Bowker, pp 144–146.)* To lock or unlock the elbow in a standard transhumeral prosthesis, the amputee must first apply tension, then, in rapid sequence, release tension on the elbow lock control cable. The amputee applies tension to the cable by slight flexion and abduction of the glenohumeral joint combined with shoulder depression. This motion, combined with rapid return of the prosthesis to the starting position, will lock or unlock the prosthetic elbow.

223. The answer is E. *(Aisen, pp 82–83.)* A spiral or hemispiral AFO is useful when weakness involves ankle dorsiflexion and plantar flexion and foot inversion and eversion, as is the case in injuries to the sciatic nerve or lumbosacral plexus. These designs are not indicated for patients with increased muscular tone or an imbalance between antagonistic groups of muscles. Spiral or hemispiral AFOs are difficult to don and doff and are not in widespread use.

224. The answer is E. *(Aisen, p 20.)* The most obvious contraindication to the use of an orthosis is the presence of adequate substitutive patterns that, although not normal, allow the safe execution of functional tasks. Another contraindication is the situation in which consumption of energy is greater when using the device for functional tasks than when not using the device. Orthoses are used effectively in blind patients, patients who cannot independently don and doff the devices, nonambulatory patients, and hemophiliacs.

225. The answer is E. *(Bowker, pp 770–772.)* The major advantage of externally powered prostheses for transradial amputees is the ability to combine cosmetic appearance with function. Other significant benefits include the absence of harnessing straps and control cables, ease of operation near the body and overhead, superior grip strength, and reduced expenditure of energy. Major disadvantages of myoelectric prostheses over mechanical prostheses for this level of amputee include increased maintenance, decreased durability, and increased weight.

226. The answer is C. *(Bunch, pp 260–261.)* The most important and frequent use for orthotics in young children with cerebral palsy is to control the tone of muscles (inhibition). It is known that the position of one joint can change the muscle tone around another joint. For example, in the young diplegic child, an ankle-foot orthosis may control tone at the ankle and foot and improve gait by improving the mechanics and tone around the knee. Orthoses are also used occasionally to prevent contractures, most often following surgical procedures.

227. The answer is D. *(Bunch, pp 289–291.)* A patient with complete paraplegia and no motor control of the hip, knee, or ankle, will require a hip-knee-ankle-foot orthosis for ambulation. With this orthosis, he will have a swing-through gait with crutch assistance. Only patients with active hip flexion and knee extension have the potential to be reciprocal walkers. The high energy cost of this mode of ambulation compared with wheelchair propulsion makes it likely that this patient will choose to sit in a wheelchair, although he may be capable of household ambulation.

228. The answer is A. *(Browner, p 589.)* Distinguishing between complete and incomplete neurologic deficits following spinal cord injury is essential to determining the prognosis for recovery. An incomplete neurologic deficit has a good prognosis for at least partial functional motor recovery. Functional motor recovery is seen in only 3 percent of patients with complete neurologic injuries present 24 h after injury. Functional motor recovery is never seen in patients with complete neurologic deficits present more than 48 h after injury.

229. The answer is C. *(Bowker, pp 470–476.)* Improper alignment of the prosthetic foot in the mediolateral plane can result in significant gait abnormalities, but the prosthetic foot can only swing laterally or medially in the initial swing phase of gait if the prosthetic socket is rotated with respect to the line of progression. Rotation of the prosthetic socket medially with respect to the line of progression will cause the prosthetic foot to swing laterally at the beginning of swing phase. A prosthesis that is too long will cause vaulting over the prosthetic limb during the stance phase of gait.

230. The answer is D. *(Bowker, pp 504–506.)* In performing a transfemoral amputation, the quadriceps must be securely fastened to the residual femur to provide good control of the residual limb in the flexion/extension plane. As such, the quadriceps should be sutured securely to the posterior aspect of the residual femur. The hip should be in extension when this is performed to prevent creation of a hip flexion contracture, which can prevent maximal use of a prosthetic limb.

231. The answer is C. *(Bowker, pp 511–515.)* Effective pelvis-trunk stabilization can only be achieved in a transfemoral prosthesis by providing adequate lateral support to the residual femur, which is accomplished by positioning the femur in slight adduction to put the abductors on stretch, allowing them to function more effectively. The socket is also aligned in flexion to avoid excessive pelvic rotation during the latter part of the stance phase.

232. The answer is C. *(Bowker, p 539.)* The rates of usage of hip disarticulation or hemipelvectomy prostheses are extremely low, in large part because the energy required to ambulate with such prostheses is approximately 200 percent of that used in normal ambulation. At the same time, the lack of muscle power in the hip, knee, and ankle results in a fixed, slow cadence. Only motivated, young, psychologically vigorous patients are likely to ambulate with these prostheses.

233. The answer is A. *(Bowker, pp 677–678.)* Terminal bony overgrowth occurs frequently in children following acquired amputations, although it usually ceases when physeal growth ceases. It is most commonly seen in the humerus, followed by the fibula, tibia, and femur. Significant overgrowth is easily treated by resection of sufficient bone to allow skin coverage with an adequate soft tissue envelope. Overgrowth may recur, however, even after adequate bony resection. Epiphysiodesis is contraindicated since this overgrowth is appositional and not related to physeal stimulation.

234. The answer is D. *(Bowker, pp 763–765.)* The design of prostheses for younger patients with transradial amputations has changed dramatically over the last decade. The development of user-friendly myoelectric controls has allowed children less than 1½ years of age to control a myoelectric prosthesis, which allows an earlier and more natural assimilation of the prosthesis. Voluntary opening and closing devices are more difficult for young children to manage.

235. The answer is D. *(Bowker, pp 135–136.)* Although glenohumeral flexion is the primary body motion required to open the terminal device of a standard transradial prosthesis, this movement cannot be performed when one is working close to the midline of the body. In this position, biscapular abduction will produce adequate tension in the control cable to operate the terminal device.

236. The answer is D. *(Bowker, pp 146–149.)* Biscapular abduction is usually strong enough to provide sufficient cable tension for full operation of the elbow and terminal device of a shoulder disarticulation prosthesis. Abduction of the scapula, however, cannot generate adequate cable excursion. Therefore, shoulder disarticulation harnesses frequently employ the addition of an excursion amplifier, in which each 1 inch of cable excursion generated by the patient causes the elbow flexion/terminal device control cable to move through an excursion of 2 inches.

237. The answer is C. *(Bowker, pp 123–124.)* Amputations immediately distal to the elbow joint require a prosthetic socket with extremely high trim lines for stability and suspension. Consequently, flexion of the anatomic elbow joint is often limited. In these situations a step-up hinge may be employed, which will amplify the excursion of the anatomic elbow joint by a ratio of approximately 2 : 1. Thus, 60° of flexion of the anatomic elbow causes 120° of flexion of the prosthetic forearm. The amputee must, however, exert twice as much force to flex the step-up hinge as to flex the anatomic elbow.

238. The answer is A. *(Bowker, pp 677–678.)* Terminal bony overgrowth occurs frequently in children, particularly those whose amputations are a result of trauma. These complications are easily treated by resection of sufficient fibula to allow coverage with an adequate soft-tissue envelope. Epiphysiodesis will not help, as the terminal overgrowth is appositional rather than physeal in origin. Resection of the entire fibula or shortening of the residual limb is not recommended, since both would decrease the patient's functional abilities.

239. The answer is B. *(Bowker, pp 239–240).* The purpose of the Krukenberg operation is to give an amputee a sensate, active pincer between the ulna and radius. It is a valuable procedure for those patients without access to prosthetic limbs and is particularly useful for the blind, bilateral, transradial amputee, since it uses sensation to enhance grasp. The power of the pincer grip is usually 2 to 3 kg when the elbow is extended and 8 to 10 kg when the elbow is flexed. Sensibility at the tips can approach normal finger sensibility in children, and adults usually achieve protective sensation. Normal skin coverage and muscle strength in the forearm are required for this operation to be successful.

Pediatric Disorders

Douglas R. Dirschl, M.D., and
Frank C. Wilson, M.D.

DIRECTIONS: Each question below contains five suggested responses. Select the **one best** response to each question.

240. A 17-year-old girl has had three stress fractures of the tibia since beginning competitive distance running at age 11. Her menstrual cycle is very irregular. The most appropriate management is to

(A) change her shoes to lightweight racing flats
(B) institute a strict diet for weight loss
(C) increase the amount of running on the road and decrease the amount on the track
(D) prescribe estrogen-containing birth control pills
(E) reduce her weekly running mileage by 15 percent

241. A 12-year-old boy collapsed during a basketball game after complaining of shortness of breath and "butterflies" in his chest. He is very tall and thin and his father has a similar habitus. This patient should be evaluated for

(A) anorexia nervosa
(B) illicit use of stimulants
(C) Marfan's syndrome
(D) Klinefelter's syndrome
(E) Larsen's syndrome

242. A slender, 14-year-old girl has had anterior knee pain for 3 months. Examination was normal except for tenderness at the medial aspect of the patella, crepitus with active knee extension, and moderate quadriceps atrophy. Radiographs of the knee were normal. The most appropriate initial management is

(A) a technetium-99 bone scan of the knee
(B) a CT scan of the patellofemoral joint
(C) isokinetic muscle testing
(D) isometric exercises and anti-inflammatory medications
(E) arthroscopy of the knee and release of the lateral retinaculum

243. A 16-year-old baseball player has had 2 weeks of aching low back pain during athletic activities. Examination was normal except for mild paraspinal muscle spasm. Radiographs showed bilateral spondylolysis at L5, with no spondylolisthesis. The most appropriate initial treatment is

(A) bed rest for 2 weeks
(B) cessation of athletic activities for 3 months
(C) immobilization in a cast or brace
(D) limitation of activity as determined by symptoms
(E) posterior spinal fusion

244. A 15-year-old wrestler noted the sudden, atraumatic onset of shoulder pain and felt as though he had "lost control" of his shoulder. Examination showed weakness of his deltoid, biceps, triceps, and wrist extensors. The most likely diagnosis is

(A) dislocation of the shoulder with injury to the axillary nerve
(B) dislocation of the shoulder with injury to the musculocutaneous nerve
(C) acute brachial neuropathy
(D) thoracic outlet syndrome
(E) acute herniation of a cervical disk

245. A 16-year-old girl thought to have an exertionally related compartmental syndrome of the leg had a postexercise pressure reading of 35 mmHg in the anterior compartment. This reading is

(A) normal
(B) above normal, but not high enough to suggest a compartmental syndrome
(C) indicative of a probable compartmental syndrome
(D) diagnostic for a compartmental syndrome
(E) an indication for immediate fasciotomy

246. An obese, 13-year-old boy complained of intermittent left knee pain of 6 weeks' duration. He denied swelling, giving way, or trauma. After examination of the knee, the most appropriate next step in evaluation is

(A) examination of the left hip
(B) anteroposterior, lateral, tunnel, and Merchant radiographs of the left knee
(C) anteroposterior, lateral, tunnel, and Merchant radiographs of the left knee; anteroposterior and frog lateral views of the pelvis
(D) an MRI scan of the left knee
(E) aspiration of the left knee

247. A 14-year-old football player had a 3-week history of sore throat, fatigue, fever, and lymphadenopathy. A serum test for mononucleosis was positive. The patient may return to football

(A) immediately
(B) when the fever and fatigue have subsided
(C) in 6 months
(D) when all clinical and hematologic signs are normal
(E) never

248. A 14-year-old had the sudden onset of heat cramps in both calves during a tennis match. The most appropriate treatment is

(A) deep massage of the cramping muscles
(B) application of a compressive wrap to the leg and ankle
(C) nonsteroidal anti-inflammatory medications
(D) replacement of fluids and electrolytes, cooling, and passive stretching
(E) application of heat to the calf and passive stretching

249. A 16-year-old girl complained of anterior knee pain that increased when she descended stairs. Examination revealed a high-riding patella, increased internal rotation of the hips, and an underdeveloped vastus medialis obliquus muscle. A sunrise radiographic view of her knee is shown in the figure. The most appropriate initial treatment is

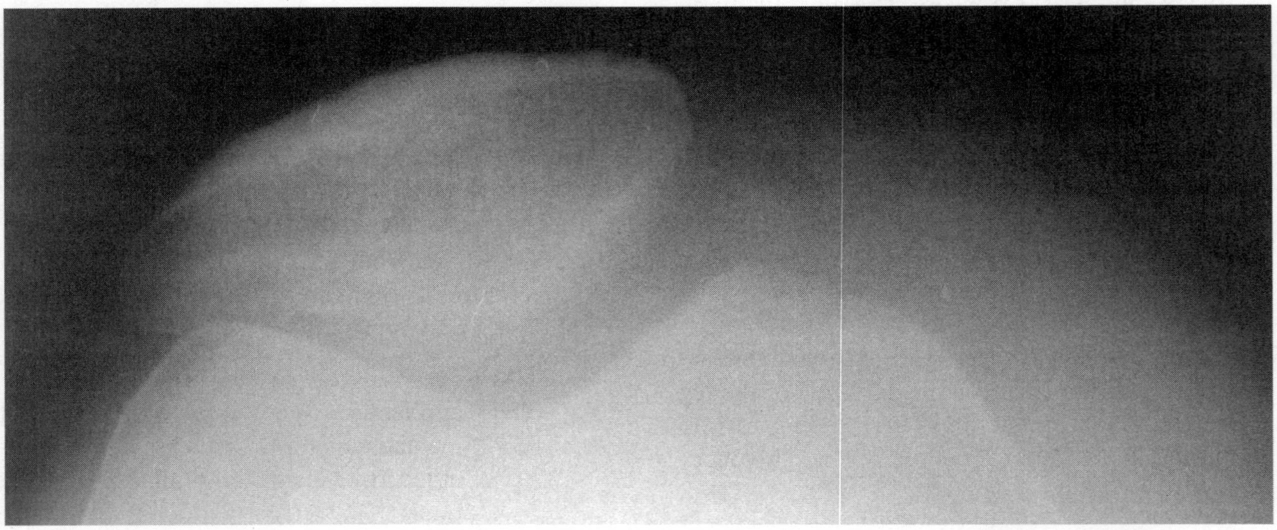

(A) observation
(B) an exercise program concentrating on the vastus medialis obliquus
(C) application of a cylinder cast
(D) arthroscopy of the knee and lateral release
(E) derotational osteotomy of the femur

250. The mode of inheritance of Duchenne's muscular dystrophy is

(A) autosomal dominant
(B) autosomal recessive
(C) sex-linked dominant
(D) sex-linked recessive
(E) multifactorial

251. An 11-year-old boy with trisomy 21 had a history of frequent falls and ankle sprains. Examination revealed generalized ligamentous laxity, normal motion of the neck, slight weakness of the gastrosoleus complex, and a hyperactive Achilles tendon reflex. The next step in management should be

(A) observation
(B) lateral flexion/extension radiographs of the cervical spine
(C) MRI scanning of the cervical spine
(D) nerve conduction studies of the peroneal and tibial nerves
(E) electromyography of the lower limbs

252. A 7-year-old girl with spastic diplegia had valgus foot deformities 3 months following lumbar selective posterior rhizotomy. The most appropriate treatment is

(A) observation
(B) application of bilateral ankle-foot orthoses
(C) lengthening of the Achilles tendon
(D) extraarticular talocalcaneal arthrodesis
(E) split transfer of the tibialis posterior tendon

253. A 6-year-old boy had a lump on the lateral aspect of his elbow. Examination was normal except for a 10° elbow flexion contracture and limitation of forearm pronation to 30°. Radiographs of the elbow are shown in the figure. The contralateral elbow was normal. The most appropriate treatment is

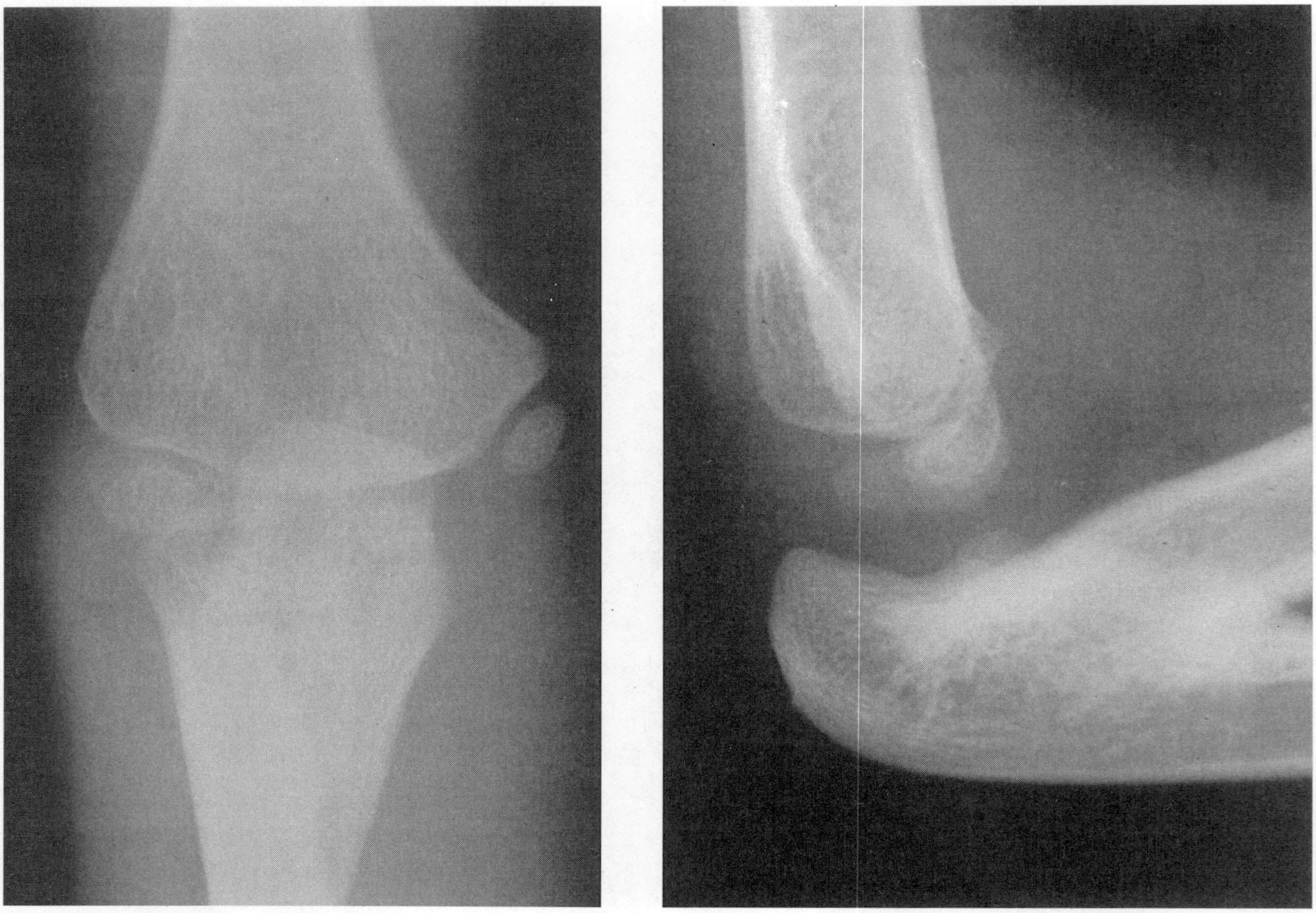

(A) observation
(B) aggressive physical therapy
(C) closed reduction and immobilization in a cast
(D) open reduction and internal fixation
(E) excision of the radial head

254. A 9-year-old girl with a lower lumbar myelomeningocele developed a 35° scoliosis between T10 and L2 during the past year and complained of intermittent low back pain after walking. She had a functioning ventriculoperitoneal shunt. Examination revealed no voluntary muscle function below the knee extensors and absent sensation below the L4 dermatome. The most likely diagnosis is

(A) juvenile idiopathic scoliosis
(B) paralytic scoliosis
(C) hydromyelia
(D) tethered spinal cord
(E) congenital scoliosis

255. A 12-year-old girl had an osteotomy of the base of the first metatarsal for symptomatic hallux valgus. She has had flexible flat feet since childhood. The most likely outcome is

(A) restoration of the longitudinal arch
(B) worsening of the pes planus deformity
(C) a recurrence rate of 5 percent or less
(D) a recurrence rate of 30 to 60 percent
(E) a recurrence rate of greater than 60 percent

256. The most important aspect of treatment in the earliest stages of Legg-Calvé-Perthes disease is

(A) frequent observation
(B) administration of anti-inflammatory medications
(C) restoration of motion in the hip
(D) containment of the femoral head within the acetabulum
(E) aspiration of the hip

257. A 4-year-old girl with a myelomeningocele had the radiograph shown in the figure. She had active hip flexors but no other voluntary motor function in the lower limbs. She also had 35° flexion contractures of both hips. The preferred treatment of the dislocated hip is

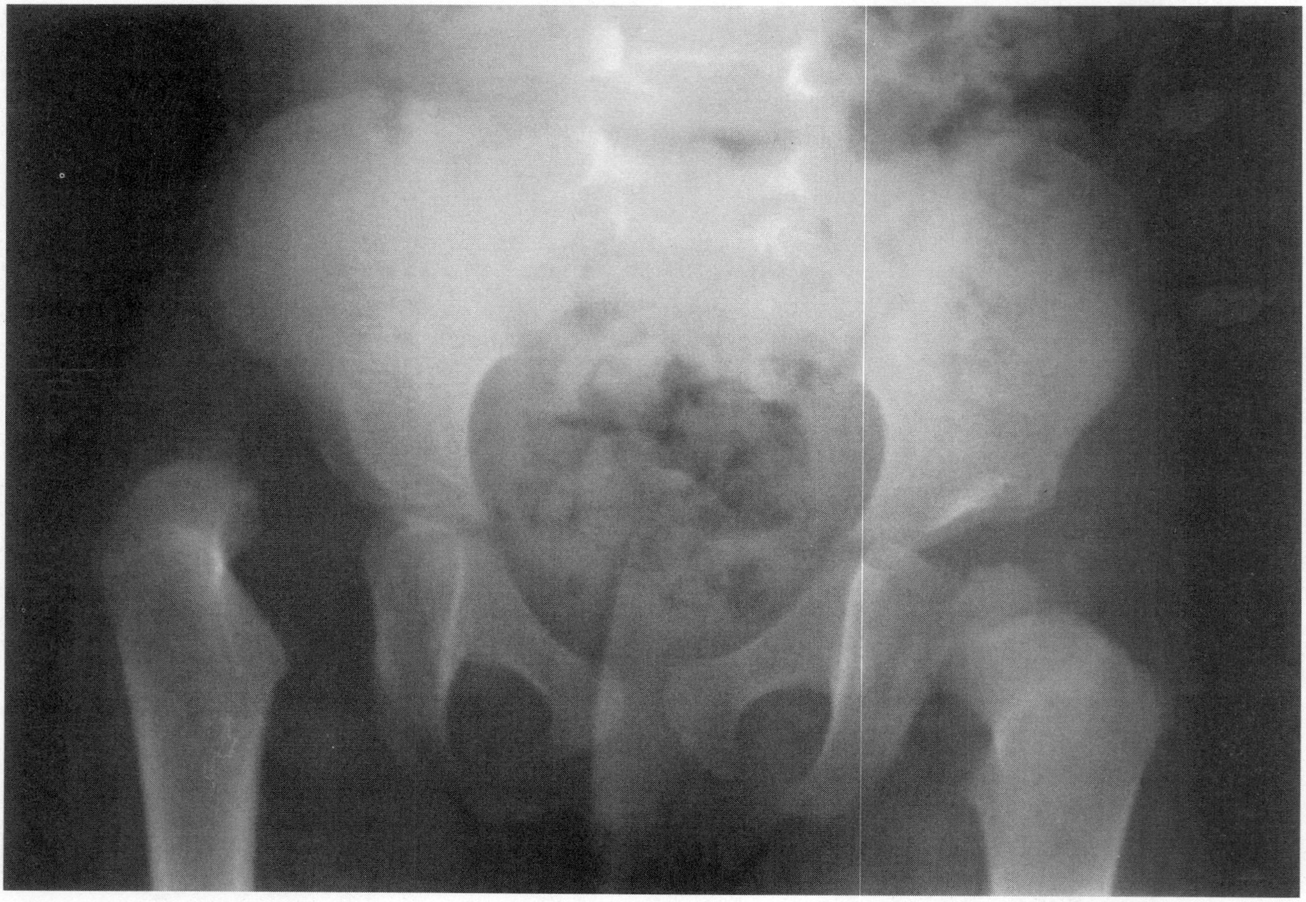

(A) observation
(B) closed reduction and cast immobilization
(C) release of the flexion contractures; application of a standing brace
(D) open reduction and varus derotation osteotomy
(E) open reduction and iliopsoas transfer

258. A 3-year-old girl recovering from an upper respiratory tract infection suddenly refused to walk. Examination revealed the right hip to be held in flexion and external rotation, and any attempt at motion caused severe pain. Her temperature was 39°C (102.2°F), WBC 17,000/mm^3, and erythrocyte sedimentation rate (ESR) 75 mm/h. The next step in management should be

(A) a CT scan of the hip
(B) an MRI scan of the hip
(C) a bone scan
(D) aspiration of the hip
(E) surgical drainage of the hip

259. A 2-year-old boy had the acute onset of pain and swelling in his left knee and refused to walk. His temperature was 39°C (102.2°F), WBC 16,000/mm^3, and ESR 90 mm/h. Aspiration of the knee yielded cloudy fluid with a nucleated cell count of 75,000/mm^3. What is the most likely cause of this infection?

(A) *Staphylococcus aureus*
(B) *Haemophilus influenzae*
(C) Streptococcus species
(D) Pneumococcus species
(E) Meningococcus species

Questions 260–261

Use the following Moseley straight-line graph in answering these questions.

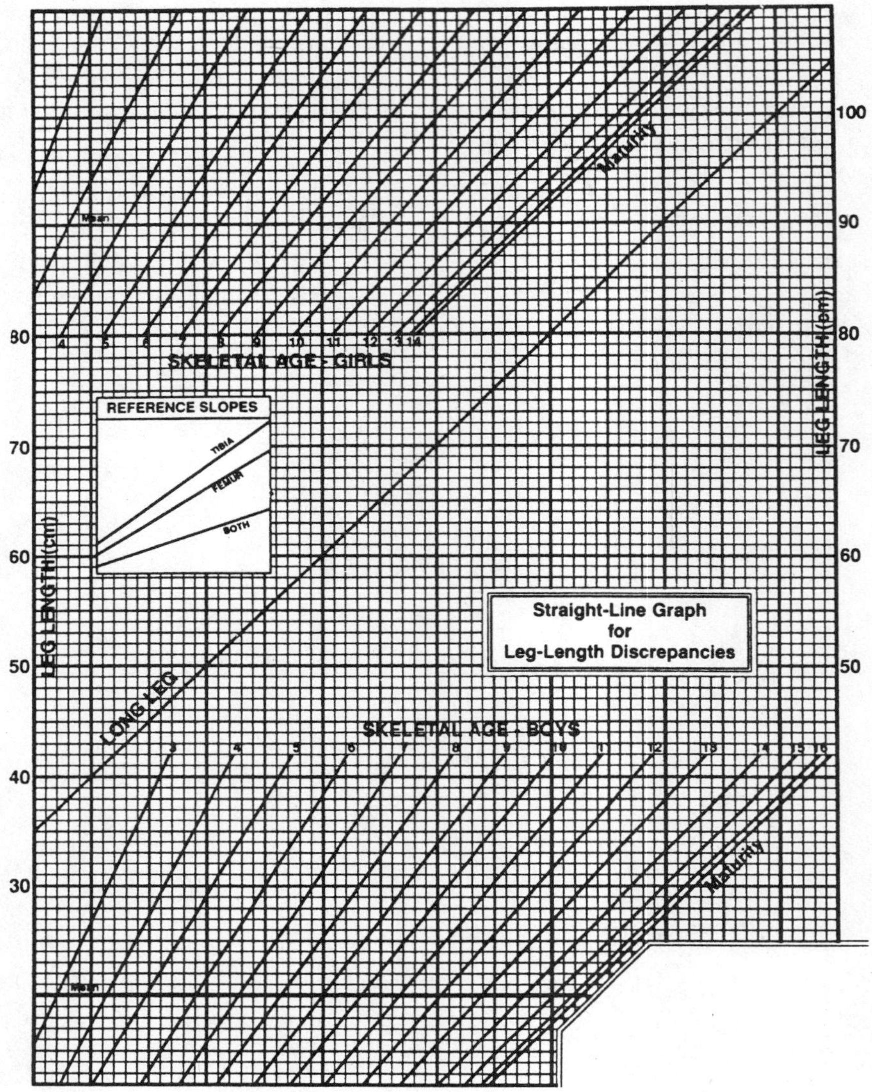

260. A 13-year-old boy had an inequality of leg length shown in the table below. Use this table and the graph to project the inequality at maturity.

Skeletal Age (yr)	Right Leg (cm)	Left Leg (cm)
9 + 0	65.0	62.0
10 + 0	69.0	65.0
11 + 0	72.5	67.8

(A) 5.0 cm
(B) 6.0 cm
(C) 7.0 cm
(D) 8.5 cm
(E) 9.5 cm

261. A 12-year-old girl had the progressive discrepancy of leg length shown in the table below. Use this table and the graph to determine the best treatment.

Skeletal Age (yr)	Right Leg (cm)	Left Leg (cm)
8 + 0	56.5	58.0
9 + 0	59.7	61.5
11 + 0	66.4	69.0

(A) Distal femoral epiphysiodesis at age 12
(B) Proximal tibial epiphysiodesis at age 12
(C) Distal femoral and proximal tibial epiphysiodeses at age 12
(D) Distal femoral and proximal tibial epiphysiodeses at age 13
(E) Lengthening of the right lower limb

262. A 6-year-old girl with a 3-week history of neck pain and torticollis had a CT scan that showed rotatory atlantoaxial subluxation. There was no history of trauma. The most appropriate treatment is

(A) application of a soft cervical collar
(B) application of a hard cervical collar
(C) application of a halo vest
(D) cervical traction
(E) C1–C2 fusion in situ

263. In a child with a cavovarus foot deformity, the standing lateral block test (Coleman block test) assesses the flexibility of the

(A) ankle
(B) hindfoot
(C) forefoot
(D) ankle and hindfoot
(E) hindfoot and forefoot

264. A 9-year-old boy complained of intermittent pain and swelling in the knee of 1 month's duration. Examination revealed tenderness over the medial femoral condyle; radiographs are shown below. The most appropriate treatment is

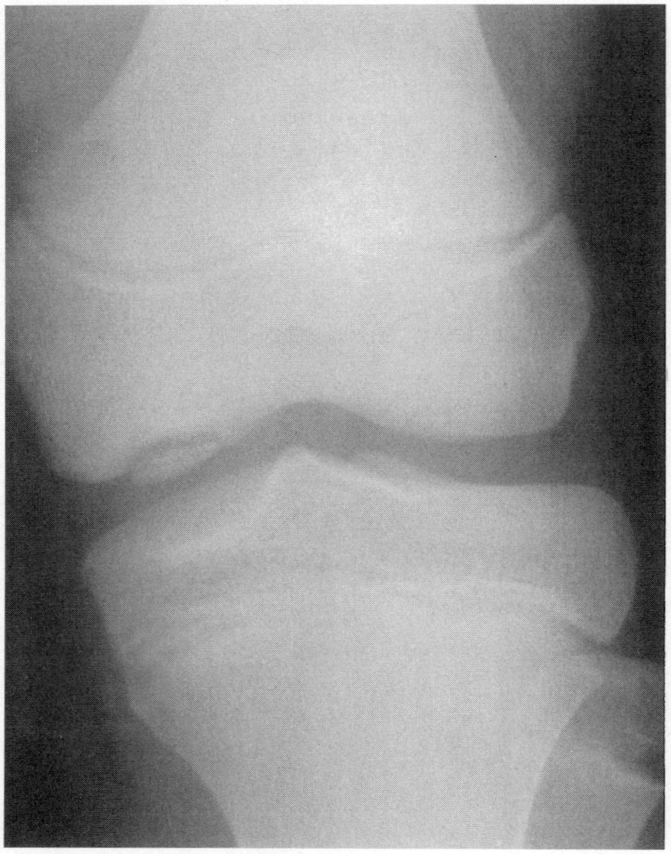

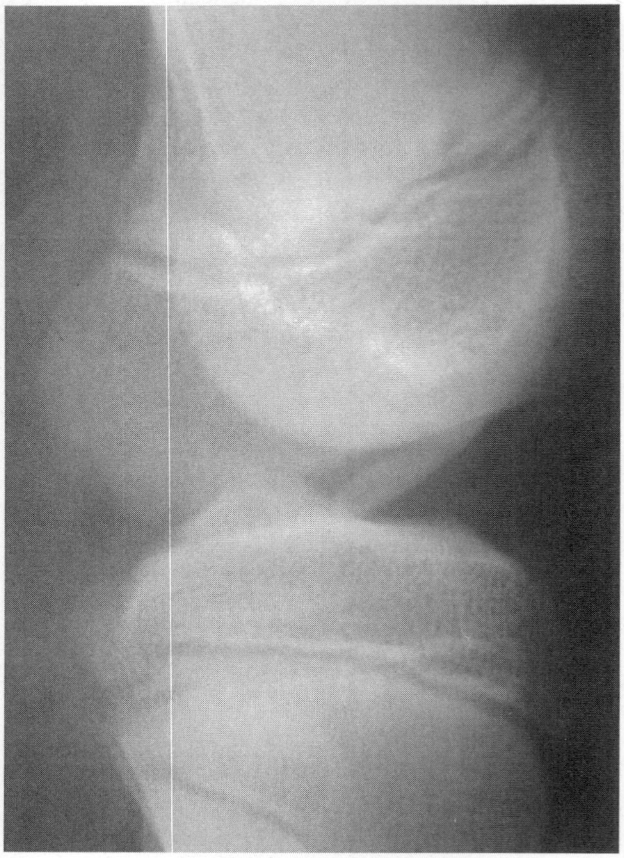

(A) limitation of activities until healing is evident
(B) immobilization in a cylinder cast for 6 weeks
(C) arthroscopy and excision of the lesion
(D) arthroscopy and pinning of the lesion
(E) arthroscopy and drilling of the lesion

265. A 13-year-old girl with no family history of scoliosis has spinal deformity. She began menstruating approximately 16 months ago and is neurologically normal. Radiographs reveal a 25° right thoracic curve from T4–T11 with a compensatory 20° left lumbar curve from T12–L3; ossification of the iliac apophysis is Risser grade III. The most appropriate treatment is

(A) observation
(B) application of a spinal orthosis
(C) electrical stimulation
(D) posterior spinal fusion with instrumentation
(E) anterior and posterior spinal fusion with instrumentation

266. The most common complication following treatment of acute slipped capital femoral epiphyses is

(A) degenerative joint disease
(B) overgrowth of the greater trochanter
(C) avascular necrosis
(D) chondrolysis
(E) coxa magna

267. An 11-year-old girl was evaluated for idiopathic scoliosis. Her neurologic examination was normal, and her anteroposterior (AP) radiograph is shown in the figure. She has not yet begun menstruating, and her skeletal maturity level is Risser O. The most appropriate management is

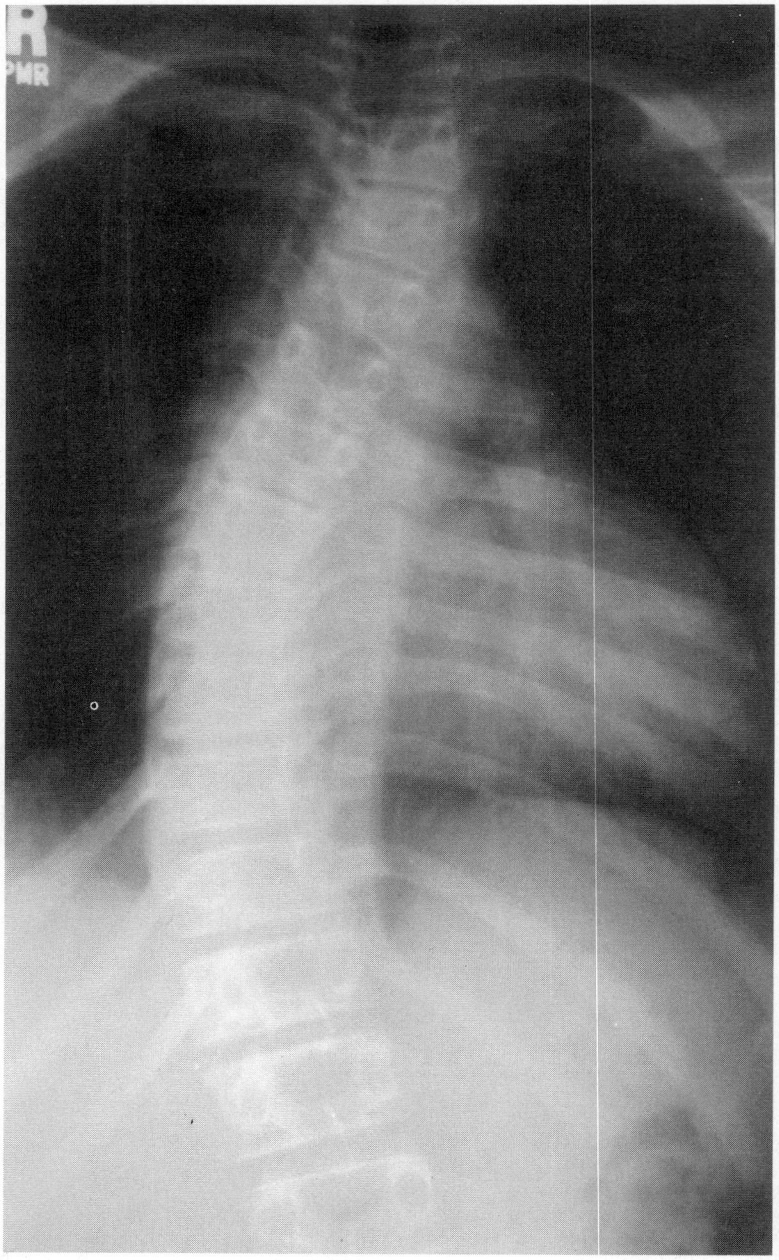

(A) reevaluation in 2 months
(B) reevaluation in 6 months
(C) reevaluation in 1 year
(D) application of a spinal orthosis
(E) posterior spinal fusion with instrumentation

268. A 12-year-old boy had a history of repeated sprains of his ankle and of foot pain aggravated by activity. Radiographs demonstrated a calcaneonavicular coalition but no other abnormalities. A period of casting relieved his symptoms, but the pain returned after removal of the cast. The most appropriate treatment is

(A) reapplication of the below-knee walking cast
(B) use of a molded arch support
(C) strengthening exercises for the peroneal muscles
(D) resection of the coalition
(E) triple arthrodesis

269. An obese, 10-year-old girl had the sudden onset of pain in the right groin when she stepped off a curb. She held the leg in external rotation, and any attempt at internal rotation reproduced the groin pain. An AP radiograph of her pelvis was obtained and is shown in the figure. The next step in management is to obtain

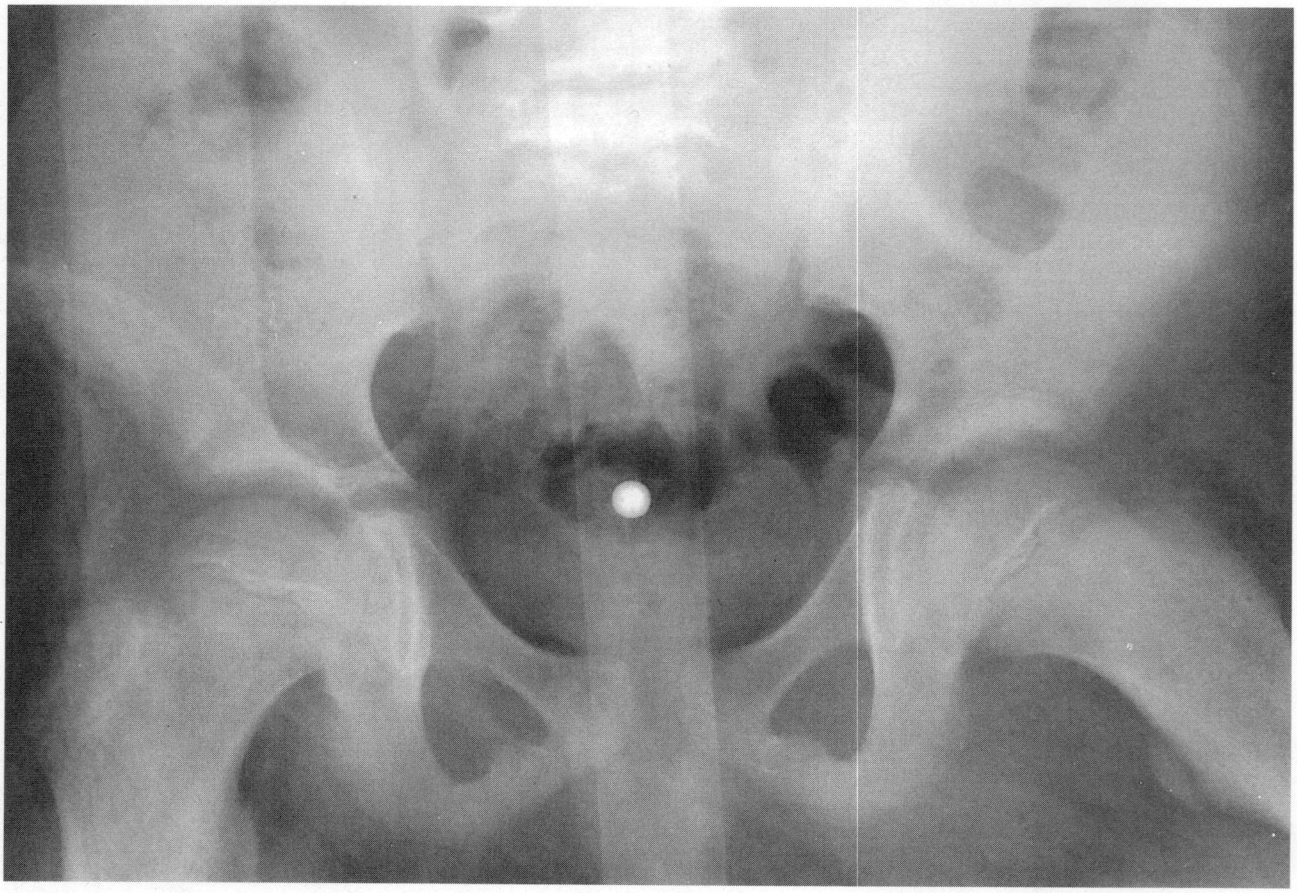

(A) a true lateral radiograph of the hip
(B) trispiral tomography
(C) a CT scan
(D) a bone scan
(E) an arthrogram of the hip

---

270. The factor most frequently associated with development of a progressively crouched gait in children with cerebral palsy is

(A) increasing body mass associated with the adolescent growth spurt
(B) progression of the neurologic lesion
(C) lack of bracing when the child was younger
(D) tightness of the hamstrings
(E) previous lengthening of the Achilles tendon

271. A 12-year-old girl concerned about the appearance of her feet had no pain and was active in athletics. Examination revealed no longitudinal arch when the patient was standing, minimal valgus of the heels, and normal ankle and subtalar motion. The most appropriate treatment is

(A) observation
(B) custom molded foot orthoses
(C) bilateral below-knee walking casts
(D) talocalcaneal arthrodeses
(E) calcaneal osteotomies

272. A 6-year-old boy had a 3-month history of a lump behind his knee that seemed to get larger with activity and smaller with rest. Examination revealed a 3-cm mass between the medial head of the gastrocnemius and the semimembranosus tendon. Radiographs were normal. The most appropriate treatment is

(A) observation
(B) application of a cylinder cast for 6 weeks
(C) aspiration of the mass and injection of corticosteroids
(D) diagnostic arthroscopy
(E) open surgical excision of the cyst

273. A 13-year-old boy with Down's syndrome is to undergo surgery for subluxation of the patella. The most important part of the preoperative evaluation is

(A) trispiral tomography of the knee
(B) a CT scan of the patellofemoral joint
(C) an MRI scan of the knee
(D) an echocardiogram
(E) lateral radiographs of the cervical spine in flexion and extension

274. In the treatment of spastic cerebral palsy, selective posterior rhizotomy

(A) is contraindicated
(B) relieves contractures of the joints
(C) increases muscular strength
(D) reduces muscular tone
(E) is not supported by clinical studies

275. A 4-year-old boy with hemihypertrophy had inequality of leg lengths. The initial evaluation of this patient should include

(A) an MRI scan of the head
(B) an MRI scan of the spine
(C) an ultrasound examination of the abdomen
(D) a CT scan of both lower limbs
(E) digital angiograms of both lower limbs

276. A 15½-year-old boy had a nonprogressive inequality of leg lengths of 2 cm. The most appropriate treatment is

(A) use of a heel lift on the shorter leg
(B) epiphysiodesis of the distal femur of the longer leg
(C) epiphysiodesis of the distal tibia of the longer leg
(D) closed femoral shortening of the longer leg
(E) one-stage femoral lengthening of the shorter leg

277. A 7-year-old boy has had a 6-month history of progressive spinal deformity. Photographs of the child 6 months previously showed no curvature of the spine. Examination revealed elevation of the right scapula and a 2-cm right thoracic rib hump on forward bending. Neurologic examination is normal. The next step in evaluation should be

(A) supine right and left side–bending radiographs
(B) serum creatine phosphokinase analysis
(C) a muscle biopsy
(D) a sural nerve biopsy
(E) an MRI scan of the spine and head

278. A 2-year-old girl with arthrogryposis and asymmetric involvement of the lower limbs had the radiograph of the pelvis shown in the figure. The most appropriate treatment of the right hip is

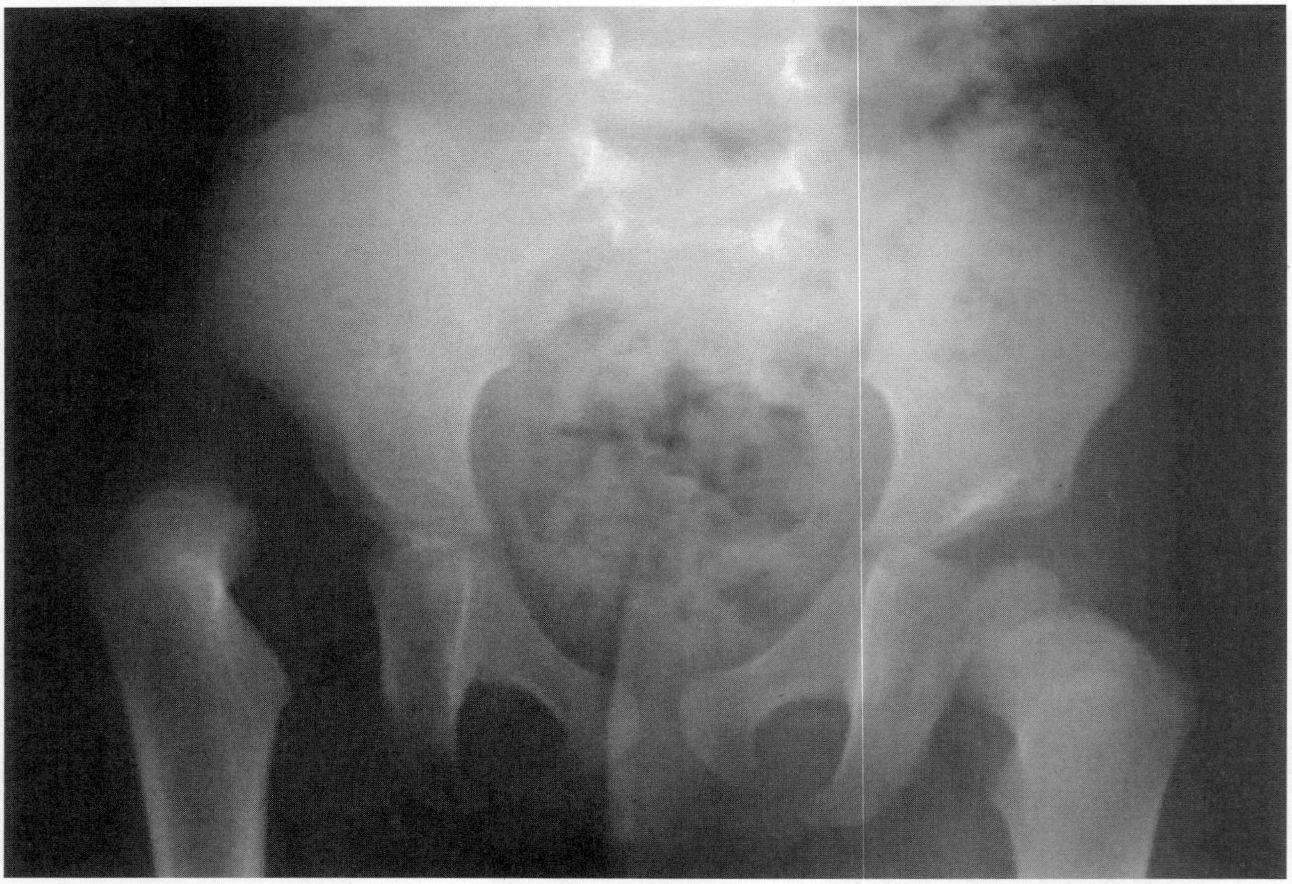

(A) observation
(B) skin traction, followed by closed reduction and application of a hip spica cast
(C) adductor tenotomy, followed by closed reduction and application of a hip spica cast
(D) open reduction and femoral shortening
(E) open reduction and innominate osteotomy

279. A 6-month-old boy had posteromedial bowing of the tibia. The most appropriate treatment is

(A) observation
(B) application of a cylinder cast
(C) application of a total contact orthosis
(D) osteotomy, intramedullary nailing, and bone grafting
(E) vascularized free fibular transfer

280. A 4-year-old girl with a myelomeningocele had the anteroposterior radiograph of the pelvis shown in the figure. The patient had full passive motion in her hips and knees, and her feet were plantigrade. She had 2/5 strength of her quadriceps and no voluntary motor function distal to the knee. The recommended treatment for the hips is

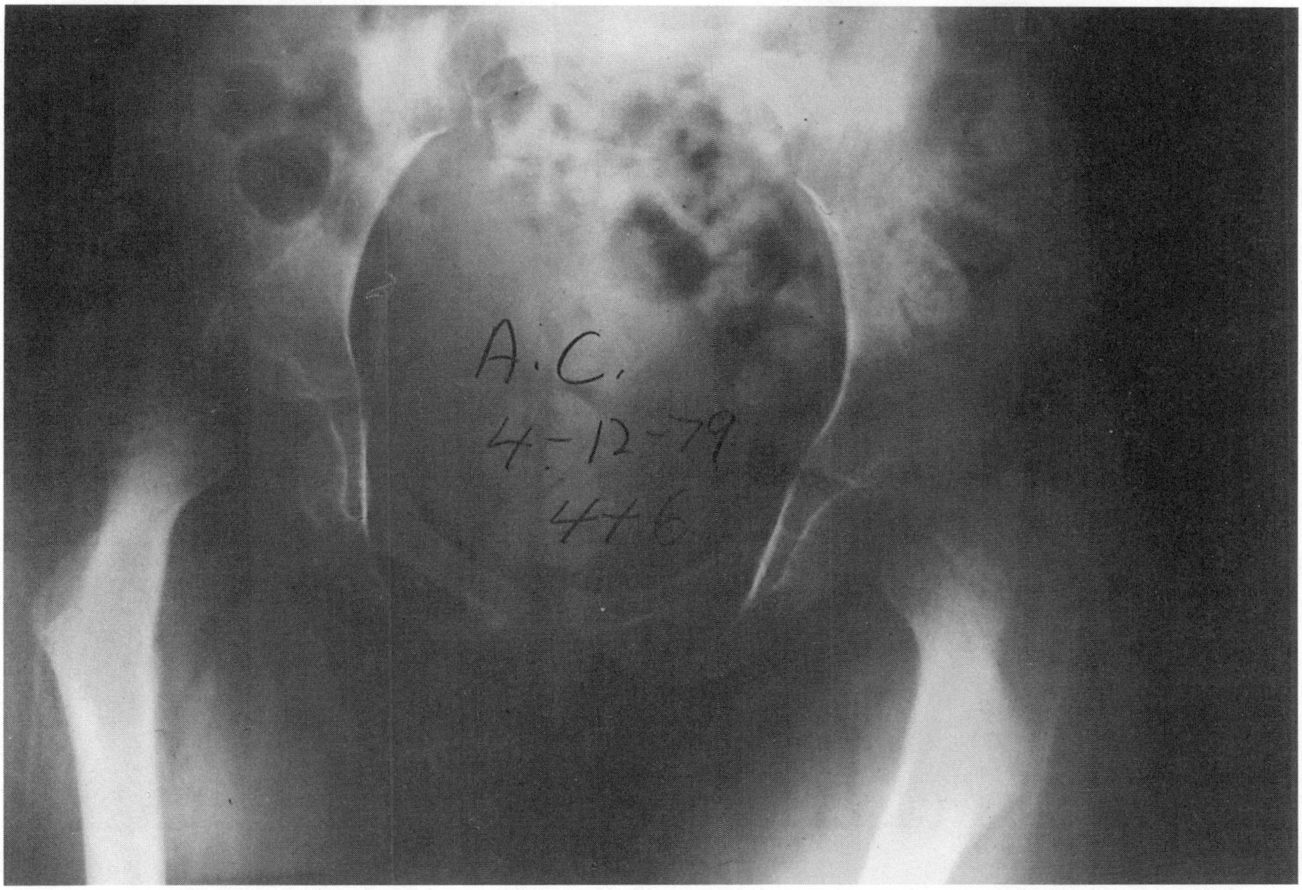

(A) observation
(B) closed reduction and application of a hip spica cast
(C) bilateral open reduction and femoral osteotomy
(D) bilateral open reduction and pelvic osteotomy
(E) bilateral open reduction, pelvic osteotomy, and femoral osteotomy

281. An 18-month-old boy has had a lump over his left clavicle since birth. A radiograph of the clavicle is shown in the figure. The most appropriate treatment is

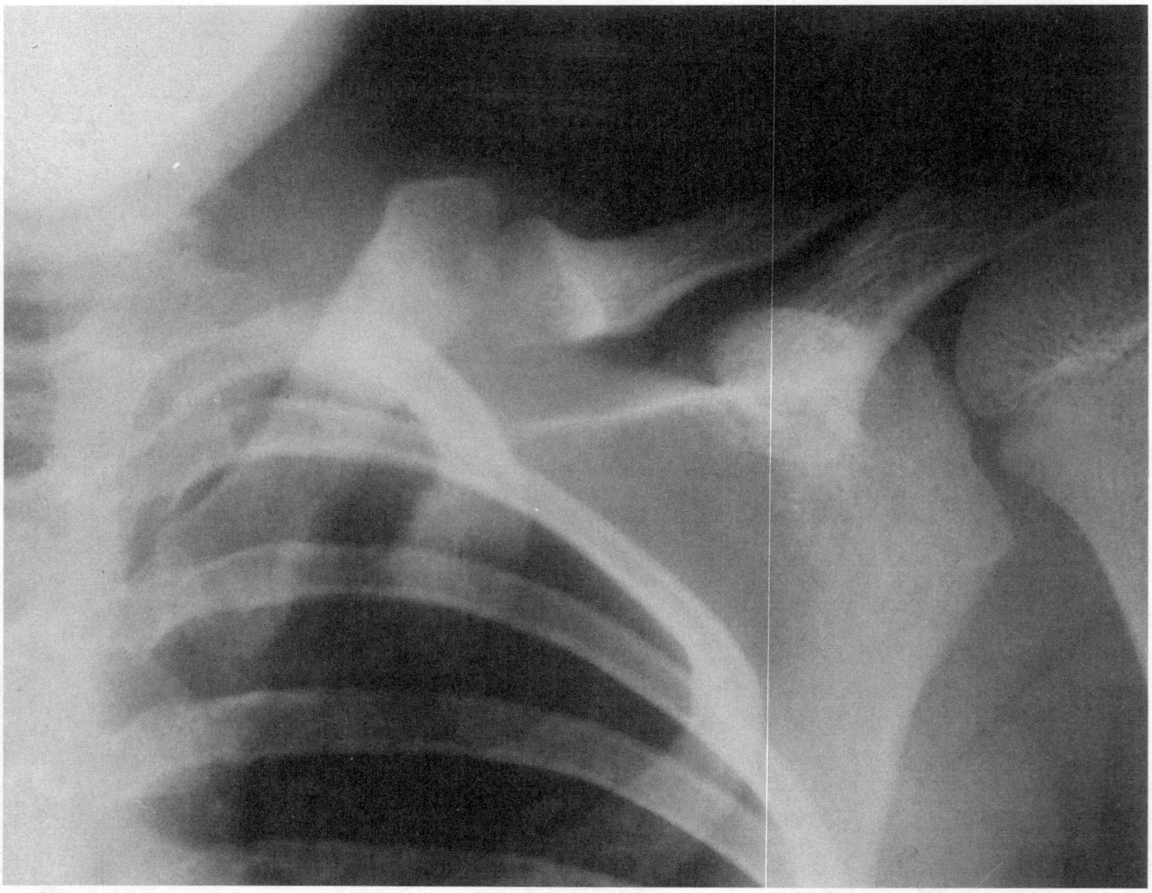

(A) observation
(B) application of a figure-of-eight bandage for 4 weeks
(C) open reduction and bone grafting
(D) open reduction, bone grafting, and internal fixation
(E) excision of the clavicle

---

282. A 2-year-old girl with spastic diplegia was evaluated for pes valgus that caused excessive medial shoe wear. Examination revealed normal passive range of motion of the subtalar joint but 20° of hindfoot valgus with weight-bearing. The most appropriate treatment is

(A) observation
(B) use of a custom molded shoe insert
(C) use of an ankle-foot orthosis
(D) transfer of the peroneal tendons
(E) a Grice procedure

283. The percentage of growth inhibition in a congenitally short femur

(A) increases during growth spurts
(B) remains constant
(C) decreases throughout growth
(D) increases throughout growth
(E) cannot be accurately predicted

284. Which of the following statements concerning congenital muscular torticollis is correct?

(A) The chin is rotated toward the side of the affected muscle
(B) The left side is involved in 75 percent of cases
(C) The torticollis may be caused by contracture of muscles other than the sternocleidomastoid
(D) Passive stretching, begun in infancy, is rarely a successful treatment
(E) Surgery is indicated if torticollis does not resolve after 3 months of passive stretching

285. Klippel-Feil syndrome results from

(A) congenital contracture of the sternocleidomastoid muscle
(B) failure of descent of the scapula
(C) failure of closure of the third branchial arch
(D) failure of segmentation of mesodermal somites
(E) arrested development of the cervical musculature

286. All the following statements regarding Sprengel's deformity are true EXCEPT that

(A) the affected scapula is abnormally high
(B) an omohyoid bone may be attached to the vertebral border of the affected scapula
(C) the affected scapula is usually smaller than the unaffected scapula
(D) the trapezius on the affected side is usually defective
(E) operative treatment is usually unnecessary

287. All the following are associated with an increased incidence of developmental dislocation of the hip (DDH) EXCEPT

(A) breech presentation
(B) polyhydramnios
(C) a parent who had developmental dislocation of the hip
(D) female sex
(E) birth in the winter months

288. A contraindication for use of a Pavlik harness in the treatment of developmental dislocation of the hip (DDH) is

(A) age over 6 months
(B) marked generalized ligamentous laxity
(C) asymmetric hip abduction
(D) a subluxatable hip
(E) a positive Ortolani sign

289. Which of the following statements regarding developmental coxa vara is correct?

(A) The incidence is greater in females
(B) Hip pain is usually present
(C) Bilateral involvement is usual
(D) The deformity corrects spontaneously with growth
(E) Epiphysiodesis of the greater trochanter is not recommended treatment

290. A newborn infant had a 60° hyperextension deformity of the knee. The knee could be flexed to 45°, and the neurovascular status of the limb was normal. A radiograph of the knee is shown in the figure. The most appropriate immediate management is

(A) application of a cylinder cast with the knee in 45° of flexion
(B) application of an above-knee cast with the knee in 45° of flexion
(C) application of skin traction with the infant supine
(D) application of skin traction with the infant prone
(E) dynamic splinting of the knee in a Pavlik harness

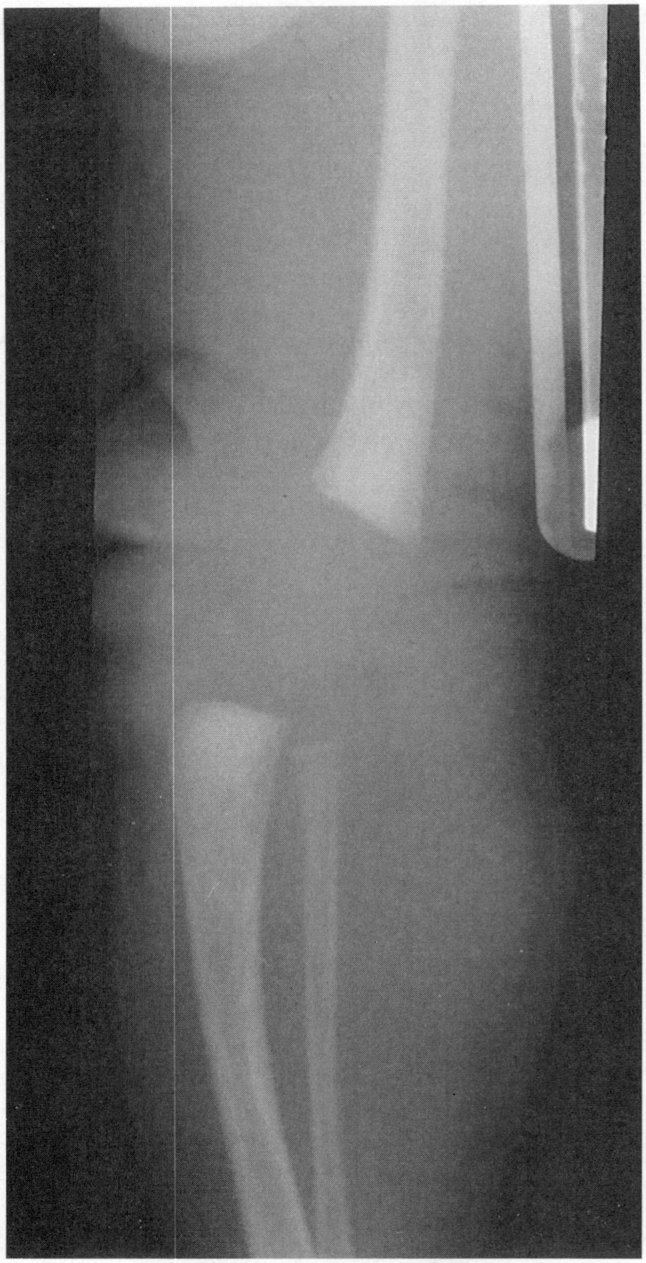

291. Which of the following statements regarding multiple epiphyseal dysplasia is correct?

(A) Inheritance is usually autosomal recessive
(B) The diagnosis is usually made in infancy
(C) Vertebral involvement is prominent
(D) Misdiagnosis as Legg-Calvé-Perthes disease is common
(E) Use of orthotic containment devices improves the outcome

292. The most common late sequela of achondroplasia is

(A) osteoarthritis
(B) hydrocephalus
(C) neurologic complications
(D) genu valgum
(E) pes planus

293. All the following are features of achondroplasia EXCEPT

(A) diminished trunk length
(B) brachycephaly
(C) exaggerated lumbar lordosis
(D) trident hand
(E) tibial bowing

294. The histologic changes in bone of hypophosphatasia most closely resemble those of

(A) osteogenesis imperfecta
(B) scurvy
(C) rickets
(D) juvenile osteoporosis
(E) achondroplasia

295. A treatment contraindicated for patients with hypophosphatasia is

(A) vitamin D
(B) calcium chelating agents
(C) enzyme replacement therapy
(D) renal dialysis
(E) osteotomy of the long bones

296. Spondyloepiphyseal dysplasia is associated with all the following EXCEPT

(A) atlantoaxial instability
(B) scoliosis
(C) coxa vara
(D) talipes equinovarus
(E) decreased lumbar lordosis

297. A 4-week-old, full-term infant had been irritable and had a swollen left shoulder for 48 h. The child was afebrile, the WBC normal, and the ESR 35 mm/h. Aspiration of the shoulder revealed cloudy, blood-tinged fluid. The organism most likely to be cultured from this fluid is

(A) group B streptococcus
(B) *Staphylococcus aureus*
(C) *Staphylococcus epidermidis*
(D) *Haemophilus influenzae*
(E) *Escherichia coli*

298. An otherwise healthy child who is suspected of having acute hematogenous osteomyelitis is allergic to penicillins and cephalosporins. The initial antibiotic administered should be

(A) ciprofloxacin
(B) gentamicin
(C) tobramycin
(D) clindamycin
(E) erythromycin

299. Patients with sickle cell hemoglobinopathy are especially predisposed to osteomyelitis caused by

(A) *Haemophilus influenzae*
(B) salmonella species
(C) *Pseudomonas aeruginosa*
(D) *Escherichia coli*
(E) enterobacter species

300. In a 4-year-old with infantile tibia vara, radiographs demonstrated a stage III Langenskiold lesion and a tibiofemoral angle of 25° varus. The most appropriate treatment is

(A) observation
(B) application of an orthosis at night
(C) application of a full-time orthosis
(D) hemiepiphysiodesis
(E) tibial osteotomy

301. A 6-year-old girl had an asymptomatic in-toeing gait. Examination revealed 15° of in-toeing relative to the angle of limb progression bilaterally. Internal rotation of the hips in extension was 80°, external rotation 5°, and the thigh-foot angles were 20° external. Neurologic examination was normal. The optimal treatment is

(A) observation
(B) physical therapy
(C) application of a Denis Browne splint
(D) application of a twister cable brace
(E) femoral osteotomy

302. A 13-year-old boy with a skeletal maturity level of Risser grade 2 had the lateral radiograph of the thoracic spine shown below. He complained of back pain and cosmetic deformity. The most appropriate treatment is

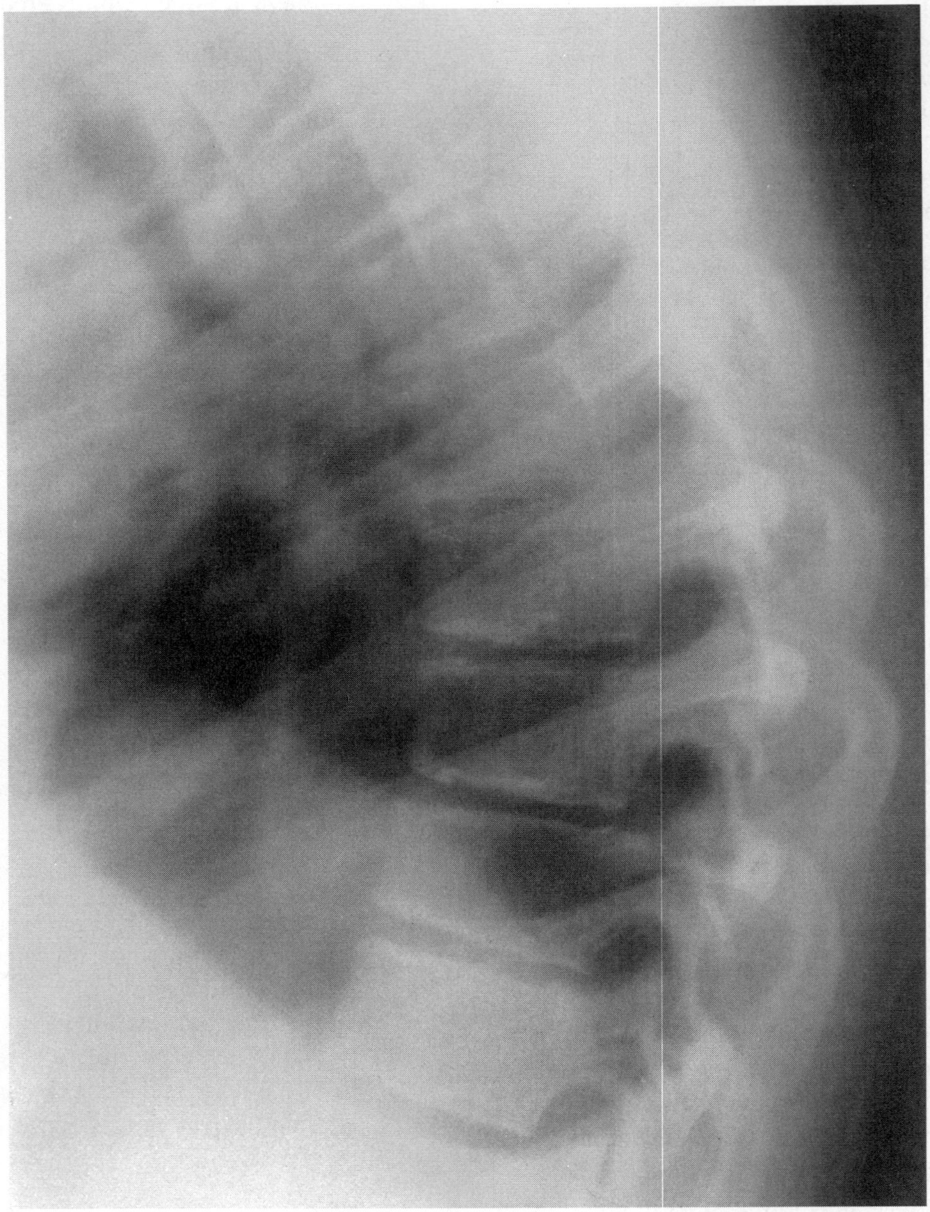

(A) observation
(B) physical therapy
(C) application of a Milwaukee brace
(D) posterior spinal fusion
(E) anterior and posterior spinal fusion

303. A 13-year-old boy was evaluated for increased difficulty running and frequent muscle cramps in his legs and feet. Examination revealed an unsteady gait, diminished vibratory sense and proprioception in both feet, symmetric muscular weakness and atrophy in the peroneal musculature, and bilateral cavovarus feet. The most likely diagnosis is

(A) Duchenne's muscular dystrophy
(B) Charcot-Marie-Tooth disease
(C) spinal muscular atrophy
(D) Friedreich's ataxia
(E) Guillain-Barré syndrome

304. The orthopaedic manifestations of Friedreich's ataxia are

(A) scoliosis and hip dislocations
(B) scoliosis and cavovarus foot deformities
(C) knee and hip flexion contractures and cavovarus foot deformities
(D) hip dislocations and cavovarus foot deformities
(E) hip dislocations and hip and knee flexion contractures

305. The most specific test for differentiating spinal muscular atrophy from muscular dystrophy is

(A) a serum creatine phosphokinase (CPK) level
(B) a serum aldolase level
(C) an electromyogram
(D) a muscle biopsy
(E) a nerve biopsy

306. The most important factor affecting the long-term ambulatory potential of a patient with a myelomeningocele is the

(A) age of the patient
(B) weight of the patient
(C) neurologic level of the lesion
(D) motor power of the muscles within the functioning neurologic levels
(E) extent and severity of musculoskeletal deformity

307. A 2-year-old child of normal intelligence was evaluated for short stature. Examination revealed scoliosis, limited motion of most joints, equinovarus feet, and bilateral hitchhiker's thumbs. The most likely diagnosis is

(A) multiple epiphyseal dysplasia
(B) achondroplasia
(C) diastrophic dwarfism
(D) Morquio's syndrome
(E) hypophosphatasia

308. An 18-month-old girl with a history of easy bruising complained of severe pain near her knee. Examination revealed multiple areas of ecchymosis, hemorrhagic gingivitis, and tenderness over the left distal femur. A radiograph is shown below. The most likely diagnosis is

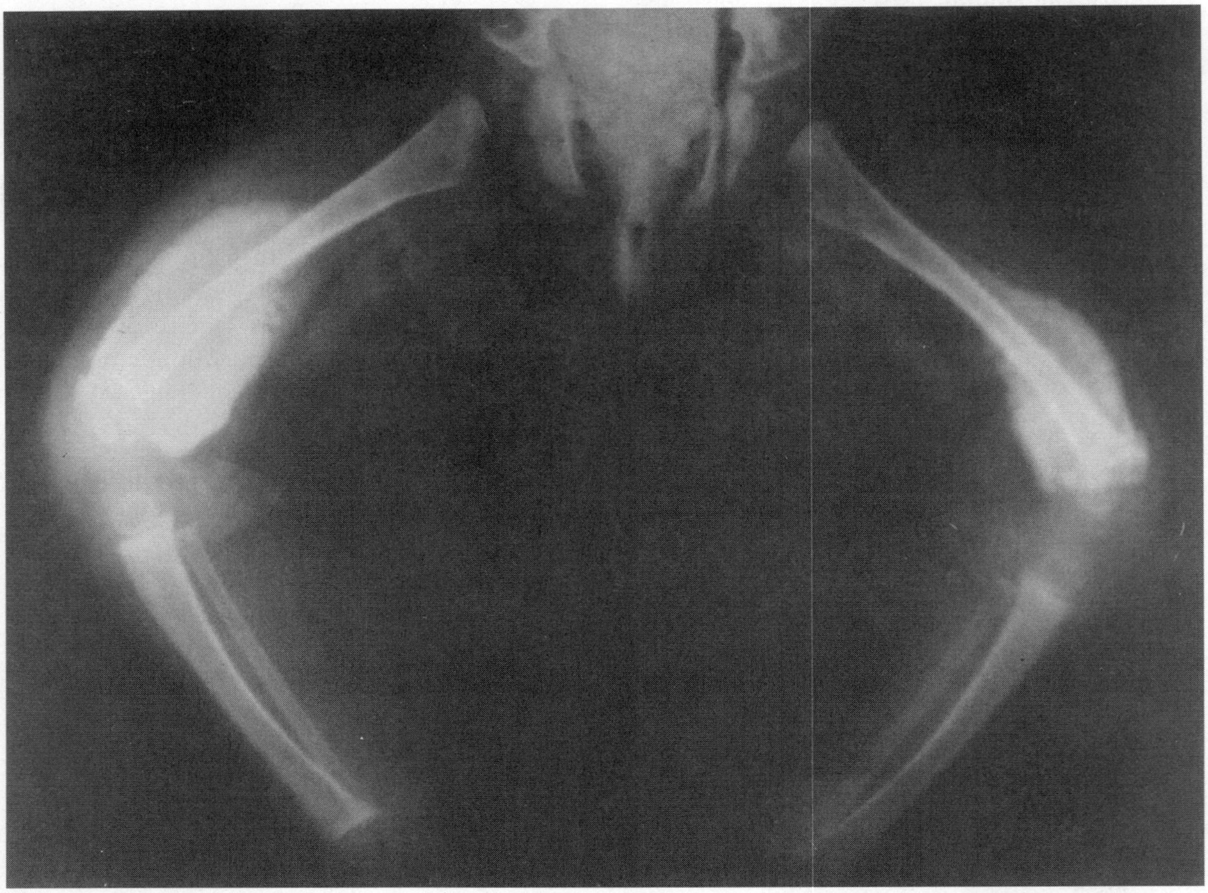

(A) osteomyelitis
(B) osteogenesis imperfecta
(C) scurvy
(D) rickets
(E) hypervitaminosis A

309. A 3-year-old girl was febrile and had refused to ambulate for 24 h. Her parents stated that she had had no recent infection or injury. Examination revealed warmth and erythema over the proximal tibia. Her temperature was 38°C (100.4°F), WBC 18,000/mm^3, and ESR 55 mm/h. Radiographs of the leg were normal. The next step in the management of this patient is

(A) a technetium-99 bone scan
(B) a CT scan
(C) a gallium scan
(D) aspiration of the proximal tibia
(E) incision and debridement of the proximal tibia

310. A 4-year-old boy with a 2-week history of malaise and back pain had refused to stand or sit for the last 24 h but was comfortable in the supine position. Examination revealed a temperature of 37.8°C (100°F), tenderness over the lumbar spine, decreased lumbar lordosis, and straight leg raising limited to 30°. Neurologic examination was within normal limits. Laboratory studies revealed a WBC of 11,000/mm^3 and an ESR of 60 mm/h. Blood cultures were negative, radiographs of the spine were normal, but a technetium-99 bone scan showed moderately increased uptake over the region of the L3 and L4 vertebrae. The most likely diagnosis is

(A) tuberculous spondylitis
(B) acute pyogenic spondylitis
(C) traumatic spondylitis
(D) discitis
(E) viral meningitis

311. A 9-year-old boy had increasing foot pain for 3 days after stepping on a nail while wearing tennis shoes. Examination revealed plantar and dorsal inflammation and tenderness of the foot, dorsal erythema, and a healed puncture wound on the sole of the foot. Laboratory studies revealed a normal WBC, and radiographs were normal. The most appropriate treatment is

(A) strict elevation; administration of oral antibiotics
(B) debridement in the emergency department; administration of oral antibiotics
(C) administration of intravenous antibiotics in the emergency department; discharge on oral antibiotics
(D) hospitalization for strict elevation; administration of intravenous antibiotics
(E) operative incision and debridement; administration of intravenous antibiotics

312. The direction of bowing most commonly associated with pseudarthrosis of the tibia is

(A) anteromedial
(B) anterolateral
(C) posteromedial
(D) posterolateral
(E) posterior

313. All the following may be seen in association with neurofibromatosis EXCEPT

(A) fibromolluscum
(B) elephantiasis
(C) focal gigantism
(D) subperiosteal bone proliferation
(E) scoliosis

314. Which of the following congenital malformations of the spine is most likely to result in progression of deformity?

(A) Klippel-Feil syndrome
(B) Fused ribs
(C) A hemivertebra
(D) A unilateral bony bar
(E) Block vertebrae

315. A 12-year-old boy had a left thoracic scoliosis caused by an unsegmented bar between T5 and T7. Over the last year, his spinal curvature increased from 35° to 45°. The most appropriate treatment is

(A) observation until spinal growth is complete
(B) electrical stimulation
(C) a thoracolumbosacral orthosis
(D) posterior spinal fusion in situ
(E) osteotomy of the bar and spinal fusion

316. Which of the following lesions has the lowest incidence of sarcomatous transformation?

(A) Solitary osteochondroma
(B) Solitary enchondroma
(C) Multiple osteochondromatosis
(D) Multiple enchondromatosis
(E) Maffucci's syndrome

317. The fundamental defect in osteogenesis imperfecta is

(A) decreased osteoblastic activity
(B) failure of mineralization of osteoid
(C) failure of maturation of collagen fibers
(D) decreased osteoclastic activity
(E) a defect in intramembranous bone formation

318. The most common mode of inheritance of Ehlers-Danlos syndrome is

(A) autosomal dominant
(B) autosomal recessive
(C) sex-linked recessive
(D) autosomal dominant with variable penetrance
(E) autosomal recessive with variable penetrance

319. A 4-year-old boy of normal intelligence was short for his age. Examination revealed splenomegaly and diffuse lymphadenopathy. A CBC showed anemia, leukocytopenia, and thrombocytopenia. A radiograph of the distal femurs is shown. The most likely diagnosis is

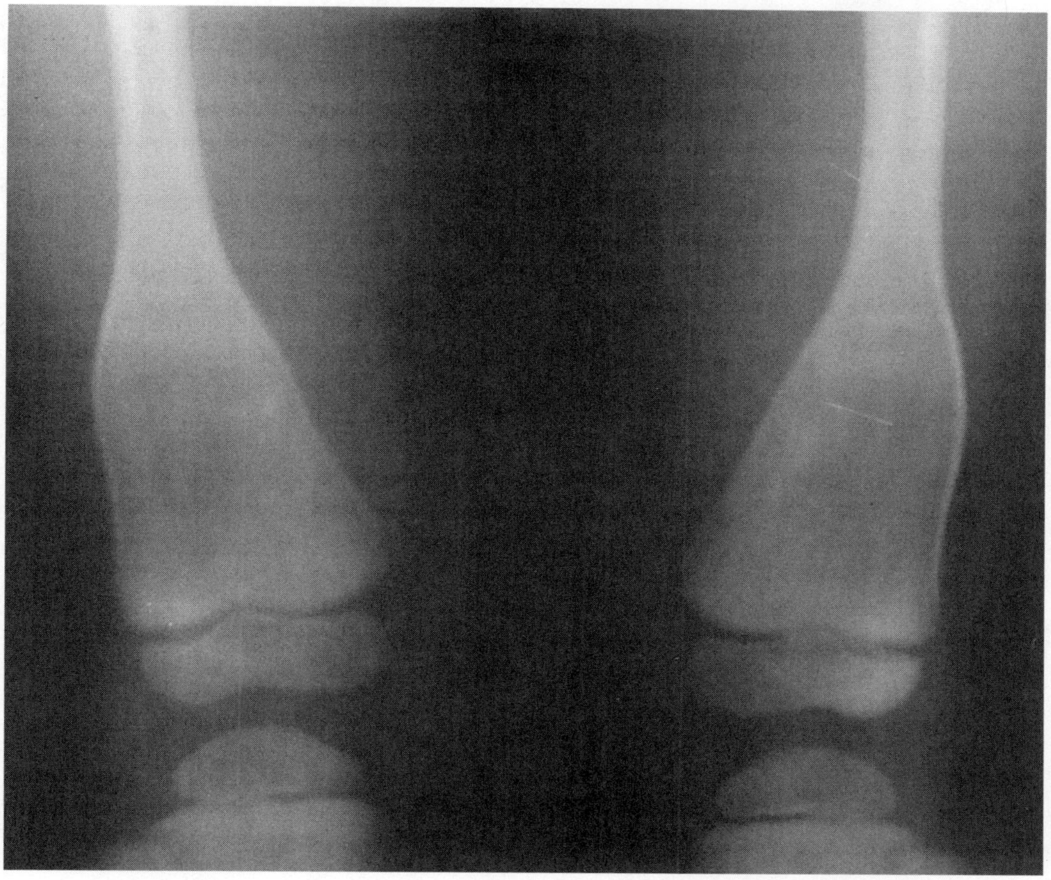

(A) homocystinuria
(B) vitamin D–resistant rickets
(C) Gaucher's disease
(D) scurvy
(E) Niemann-Pick disease

320. The most common osseous lesions in the leukemias of early childhood are

(A) osteolytic lesions in the metaphyseal-diaphyseal areas of long bones
(B) osteolytic and osteoblastic lesions in the centra of the vertebrae
(C) osteoblastic lesions in the diaphyses of short tubular bones
(D) osteoblastic lesions in the skull
(E) premature closure of cranial sutures and epiphyses

321. Appropriate initial treatment of a child with severe factor VIII hemophilia and high titer inhibitor who has an acute hemarthrosis of the knee is

(A) administration of heat-treated factor VIII concentrate, aspiration, and splinting of the knee in maximum extension
(B) administration of fresh-frozen plasma, aspiration, and casting of the knee in 25° of flexion
(C) administration of desmopressin (DDAVP) and splinting of the knee in maximum extension
(D) splinting of the knee in the position of comfort and observation
(E) administration of heat-treated cryoprecipitate, aspiration, and splinting in maximum extension

322. An 18-year-old with severe classic hemophilia, no inhibitor, and a history of recurrent hemarthroses and pain in the left elbow has 20° to 100° of motion in that joint. Radiographs are shown below. The most appropriate treatment is

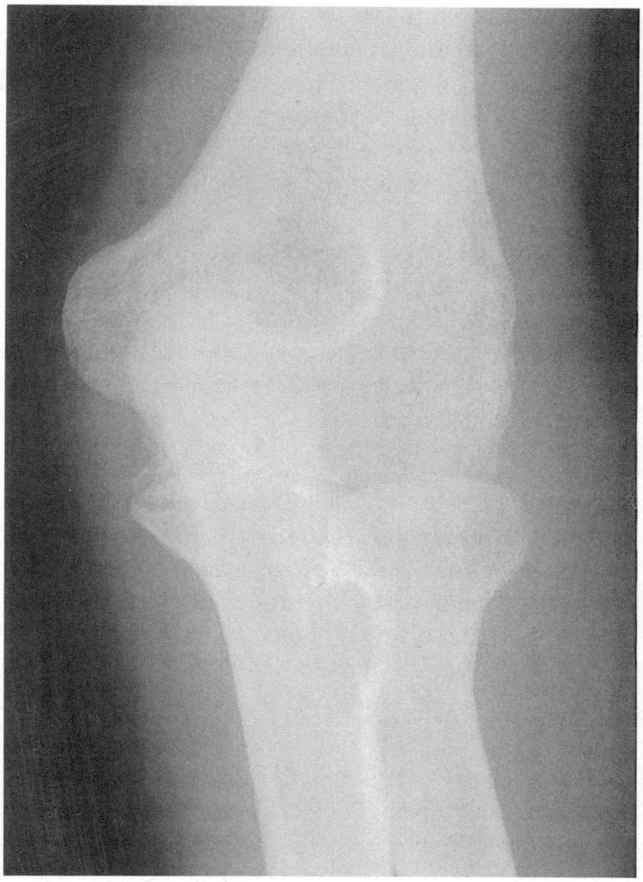

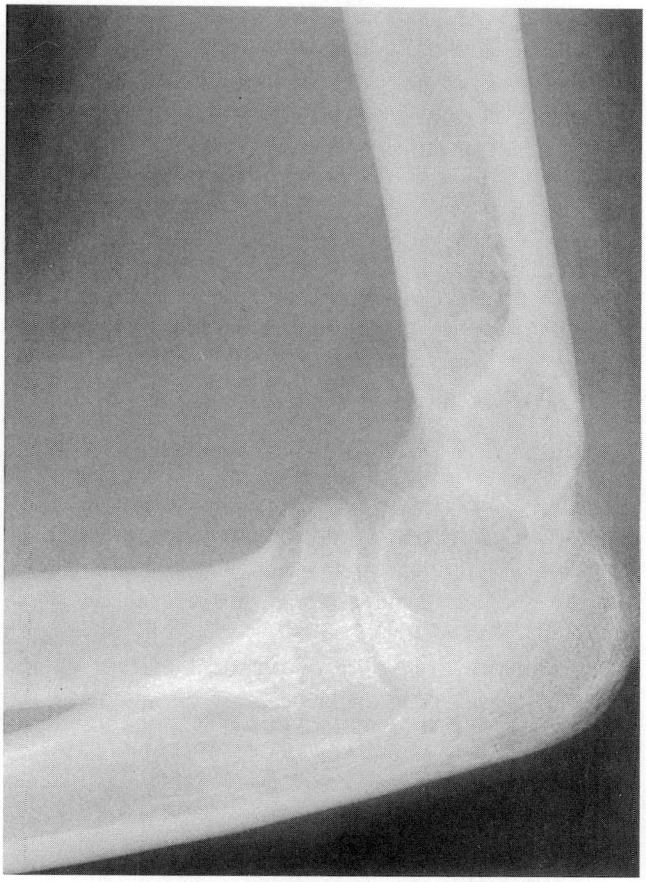

(A) home treatment with factor VIII at the earliest sign of an elbow bleed
(B) application of a hinged elbow brace
(C) synoviorthesis (chemical synovectomy)
(D) surgical synovectomy with excision of the radial head
(E) total elbow replacement

323. The single most frequent finding in patients infected with human immunodeficiency virus (HIV) is

(A) lymphadenopathy
(B) Kaposi's sarcoma
(C) *Pneumocystis carinii* pneumonia
(D) thrombocytopenia
(E) psoriatic arthritis

324. A child with cerebral palsy and spastic equinus will be unable to walk on tip-toe following lengthening of the Achilles tendon owing to

(A) a decrease in the cross-sectional diameter of the calf muscle
(B) an increase in the cross-sectional diameter of the calf muscle
(C) a reduction in the excursion of the calf muscle
(D) damage to proprioceptive receptors in the tendon
(E) loss of the stretch reflex

325. The primary value of physical therapy in the young child with spastic cerebral palsy is

(A) to enhance walking
(B) to improve grasp
(C) to prevent contracture
(D) to improve sitting balance
(E) unknown

326. Improved ambulation in a 3-year-old child with cerebral palsy and a mild, fixed, spastic equinus deformity is best achieved by

(A) inhibitive casting
(B) corrective casting
(C) double upright, below-knee bracing
(D) biofeedback
(E) electrical stimulation

327. The most important principle to observe when lengthening a tendon in a spastic child is to

(A) release the tendon completely
(B) perform the lengthening at the musculotendinous junction
(C) lengthen the tendon so that full passive motion of the joint places no tension on the muscle repair
(D) immobilize the lengthened muscle under tension
(E) begin passive stretching of the lengthened muscle as soon as the incision has healed

328. Which of the following clinical pictures is most compatible with juvenile pauciarticular rheumatoid arthritis?

(A) Age 3, female, involvement of hips and knees, normal ESR, no fevers, negative rheumatoid factor
(B) Age 1, male, involvement of feet, hands, and wrists, slight elevation of ESR, low-grade fevers, negative rheumatoid factor
(C) Age 13, female, involvement of hips and hands, moderate elevation of ESR, high fevers, rash, positive rheumatoid factor
(D) Age 10, male, involvement of the knees, normal ESR, no fevers, negative rheumatoid factor
(E) Age 4, female, involvement of hands and feet, slight elevation of ESR, positive rheumatoid factor

329. The earliest radiographic findings in ankylosing spondylitis are

(A) marginal erosions of the apophyseal joints
(B) narrowing of the apophyseal joints
(C) flattening of the cervical lordosis
(D) symmetric narrowing of the sacroiliac joints
(E) subchondral erosions of the sacroiliac joints

330. The etiology of juvenile chronic arthritis (JCA) is

(A) unknown
(B) genetic
(C) postinfectious
(D) an autoimmune response
(E) vasculitic

331. The most predictable benefit from synovectomy in patients with JRA is

(A) increased motion
(B) reduction of pain and swelling
(C) slowing of radiographic progression
(D) decreased stimulation of adjacent physes
(E) prevention of recurrent episodes of acute synovitis

332. The earliest manifestation of involvement of the cervical spine in polyarticular JRA is usually

(A) neck pain
(B) torticollis
(C) stiffness
(D) brachial hypesthesia
(E) weakness in elbow flexion

333. Isolated congenital talipes equinovarus is most likely to be the result of

(A) maternal trauma in the first trimester
(B) maternal ingestion of an abortifacient in the first trimester
(C) Mendelian inheritance
(D) a cytogenetic abnormality
(E) multifactorial inheritance

334. The most useful radiographic technique for assessment of the severity and response to treatment of congenital talipes equinovarus in an infant is

(A) arthrography
(B) computerized tomography
(C) magnetic resonance imaging
(D) measurement of the talocalcaneal angles in standard AP and lateral radiographs
(E) measurement of the talar–first metatarsal angle on standard AP and lateral radiographs

335. Following 6 months of manipulation and casting, an infant with talipes equinovarus has residual, fixed equinus and approximation of the navicular to the medial malleolus. The midfoot is supple, but there is posterior displacement of the fibular malleolus. Preferred treatment is

(A) continued manipulation and casting
(B) use of a Denis Browne splint 23 h per day
(C) use of a hinged ankle-foot orthosis
(D) medial and posterior release
(E) posterior, plantar, and lateral release

336. The most likely cause of persistent or increasing cavus deformity following surgery for congenital talipes equinovarus is

(A) failure to correct dorsal subluxation of the talonavicular joint
(B) incomplete medial release
(C) failure to correct forefoot supination
(D) failure to include release of tight plantar structures
(E) excessive medial scarring following initial surgery

337. Preferred treatment of a 13-year-old, otherwise healthy boy with an untreated congenital vertical talus is

(A) open reduction of the talonavicular and talocalcaneal joints
(B) open reduction of the talonavicular and talocalcaneal joints, followed in 6 weeks by talocalcaneal fusion
(C) talocalcaneal and calcaneocuboid releases, followed in 3 weeks by lengthening of the Achilles tendon and posterior capsulotomy of the ankle
(D) serial manipulation and casting for 3 months, followed by open reduction of the talonavicular joint if necessary
(E) triple arthrodesis

338. The pathognomonic clinical feature of congenital vertical talus is

(A) contracture of the Achilles tendon
(B) contracture of the extensor digitorum longus tendons
(C) hypoplasia of the talus
(D) plantar flexion of the talus and calcaneus
(E) fixed dorsal dislocation of the talonavicular joint

339. Which of the following best describes the bony changes in congenital talipes equinovarus?

(A) Talus: medial rotation in the ankle mortise
Calcaneus: lateral rotation
Cuboid: medial displacement in relation to the long axis of the calcaneus

(B) Talus: medial rotation in the ankle mortise
Calcaneus: medial rotation
Cuboid: medial displacement in relation to the long axis of the calcaneus

(C) Talus: lateral rotation in the ankle mortise
Calcaneus: medial rotation
Cuboid: lateral displacement in relation to the long axis of the calcaneus

(D) Talus: lateral rotation in the ankle mortise
Calcaneus: lateral rotation
Cuboid: lateral displacement in relation to the long axis of the calcaneus

(E) Talus: medial rotation in the ankle mortise
Calcaneus: medial rotation
Cuboid: lateral displacement in relation to the long axis of the calcaneus

340. The effect of JCA on limb length (overgrowth or shortening) is related primarily to the

(A) involvement of the hip joints
(B) presence or absence of systemic manifestations
(C) presence or absence of rheumatoid factor in the serum
(D) age of onset
(E) gender of the patient

341. The indications for calcaneocuboid fusion in surgery for talipes equinovarus are

(A) age over 3 years; residual varus; short medial and long lateral columns of the foot
(B) age over 6 years; residual varus; equal length of the medial and lateral columns of the foot
(C) age over 3 years; residual supination and adduction of the forefoot
(D) age over 6 years; failed lateral release; medially curved outer border of the foot
(E) age over 1 year; hindfoot valgus resulting from overcorrection during initial surgery

Pediatric Disorders

Answers

240. The answer is D. *(Barrow, Am J Sports Med 16:209–216, 1988.)* Stress fractures are frequently associated with menstrual irregularity in female distance runners. Female runners who use birth control pills for more than 1 year have a lower rate of stress fractures than runners who do not use birth control pills. Poorly cushioned shoes, increased road running, and eating disorders have all been implicated as potential causes of stress fractures.

241. The answer is C. *(Tachdjian, pp 829–833.)* Marfan's syndrome is an autosomal dominant condition leading to the production of abnormal connective tissue, which causes abnormalities in a variety of organ systems, including the eye, heart, skeleton, and skin. The spectrum of cardiac disease in Marfan's syndrome ranges from minimal to lethal. These patients are at risk for arrhythmia and should undergo cardiac evaluation prior to participation in athletic activities.

242. The answer is D. *(Yates, Orthopaedics 9:663, 1986.)* For a patient with anterior knee pain, a relatively normal examination, and normal radiographs, the initial treatment should be conservative. Pain will resolve in 75 percent of patients treated with isometric exercises and anti-inflammatory medications; further diagnostic work-up is unnecessary unless this regimen fails. Active knee extension exercises, even if isokinetic, may aggravate retropatellar pain.

243. The answer is D. *(Poss, p 416.)* Symptoms caused by spondylolysis will frequently resolve with limitation of activity, making bed rest and cessation of athletic activities unnecessary. Bracing or surgical treatment may be needed if symptoms persist in spite of modifications in activity, but are not appropriate initial treatment modalities.

244. The answer is C. *(Hershman, Am J Sports Med 17:655–659, 1989.)* Acute brachial neuropathy appears sporadically, occurs spontaneously, usually involves multiple nerves, and is of unknown etiology, although it occasionally follows immunization or viral illness. The distribution of weakness is variable, but motor findings are predominant, with sensory findings usually limited to hypesthesias over the lateral shoulder. Since more than one root or nerve is involved here, none of the other choices is correct.

245. The answer is C. *(Poss, p 567.)* Normal resting compartmental pressure is 0 to 4 mmHg. A postexercise compartmental pressure of 40 mmHg or higher is diagnostic of an exertional compartmental syndrome, while a postexercise reading of 35 mmHg is highly indicative of a compartmental syndrome. Emergency fasciotomy is rarely necessary for exertional compartmental syndromes.

246. The answer is A. *(Morrissy, pp 741–750.)* In addition to knee pathology, slipped capital femoral epiphysis must be considered in this patient. A careful examination of the hip is vital to the initial evaluation of the adolescent with knee pain and should precede radiographs, MRI scans, or joint aspiration.

247. The answer is C. *(Kuland, p 43.)* Mononucleosis results in an enlarged spleen surrounded by a weakened capsule. An increased risk of splenic rupture following trauma is present for approximately 6 months, which often extends beyond the time when clinical, hematologic, and serologic signs have returned to normal.

248. The answer is D. *(Allison, p 530.)* Heat cramps are caused by excessive fluid loss and electrolyte imbalance in muscle. They are often preceded by profuse sweating and occur most frequently when an athlete is not acclimated to a hot, humid climate. They are best treated with passive stretching, cooling, and rapid replacement of fluids and electrolytes.

249. The answer is B. *(Henry, Am J Sports Med 14:221, 1986.)* Most patients with patellofemoral syndrome can be treated successfully with a program of stretching, strengthening of the vastus medialis obliquus, and modification of activity. Casting or bracing is generally ineffective. Initial nonoperative management is indicated even in the presence of mild lateral subluxation on the sunrise view of the knee. Surgical management is indicated only if nonoperative treatment fails.

250. The answer is D. *(Shapiro, J Bone Joint Surg 75-A:439–454, 1993.)* The sex-linked recessive muscular dystrophies include the Duchenne and Becker types. The autosomal recessive forms include limb-girdle and childhood muscular dystrophies. The facioscapulohumeral type of muscular dystrophy is characterized by an autosomal dominant pattern of inheritance.

251. The answer is B. *(Poss, p 379.)* Atlantoaxial instability is common in patients with Down's syndrome and is often manifest by frequent falls or ankle sprains. These children should be screened with lateral flexion/extension radiographs of the cervical spine. Minimal to moderate instability is usually managed with a cervical orthosis and avoidance of contact sports. Marked instability with progressive neurologic signs or symptoms may warrant surgical stabilization.

252. The answer is B. *(Oppenheim, Clin Orthop 253:20–29, 1990.)* When spasticity is alleviated by lumbar selective posterior rhizotomy, the resulting limb weakness may cause valgus foot deformities, which are best treated by bracing. Strength in the limb will return within 1 year of posterior rhizotomy, so further surgery should be deferred for at least 1 year after rhizotomy.

253. The answer is A. *(Morrissy, pp 576–577.)* Congenital dislocation of the radial head usually causes minimal loss of motion but no pain. Radiographs reveal a hypoplastic capitellum and a dome-shaped radial head. Treatment is directed at increasing motion and improving cosmetic appearance. Because this patient is asymptomatic and functions well, observation is the most appropriate treatment. Excision of the radial head is contraindicated in the skeletally immature patient.

254. The answer is D. *(Morrissy, p 517.)* The scoliosis in this patient is above the level of paralysis and above the spina bifida, making paralytic scoliosis an unlikely diagnosis. Both hydromyelia and tethered cord may cause scoliosis, but scoliosis secondary to hydromyelia is rare with a functioning ventriculoperitoneal shunt. Symptoms of a tethered spinal cord include increased lumbar lordosis, back and buttock pain, and spasticity in the sacral nerve roots.

255. The answer is D. *(Mann, Instr Course Lect 39:3–13, 1990.)* A 36 percent failure rate was reported in a series of adolescents who had surgical correction of hallux valgus, with the recurrence rate increasing to 56 percent for adolescents with flexible pes planus. Regardless of the surgical procedure used for correction of hallux valgus, the longitudinal arch of the foot will not be restored.

256. The answer is C. *(Morrissy, pp 831–833.)* Treatment of patients with Legg-Calvé-Perthes disease should begin in the initial or fragmentation stage of the disease. Restoration of motion in the hip is the earliest and most important aspect of treatment. After motion in the hip is restored, the next step is obtaining and maintaining containment of the femoral head within the acetabulum by bracing or surgery.

257. The answer is C. *(Tachdjian, pp 1821–1824.)* Although unlikely to walk as adults, children with myelomeningoceles who walk and stand are more independent as adults than those who do not walk or stand as children. Releasing hip flexion contractures and placing the child into the standing position during preschool and early school-age years are recommended. Reduction of the dislocated hip is not necessary for standing, and attempts at reduction usually fail. Transfer of the iliopsoas in a patient with this level of paraplegia is not recommended.

258. The answer is D. *(Dirschl, Orthop Rev 23:305–312, 1994.)* Approximately 50 percent of children with septic arthritis have infection elsewhere. The erythrocyte sedimentation rate is a useful, but nonspecific test; only demonstration of organisms by Gram stain and culture is diagnostic of infection. It is imperative that material from aspiration of the involved joint be obtained. Positive bone scans are not diagnostically specific for acute septic arthritis.

259. The answer is B. *(Dirschl, Orthop Rev 23:305–312, 1994.)* In children 1 month to 3 years of age, the predominant cause of hematogenous septic arthritis is *Haemophilus influenzae*, followed by staphylococci and streptococci. However, initial antibiotic treatment should cover all three of these pathogens.

260. The answer is D. *(Tachdjian, pp 2871–2876.)* With three or more points to plot, the Moseley straight-line graph method is highly accurate for estimating inequality of leg length. For this patient, the projected discrepancy at maturity is 8.5 cm.

261. The answer is C. *(Tachdjian, pp 2871–2876.)* From the Moseley graph, distal femoral and proximal tibial epiphysiodeses would be required immediately in this 12-year-old patient to obtain equality of leg length at maturity. The estimated inequality of leg length at maturity is 3.5 cm; leg lengthening is not indicated for discrepancies of less than 5 cm at maturity.

262. The answer is D. *(Phillips, J Bone Joint Surg 71-A:664–668, 1989.)* Since the atlantoaxial rotary subluxation has been present for 3 weeks, successful treatment entails more than a cervical collar. Cervical traction, anti-inflammatory medications, and muscle relaxants will usually reduce the subluxation. Cervical fusion is reserved for patients refractory to traction.

263. The answer is B. *(Coleman, Clin Orthop 123:60–68, 1977.)* The standing lateral block test is used to evaluate hindfoot flexibility. It is performed by placing the heel and lateral border of the patient's foot on a wooden block 2 to 4 cm thick, while the medial border of the foot is allowed to hang freely. This test negates any effect the forefoot may have on the hindfoot in stance. If the heel varus corrects with the patient standing on the block, the hindfoot is considered flexible.

264. The answer is A. *(Morrissy, pp 2761–2763.)* Osteochondritis dissecans is most common in the knee, particularly in the posterolateral aspect of the medial femoral condyle. Nonsurgical management is effective in children under 10 years of age since the lesion will usually heal spontaneously if it has not become completely detached. Studies showing the importance of joint motion in the healing of cartilage have led to the recommendation of limited activity rather than immobilization in a cylinder cast.

265. The answer is A. *(Lonstein, J Bone Joint Surg 66-A:1061–1071, 1984.)* A patient who is 16 months post menarche and whose iliac apophyses are nearly fused (Risser III) has nearly reached skeletal maturity. The probability that the scoliosis will progress is less than 20 percent. It is unlikely that treatment will be necessary, but further observation is prudent.

266. The answer is C. *(Tachdjian, pp 1062–1073.)* Although chondrolysis and late degenerative joint disease occur following treatment of acute slipped capital femoral epiphyses, aseptic necrosis is the most common complication. Overgrowth of the greater trochanter and coxa magna are rare outcomes of this condition.

267. The answer is B. *(Lonstein, J Bone Joint Surg, 66-A:1061–1071, 1984.)* The probability of progression of this spinal deformity in this premenarchal child with skeletal maturity of Risser 0 is approximately 70 percent. The patient should be observed and reevaluated in 4 to 6 months. Earlier follow-up might yield a result for curve progression that would still be within the error of measurement. If reevaluation were delayed for 1 year, the curve might have progressed too far for bracing to be effective.

268. The answer is D. *(Gonzales, J Bone Joint Surg 72-A:71–79, 1990.)* All tarsal coalitions—osseous, cartilaginous, or fibrous—cause progressive restriction of motion in the subtalar joint, leading to lateral ligamentous laxity and pain. When nonoperative treatment of a calcaneonavicular coalition has failed, resection of the coalition is indicated, provided there are no degenerative changes in the other tarsal joints. Triple arthrodesis is reserved for patients with extensive degenerative changes.

269. The answer is A. *(Tachdjian, pp 1026–1028.)* The patient has a typical history and physical findings for slipped capital femoral epiphysis. Although the AP radiograph of the pelvis shows no abnormality, a true lateral radiograph of the hip is often necessary to make the diagnosis. A frog-leg lateral should be avoided because placing the hip in this position can increase the displacement. Although tomography and CT scanning will show the slipped capital femoral epiphysis, these tests are expensive and are usually not necessary for diagnosis.

270. The answer is E. *(Tachdjian, pp 1665–1680.)* Cerebral palsy is a static neurologic lesion, so progression does not occur. Increased body mass makes walking more difficult but does not usually increase deformities. Nor has postoperative bracing been clearly related to an increasingly crouched gait. Overlengthening of the Achilles tendon allows increased dorsiflexion of the ankle during gait, which must be compensated for by more flexion of the knee and hip to maintain balance.

271. The answer is A. *(Tachdjian, pp 2728–2734.)* There is no indication for operative treatment of an asymptomatic, flexible flatfoot. A custom molded orthosis may relieve symptoms in a patient with a *painful* flexible flatfoot. Surgical treatment is reserved for the rare patient who has continued pain despite an adequate period of nonoperative treatment.

272. The answer is A. *(Tachdjian, pp 1582–1593.)* Popliteal cysts are common in children, occur more frequently in boys than in girls, and are usually found on the medial aspect of the popliteal fossa. In children, the cysts are rarely associated with intraarticular pathology. The cyst is likely to disappear spontaneously in 10 to 20 months, so a prolonged period of observation is recommended prior to considering surgical excision.

273. The answer is E. *(Morrissy, pp 724–725.)* Atlantoaxial instability occurs in up to 20 percent of children with Down's syndrome. Since only a small percentage have neurologic symptoms, it is important to perform lateral flexion/extension radiographs of the cervical spine in those children who may participate in athletics or undergo general anesthesia. At atlas-dens interval of 5 mm or less is considered normal. Down's syndrome is not characteristically associated with cardiac abnormalities.

274. The answer is D. *(Oppenheim, Clin Orthop 253:20–29, 1990.)* Selective posterior rhizotomy is a procedure in which certain posterior nerve roots are divided within the dural sac. This procedure decreases muscle spasticity, whereas soft tissue releases relieve joint contractures. Published studies support clinical improvement in children undergoing posterior rhizotomy.

275. The answer is C. *(Tachdjian, pp 2850–2852.)* Wilms' tumor of the kidney is associated with hemihypertrophy in a significant percentage of cases and can be easily diagnosed by abdominal ultrasonography. This study should be performed initially and yearly during growth.

276. The answer is A. *(Poss, p 551.)* A 15½-year-old boy has essentially reached skeletal maturity, and an inequality of 2.0 to 2.5 cm in leg length will not interfere with athletic activities. There is no evidence to support the claim that inequalities of limb length of this magnitude cause arthritis of the spine or lower extremities. Therefore, nonoperative management is indicated. A heel lift will level the pelvis and may decrease the slight limp that can result from this amount of inequality.

277. The answer is E. *(Baker, J Bone Joint Surg 65-B:472–473, 1983.)* This patient has had rapid development of a spinal deformity, and an underlying cause must be identified. A syrinx (cystic cavity) within the spinal cord leads to progressive myopathy and scoliosis in 25 to 80 percent of patients. Syringomyelia, with or without the Chiari malformation, should be suspected in any child with the sudden onset or rapid progression of scoliosis. An MRI scan is the preferred imaging modality.

278. The answer is D. *(Poss, pp 252–253.)* Since a closed reduction is seldom achievable, unilateral hip dislocation in a patient with arthrogryposis is best managed by open reduction. To avoid excess pressure across the hip joint, as well as to correct proximal femoral malalignment, femoral shortening is often required. Innominate osteotomy increases pressure between the articular surfaces of the proximal femur and acetabulum.

279. The answer is A. *(Pappas, Pediatr Orthop 4:525–531, 1984.)* Posteromedial bowing of the tibia is not associated with other musculoskeletal conditions and is not likely to result in fracture or pseudarthrosis. The posterior bowing eventually corrects, while the medial bowing may persist. In the older child, osteotomy is occasionally necessary to correct residual medial bowing. Orthotics are unnecessary.

280. The answer is A. *(Samuelsson, J Pediatr Orthop 8:569–575, 1988.)* With only grade 2/5 quadriceps strength, the patient's neurologic level is high lumbar, and she will be a nonambulator. In nonambulatory patients with a myelomeningocele and bilateral hip instability, no treatment is advised. If this patient had ambulatory potential, bilateral hip reconstruction would be considered.

281. The answer is A. *(Tachdjian, pp 168–174.)* Since there is no radiographic healing of the clavicle at 18 months of age, the lesion is probably a congenital pseudarthrosis of the clavicle, rather than a birth fracture. Such lesions rarely cause symptoms, so observation is the recommended treatment. If the cosmetic deformity is significant, excision of the pseudarthrosis, bone grafting, and internal fixation yields excellent results.

282. The answer is A. *(Tachdjian, pp 1692–1693.)* Up to 64 percent of children with spastic diplegia have pes valgus. This deformity is flexible until adolescence and generally decreases with growth. Surgical treatment is best delayed until at least 7 years of age, when mature gait parameters emerge. An ankle-foot orthosis is not an inappropriate treatment at any time, but it is desirable to keep these children brace-free as long as possible.

283. The answer is B. *(Tachdjian, pp 582–583.)* The percentage of growth inhibition remains constant throughout development in patients with congenitally short femurs. For example, if the affected femur is 25 percent shorter than the normal femur at birth, it will be 25 percent shorter at maturity. Predictions such as this may be helpful in surgical planning.

284. The answer is C. *(Tachdjian, pp 112–117.)* Congenital muscular torticollis, though nearly always caused by contracture of the sternocleidomastoid, may also be caused by contracture of the omohyoid or scalenus anterior. The right side is involved in 75 percent of cases, and the head is tilted toward the affected side while the chin is rotated away from the affected side. Passive stretching, begun in infancy, is successful in up to 86 percent of cases. Surgery is reserved for patients whose contracture persists beyond 1 year of age.

285. The answer is D. *(Tachdjian, pp 128–133.)* Klippel-Feil syndrome, congenital fusion of two or more cervical vertebrae, results from failure of normal segmentation of mesodermal somites during the 3rd to 8th weeks of fetal life. The exact cause of this failure of segmentation is still unknown. Although torticollis, Sprengel's deformity, and scoliosis often accompany Klippel-Feil syndrome, they do not cause it.

286. The answer is B. *(Tachdjian, pp 136–145.)* The affected scapula in Sprengel's deformity is abnormally high, is usually smaller than the unaffected scapula, and often has an *omovertebral* bone attached to its vertebral border. The shoulder musculature, most often the trapezius, is usually defective. Except in the most severe cases, function is minimally affected and surgical treatment is usually unnecessary. The omohyoid muscle is located in the anterior triangle of the neck.

287. The answer is B. *(Tachdjian, pp 302–306.)* Although the exact etiology is unclear, many factors have been shown to be associated with an increased risk of developmental dislocation of the hip. These factors include breech presentation, a firstborn child, oligohydramnios, female sex, and a family history of DDH. The left hip is involved three times as often as the right hip, and a higher percentage of infants born in the winter months have DDH.

288. The answer is B. *(Tachdjian, pp 333–336.)* The Pavlik harness may be used up to the age at which the child can stand. It also provides stability to the subluxatable hip. Asymmetric hip abduction is a common finding in DDH and is not a contraindication for use of the Pavlik harness. Contraindications for use of the Pavlik harness include a child strong enough to stand (usually 9 months and older) and severe generalized ligamentous laxity, as seen in Down's or Marfan's syndromes.

289. The answer is E. *(Tachdjian, pp 583–591.)* In developmental coxa vara, there is a decrease in the normal femoral neck-shaft angle and progressive shortening of the affected lower limb with growth. The condition is equally distributed among males and females, is unilateral in two-thirds of cases, and rarely causes hip pain. Although operative treatment is often indicated, the results of epiphysiodesis of the greater trochanter are unreliable, so this procedure is not recommended for the treatment of coxa vara. When operative treatment is necessary, a valgus-producing proximal femoral osteotomy is recommended.

290. The answer is B. *(Tachdjian, pp 609–615.)* In grade I congenital dislocation of the knee, the knee can be passively manipulated into 45° to 90° of flexion and shows only subluxation on the lateral radiograph. Treatment is begun as early as possible and consists of immobilization in an above-knee cast with the knee in maximal flexion. The cast is changed and flexion increased at 2-week intervals. Range of motion exercises are ordinarily not begun for 4 to 6 weeks. Skin traction is indicated only if the subluxation cannot be reduced immediately by gentle stretching.

291. The answer is D. *(Tachdjian, pp 701–707.)* Multiple epiphyseal dysplasia is an autosomal dominant condition characterized by irregularity of the epiphyses. The condition is not obvious in infancy; as a result, the diagnosis may not be made until early adolescence. In contrast to spondyloepiphyseal dysplasia, vertebral involvement is not seen. As involvement is usually bilateral, differentiation from Legg-Calvé-Perthes disease is a common problem. There is no evidence that orthotic devices improve the outcome.

292. The answer is C. *(Tachdjian, pp 726–727.)* Neurologic complications are common in the adult with achondroplasia owing to the small diameter of the spinal canal and to multiple herniations of intervertebral disks. Paraplegia occurs in 11 percent of patients. Hydrocephalus can be present but is nonprogressive. Osteoarthritis is not a frequent sequela, since the epiphyses are normal. Genu valgum is rare.

293. The answer is A. *(Tachdjian, pp 721–726.)* Although the limbs are short in achondroplasia, trunk length (crown to pubis) is normal. The skull is brachycephalic, the face broad, and the bridge of the nose flattened. There is exaggeration of the normal lordotic curve of the lumbar spine. The digits of the hand are of equal length, with the long and ring fingers spread, forming a trident hand. Tibial and, less commonly, femoral bowing are also seen.

294. The answer is C. *(Tachdjian, pp 741–745.)* Hypophosphatasia is an autosomal recessive, inborn error of metabolism characterized by low alkaline phosphatase activity, which results in disturbances of ossification of bone and cartilage. In the skeleton, there is an excessive amount of unmineralized osteoid tissue, which produces a histologic picture similar to that of rickets.

295. The answer is A. *(Tachdjian, pp 242–245.)* There is no specific treatment for infantile hypophosphatasia. Enzyme replacement therapy has been attempted but does not seem to improve the outcome. Calcium chelating agents may decrease hypercalcemia, and renal dialysis may be necessary if renal failure occurs. Vitamin D should not be administered because it will increase the hypercalcemia and may cause metastatic calcification. Osteotomy of the long bones may be necessary to correct severe angular deformities.

296. The answer is E. *(Tachdjian, pp 746–748.)* Spondyloepiphyseal dysplasia congenita is characterized by flattened vertebral bodies, hyperlordosis of the lumbar spine, and a dysplastic odontoid process, which can lead to atlantoaxial instability. Coxa vara is frequently seen and may be severe. Scoliosis and kyphosis develop in late childhood or early adolescence. Talipes equinovarus is also associated with this syndrome.

297. The answer is A. *(Dirschl, Orthop Rev 23:305–312, 1994.)* Osteomyelitis and septic arthritis in neonates are most frequently caused by group B streptococci, followed by *Staphylococcus aureus*. Neonates may have few clinical or laboratory signs of infection, making diagnosis difficult. Initial antibiotic therapy should cover group B streptococci, *S. aureus*, and *E. coli*. *Candida albicans* infection must also be considered in neonates with indwelling intravenous catheters.

298. The answer is D. *(Dirschl, Orthop Rev 23:305–312, 1994.)* Since 90 percent of cases of acute hematogenous osteomyelitis in otherwise healthy children are caused by coagulase-positive staphylococci, initial antibiotic therapy should consist of a beta-lactamase–resistant semisynthetic penicillin. Cephalosporins are administered to children who are allergic to penicillin. Clindamycin is the antibiotic of choice in children allergic to both penicillins and cephalosporins. Ciprofloxacin is not approved for use in children.

299. The answer is B. *(Dirschl, Orthop Rev 23:305–312, 1994.)* Osteomyelitis in patients with sickle cell disease is frequently caused by salmonella species, although staphylococcal infections are also common. It is postulated that microinfarcts in the bowel from sickle cell disease allow salmonella bacteremia, which may then seed bone. Initial antibiotic therapy for acute osteomyelitis in patients with sickle cell disease includes a semisynthetic penicillin in combination with an aminoglycoside.

300. The answer is E. *(Tachdjian, pp 2842–2845.)* In infantile tibia vara, surgery is recommended for a child 4 years or older with stage II or stage III deformity, a tibiofemoral angle greater than 15° varus, and a metaphyseal-diaphyseal angle over 14°. Orthotic management may be successful up to 36 months of age. Osteotomy should be performed prior to 8 years of age to optimize the surgical result. Hemiepiphysiodesis is not indicated for a 4-year-old child.

301. The answer is A. *(Tachdjian, pp 2805–2810.)* Spontaneous improvement of excessive femoral anteversion may occur until the age of 7 or 8 years. Nonoperative measures are ineffective in the treatment of femoral anteversion, so physical therapy, Denis Browne splints, or twister cable braces should be not used. Although derotation femoral osteotomy is the only effective method of correcting excessive femoral anteversion, surgery should not be performed before the age of 8 years.

302. The answer is C. *(Tachdjian, pp 2386–2388.)* The most effective method of treating Scheuermann's kyphosis is a Milwaukee brace with two posterior kyphosis pads and a neck ring. The results of this treatment have been excellent, but treatment for up to 18 months is required to obtain good results. Operative correction of kyphotic deformity in Scheuermann's disease is performed only in a skeletally mature patient with chronic pain and a kyphotic deformity greater than 70°.

303. The answer is B. *(Tachdjian, pp 1982–1986.)* Charcot-Marie-Tooth disease is a disorder of peripheral nerves in which there are neuronal degenerative changes, most prominently in the lower limbs and feet. Muscle cramps and difficulty running or walking are the most common presenting complaints. Muscular atrophy and loss of proprioception and vibratory sense are symmetric in the lower limbs, and pes cavovarus is an early deformity. Friedreich's ataxia is characterized by cerebellar signs, speech disturbances, and a positive Babinski's response.

304. The answer is B. *(Shapiro, J Bone Joint Surg 75-A:1699–1714, 1993.)* Friedreich's ataxia is a rare, autosomal recessive, spinocerebellar disorder with a slow, degenerative course. The orthopaedic hallmarks of this condition, which become most apparent during the second decade of life, are scoliosis and cavovarus foot deformities. Dislocations of the hip and flexion contractures of the lower limb are not commonly seen in this condition.

305. The answer is D. *(Shapiro, J Bone Joint Surg 75-A:438–454, 1993.)* Although Duchenne's muscular dystrophy can be easily differentiated from spinal muscular atrophy because of the markedly elevated serum CPK, other forms of muscular dystrophy may have only mildly elevated levels of CPK. Spinal muscular atrophy is primarily a neurogenic disorder; as such, muscle biopsy will reveal atrophy of muscle fibers, with all fibers in an abnormal group having uniformly small diameter. Muscle biopsy in patients with muscular dystrophy shows variation in the size of the fibers, centrally located nuclei, and degeneration and regeneration of fibers. Although there are electromyographic differences between muscular dystrophies and neurogenic disorders, muscle biopsy remains the most specific test for differentiating these conditions.

306. The answer is C. *(Tachdjian, pp 1792–1795.)* All the listed factors affect the long-term ambulatory potential of a patient with a myelomeningocele, but the level of the neurologic lesion is by far the most important factor. Patients with sacral and L5 lesions are almost always independent community ambulators; patients with L4 lesions are usually community ambulators with orthoses; patients with upper lumbar and thoracic level lesions are usually not functional ambulators. Other factors affecting ambulatory potential include patient motivation, the presence of spasticity, and the effectiveness of the orthoses used.

307. The answer is C. *(Tachdjian, pp 752–756.)* Diastrophic dwarfism is an autosomal recessive skeletal dysplasia characterized by normal intelligence, short stature, equinovarus feet, and very short limbs. Two distinctive features of this condition are hitchhiker's thumbs and a "cauliflower" appearance of the earlobes. Scoliosis is almost always present, and stiffness of all major joints is common.

308. The answer is C. *(Tachdjian, pp 918–920.)* Ascorbic acid deficiency causes dysfunction of osteoblasts and interferes with collagen biosynthesis. Clinical features include easy bruising, gingival hemorrhage, subperiosteal hemorrhages with calcification, short stature, anemia, and delayed wound healing. Rapid recovery of normal clinical and radiologic features occurs following daily administration of vitamin C.

309. The answer is D. *(Dirschl, Orthop Rev 23:305–312, 1994.)* The diagnosis of acute osteomyelitis in children is a clinical as well as a laboratory one. Children with signs, symptoms, and laboratory studies consistent with osteomyelitis should have aspiration of the affected site. Aspiration is desirable both to establish a bacteriologic diagnosis and to determine whether an abscess is present. Technetium-99 bone scanning is less than 80 percent accurate in diagnosing acute hematogenous osteomyelitis; gallium scintigraphy is not universally available and is associated with large doses of radiation. CT scanning is not a useful tool for establishing the diagnosis of acute osteomyelitis but may be helpful in searching for extraosseous collections of pus.

310. The answer is D. *(Tachdjian, pp 2394–2401.)* Discitis is a nonspecific inflammatory or infectious lesion of the intervertebral disk with minimal or no evidence of primary bone involvement. It occurs primarily in infants and young children under the age of 5. Radiographs are generally normal, although narrowing of the disk space may be seen 2 to 3 weeks after the onset of symptoms. Tuberculous spondylitis occurs more commonly in the thoracic spine and is associated with bony destruction. Acute pyogenic spondylitis is characterized by fulminant systemic signs, rapidly progressive bone destruction, and markedly increased uptake on bone scan.

311. The answer is E. *(Dirschl, Orthop Rev 23:305–312, 1994.)* Infection following puncture wounds of the foot are caused by *Pseudomonas aeruginosa* in approximately 95 percent of cases. Antibiotic treatment alone does not eradicate the infection, does not remove foreign material from the foot, and allows the infection to destroy more tissue. Thorough surgical debridement should be performed, deep intraoperative cultures obtained, and intravenous antibiotic therapy begun with tobramycin.

312. The answer is B. *(Tachdjian, pp 656–658.)* Anterolateral bowing of the tibia is most frequently associated with subsequent pseudarthrosis. This pseudarthrosis may be present at birth, but more commonly it develops at about 12 months of age. Over 40 percent of cases of tibial pseudarthroses are caused by neurofibromatosis.

313. The answer is D. *(Tachdjian, pp 1289–1294.)* Cutaneous manifestations of neurofibromatosis include *café au lait* spots, fibromolluscum (dermal neurofibromas), nevi, verrucous hyperplasia, and elephantiasis. Skeletal findings include focal gigantism, focal defects in the cortices of bone, scoliosis, pseudarthrosis, and alterations in the internal structure of bone. Subperiosteal new bone formation is not a feature of neurofibromatosis.

314. The answer is D. *(Tachdjian, pp 2201–2202.)* Unilateral, unsegmented bony bars are common anomalies that occur most often in the thoracic area and are very likely to cause progression of scoliosis. Circumferential symmetric failure of segmentation (block vertebra) does not cause angular or rotatory spinal deformity. Klippel-Feil syndrome does not result in scoliosis. Hemivertebrae and fused ribs may result in scoliosis, but the likelihood of progression is less than with a unilateral bony bar.

315. The answer is D. *(Tachdjian, pp 2202–2205.)* Nonoperative treatment is ineffective in the adolescent child with congenital scoliosis. In situ posterior fusion is recommended when the deformity is minimal to moderate and cosmetically acceptable. The natural history of the deformity is relentless progression, which is the case in this patient with a unilateral bony bar. Osteotomy of the bar and spinal fusion are indicated in an adolescent with a rigid, severe scoliosis that is cosmetically unacceptable and unbalanced.

316. The answer is A. *(Tachdjian, pp 1163–1195.)* Since the osseous tissue produced is normal in every respect, an osteochondroma is not a true neoplasm. It should be considered a developmental defect. Sarcomatous transformation occurs in less than 0.5 percent of lesions. The incidence of sarcomatous transformation is slightly higher in solitary enchondromas and much higher in multiple osteochondromatosis, Ollier's disease, and Maffucci's syndrome.

317. The answer is C. *(Tachdjian, pp 758–761.)* The fundamental defect in osteogenesis imperfecta is failure of maturation of collagen fibers beyond the reticulin fiber stage. The osteoblasts demonstrate normal or increased activity, but organization and maturation of collagen chains after synthesis is defective. Mineralization of osteoid, osteoclastic activity, and intramembranous bone formation are not impaired.

318. The answer is A. *(Tachdjian, pp 861–864.)* Ehlers-Danlos syndrome is a group of related disorders caused by defective collagen metabolism and characterized by skin changes consisting of hyperextensibility, fragility, and easy bruising. Ligamentous laxity and bone fragility are also seen. A rare disease, it is inherited as an autosomal dominant trait.

319. The answer is C. *(Tachdjian, pp 882–886.)* The figure shows expansion of the distal femoral metaphyses, giving the bones the appearance of Erlenmeyer flasks on the radiograph. This is seen in Gaucher's disease, Niemann-Pick disease, and osteopetrosis. Gaucher's disease is an inherited inborn disturbance of lipid metabolism, which results in infiltration of the reticuloendothelial system and bone by cells containing accumulated glucocerebrosides. This is manifested clinically by hepatosplenomegaly and on a CBC by pancytopenia. Niemann-Pick disease can have the same clinical manifestations as Gaucher's disease, but is universally associated with profound mental retardation. Osteopetrosis is characterized by extensive osteosclerosis, which is not evident in the figure.

320. The answer is A. *(Morrissy, p 268.)* Some two-thirds of infants with leukemia will display diffuse osteolysis in the metaphyseal-diaphyseal regions of long bones. The finding seen most often in the skull is widening of the cranial sutures. Vertebral changes usually take the form of radiolucencies adjacent to the end plates of the bodies.

321. The answer is D. *(Morrissy, p 282.)* In severe hemophiliacs with inhibitors, the joints should be splinted in the position of maximum comfort and observed. Given the presence of an inhibitor, raising the level of factor VIII activity to the 25 percent level necessary for aspiration is impossible. Desmopressin is used only for the treatment of mild or moderate hemophilia. While initial splinting should be in the position of maximum comfort, as discomfort subsides, usually within 48 h or so, further extension can be obtained safely and comfortably.

322. The answer is D. *(Morrissy, p 291.)* Even with the arthropathy evident in this patient, synovectomy with radial head excision is effective in relieving pain and reducing the frequency of hemarthroses. The arthropathy is too advanced for home replacement therapy or bracing to be effective. Joint replacement, a more complex but no more reliable procedure, should be reserved for failure of synovectomy and radial head excision. Synovectomy alone (chemical or surgical) would not address the significant arthropathy in this patient.

323. The answer is A. *(Morrissy, p 291.)* Lymphadenopathy is generalized and consistent even in the early stages of HIV infection. The other choices listed occur less frequently and later in the course of the disease.

324. The answer is C. *(Morrissy, p 476.)* In spastic cerebral palsy, contractures result from shortening of muscle fiber length. Lengthening of the musculotendinous unit eliminates the contracture but also decreases excursion of the muscle, which would prevent tip-toeing. Neither the fiber length nor the cross-sectional area of the muscle changes significantly.

325. The answer is E. *(Morrissy, p 479.)* The value of physical therapy in the management of spastic cerebral palsy is unproven. The physical therapist, in his or her role as counselor, advisor, and cheerleader, may be more important than the specific therapy. Certainly this is an area in which there exists more dogma than data.

326. The answer is B. *(Morrissy, p 480.)* With mild, fixed deformity (ankle cannot be dorsiflexed past 0°), muscle growth can be stimulated by stretching, which is best accomplished by corrective casting. Inhibitive casting, which has given way to fiberglass orthotics, is used to facilitate standing rather than walking. Neither braces nor biofeedback has value in the treatment of fixed deformity. Electrical stimulation is used to strengthen muscles rather than correct deformity.

327. The answer is D. *(Morrissy, p 484.)* Immobilization under some tension minimizes shortening of muscle bellies, which may cause a decrease in excursion of the muscle. The muscle should not be released completely. The site of the lengthening does not usually affect the result, although lengthening at the musculotendinous junction results in a higher rate of recurrent contracture.

328. The answer is A. *(Morrissy, p 298.)* Juvenile pauciarticular chronic arthritis (the most common form of JCA) typically involves less than five (large) joints in females under age 4. The ESR is normal or low, systemic signs are absent, and the rheumatoid factor is negative. The polyarticular form is similar except that it involves more than four joints (which may be large or small) and is more likely to have systemic signs and a positive rheumatoid factor. Systemic JCA involves any age, has no sex predilection, and is associated with striking systemic signs, such as high fevers, rash, and lymphadenopathy. The rheumatoid factor is infrequently positive. Seronegative spondyloarthropathies most commonly affect males over age 8 and usually involve the lower limbs. Systemic signs are minimal, although the ESR may be moderately elevated.

329. The answer is E. *(Morrissy, p 303.)* In ankylosing spondylitis, there are ascending changes in the spine, usually culminating in ankylosis. The earliest radiographic findings are symmetric, bilateral erosions of the sacroiliac joints. Inflammatory changes subsequently cause destruction and ankylosis of the apophyseal joints.

330. The answer is A. *(Morrissy, p 302.)* The etiologies of both JCA and the seronegative spondyloarthropathies are unknown. Familial clustering suggests genetic influences. Although rubella, varicella, and Epstein-Barr viruses have been cultured from patients with JCA, the majority of patients have no evidence of chronic infection. Some children with JCA also have anticollagenous antibodies, suggesting an element of autoimmunity, but this is also an inconsistent finding.

331. The answer is B. *(Morrissy, p 313.)* The most consistent benefits from synovectomy in JRA are in reduction of pain and swelling. Results are better following synovectomy of large rather than small joints. Motion is rarely improved, and there is no predictable effect on radiographic progression, physeal growth, or prevention of recurrence.

332. The answer is C. *(Morrissy, p 320.)* The cervical spine is involved in up to 60 percent of patients with polyarticular JRA. Torticollis is infrequent. Neurologic findings are also uncommon, probably because basilar invagination is much rarer in the juvenile than in the adult form of RA. Stiffness is more common than pain in the early stages of the disease.

333. The answer is E. *(Morrissy, p 928.)* Maternal trauma can result in rupture of the amnion, with encirclement of the limb by strings of amniotic tissue. Clubfoot in these patients is associated with congenital constricting bands. Clubfoot associated with Mendelian inheritance patterns or excessive cytogenetic material is part of a symptom complex. Isolated, idiopathic talipes equinovarus is thought to result primarily from a multifactorial inheritance pattern.

334. The answer is D. *(Morrissy, pp 937–938.)* Arthrographic techniques have not been sufficiently evaluated in clubfeet and are difficult to perform. Computerized tomography does not adequately determine positional relationships of the bones, since it cannot distinguish cartilaginous "bone" from the beginnings of ligaments. MRI findings may be valuable with further accumulation of data, especially if three-dimensional reconstruction becomes widely available. The most valuable technique currently is measurement of the talocalcaneal angles on standardized AP and lateral radiographs.

335. The answer is D. *(Morrissy, pp 941–942.)* If correction of equinus and varus has not been achieved after 6 months of appropriate nonoperative treatment, surgical release is indicated. Since no cavus exists and the midfoot is supple, plantar and lateral releases are unnecessary. The posterior release includes division of the calcaneofibular and posterior talofibular ligaments.

336. The answer is D. *(Morrissy, p 952.)* Failure to include release of the plantar fascia and the short and long plantar ligaments during the initial posteromedial release is a common cause of persistent cavus deformity. Inadequate plantar release may, with further growth, lead eventually to dorsal subluxation or extrusion of the navicular. Failure to position the cuboid anatomically at the end of the calcaneus contributes to residual cavus.

337. The answer is E. *(Morrissy, pp 960–962.)* Correction of congenital vertical talus in an adolescent can be accomplished only by triple arthrodesis, usually with sacrifice of a significant portion of the talar head and neck. The other surgical procedures listed above may be useful in the treatment of this condition in younger children. Manipulation and casting in equinus are useful only to stretch contracted anterior soft tissues prior to open reduction.

338. The answer is E. *(Morrissy, p 958.)* Irreducible dorsal dislocation of the talonavicular joint is the hallmark of congenital vertical talus. Contractures of the Achilles and extensor digitorum longus tendons occur in the hypermobile flatfoot as well, but plantar flexion of the foot and ankle in the latter condition reduces talonavicular displacement. Hypoplasia and plantar flexion of the talus are present in congenital vertical talus, but these changes are undetectable clinically.

339. The answer is B. *(Morrissy, pp 933–934).* Pathoanatomic changes in talipes equinovarus include medial rotation of the talus in the ankle mortise, medial rotation of the calcaneus, and medial displacement of the cuboid in relation to the long axis of the calcaneus. In addition, the anterior tarsals and metatarsals are supinated and adducted, and the lateral malleolus is displaced posteriorly.

340. The answer is D. *(Morrissy, p 303.)* The inflammatory hyperemia of JCA may either stimulate bony overgrowth or cause premature closure of the physes with shortening. Both changes are more frequent with involvement of the knee. Overgrowth is usual when the age of the patient is under 9; shortening follows in patients over the age of 9. Overgrowth rarely exceeds 3 cm, whereas shortening may be as marked as 6 cm.

341. The answer is A. *(Morrissy, p 953.)* The indications for calcaneocuboid fusion (Dillwyn Evans' procedure) are a child 4 years of age or older with residual varus, a short medial column, and a long lateral column of the foot. Earlier fusion results in loss of lateral growth that may lead to overcorrection. The procedure has no place in the correction of forefoot deformities.

Pediatric Trauma

Douglas R. Dirschl, M.D.

DIRECTIONS: Each question below contains five suggested responses. Select the **one best** response to each question.

342. The front tooth of an 11-year-old boy was knocked out during a baseball game. The most appropriate management for this injury is to

(A) discard the tooth; consult a dentist
(B) wrap the tooth in dry gauze; consult a dentist
(C) place the tooth in saline solution; go to the emergency room following the game
(D) place the tooth in ice; go to the emergency room following the game
(E) replace the tooth in the socket; consult a dentist immediately

343. The most appropriate treatment for a 6-year-old boy with a displaced fracture of the lateral humeral condyle is

(A) closed reduction and application of an above-elbow cast
(B) a collar and cuff
(C) skeletal traction
(D) open reduction and internal fixation
(E) excision of the fracture fragment

344. An 11-year-old boy seen 48 h after stepping on a nail had a puncture wound beneath the second metatarsal head and erythema on the dorsum of the foot. His temperature was normal. Radiographs revealed only soft-tissue swelling. In conjunction with thorough debridement, the antibiotic of choice is

(A) oral amoxicillin–clavulanic acid
(B) parenteral cefazolin
(C) oral ciprofloxacin
(D) parenteral ciprofloxacin
(E) parenteral tobramycin

345. All the following statements concerning child abuse are true EXCEPT that

(A) most cases involve children under 3 years of age
(B) handicapped children are at greater risk for abuse than normal children
(C) nearly half of abused children come from a single-parent home
(D) first-born children are at less risk for abuse than their siblings
(E) relatives are frequent abusers

346. The most commonly fractured bone in cases of child abuse is the

(A) rib
(B) humerus
(C) femur
(D) tibia
(E) skull

347. A 4-year-old girl sustained an isolated, closed, diaphyseal fracture of her left femur in a motor vehicle accident. The fracture was transverse with approximately 1.5 cm of shortening. The most appropriate definitive management of this fracture is

(A) skeletal traction
(B) immediate application of a hip spica cast
(C) skeletal traction for 2 weeks followed by application of a hip spica cast
(D) external skeletal fixation
(E) intramedullary nailing

348. Initial management of a pediatric patient in posttraumatic shock consists of insertion of at least two peripheral intravenous catheters and resuscitation with a bolus of

(A) lactated Ringer's, 15 mL/kg
(B) 5% dextrose in one-half normal saline (D-5 ½NS), 15 mL/kg
(C) lactated Ringer's, 30 mL/kg
(D) D-5 ½NS, 30 mL/kg
(E) lactated Ringer's, 2 L

349. All the following statements regarding fractures in children are correct EXCEPT that

(A) they are more common than fractures in adults
(B) physeal disruptions constitute 15 percent of skeletal injuries
(C) they may result in disturbances of growth
(D) the periosteum is less likely to be stripped from the bone than in the adult
(E) Salter type I injuries are more common in infants than in older children

350. All the following statements regarding fracture healing in children are correct EXCEPT that

(A) the thickened periosteum contributes to rapid healing
(B) fracture union is more rapid in younger children than in older children
(C) physeal injuries heal more slowly than injuries through the metaphysis or diaphysis
(D) fractures may stimulate excessive longitudinal growth
(E) nonunion rarely occurs

351. The degree of remodeling of fracture deformities in children is dependent on all the following EXCEPT the

(A) age of the child
(B) distance of the fracture from the physis
(C) skeletal maturity of the child
(D) degree of angulation
(E) amount of rotational deformity

352. A 16-year-old soccer player sustained a closed, blunt head injury that caused him to lose consciousness for 10 min. The player should be

(A) allowed to return to the game if he is lucid
(B) restricted from practice and competition for 3 days
(C) restricted from practice and competition for 1 month
(D) restricted from practice and competition for 6 months
(E) restricted from practice and competition for 1 year

353. Nine months following treatment of a Salter type II distal femoral fracture in a 9-year-old boy, routine radiographs reveal "tenting" of the physis. You suspect a central growth arrest. The best imaging modality to confirm this impression is

(A) oblique radiography of the knee
(B) polytomography
(C) hypocycloidal motion tomography
(D) CT
(E) MRI

354. The most common site of *epiphyseal* injury associated with birth trauma is the

(A) clavicle
(B) proximal humerus
(C) distal humerus
(D) proximal femur
(E) distal femur

355. The most common cause of a fracture of the hand in toddlers is

(A) a fall onto the outstretched hand
(B) a twisting injury
(C) a crushing injury
(D) a motor vehicle accident
(E) an axial loading injury

356. The most common complication following open Salter type I or II fractures of the distal phalanx in the hand is

(A) nonunion
(B) growth arrest
(C) persistent mild deformity
(D) infection
(E) joint stiffness

357. A 7-year-old girl sustained the injury to her middle finger shown in the figure. The most appropriate treatment is

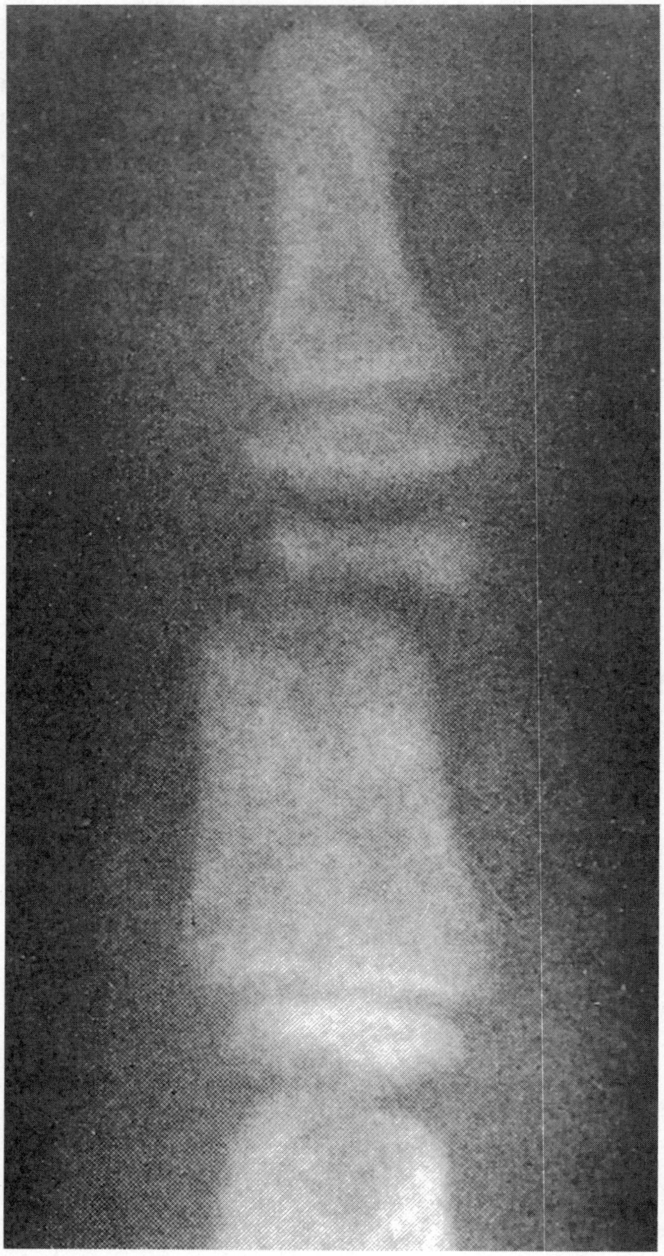

(A) "buddy-taping" to the adjacent digit
(B) closed reduction and splinting
(C) closed reduction and "buddy-taping" to the adjacent digit
(D) closed reduction and percutaneous pinning
(E) open reduction and plate fixation

358. The most commonly dislocated joint in the child's hand is the

(A) distal interphalangeal joint
(B) proximal interphalangeal joint
(C) metacarpophalangeal joint
(D) carpometacarpal joint
(E) radiocarpal joint

359. All the following statements regarding fractures of the scaphoid in children are true EXCEPT that

(A) they are less common than in adults
(B) displacement is infrequent
(C) the waist is the most common site of injury
(D) fractures of the proximal pole are almost never seen
(E) the primary cause of nonunion is delay in diagnosis

---

360. A 9-year-old girl seen 2 weeks following an injury to her wrist has had no prior treatment. Radiographs are shown on the following page. The most appropriate management is

(A) application of a below-elbow cast
(B) closed reduction and application of a below-elbow cast in the office
(C) closed reduction and application of a below-elbow cast under general anesthesia
(D) closed reduction and application of an above-elbow cast under general anesthesia
(E) open reduction and internal fixation

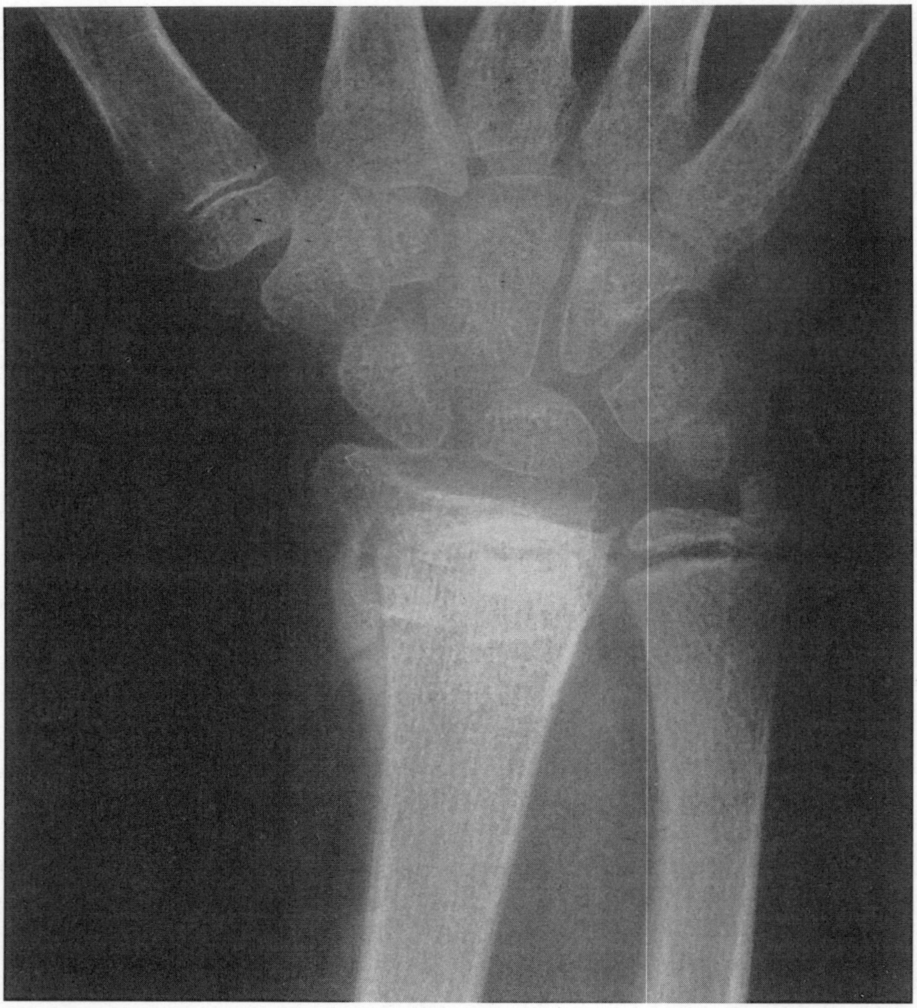

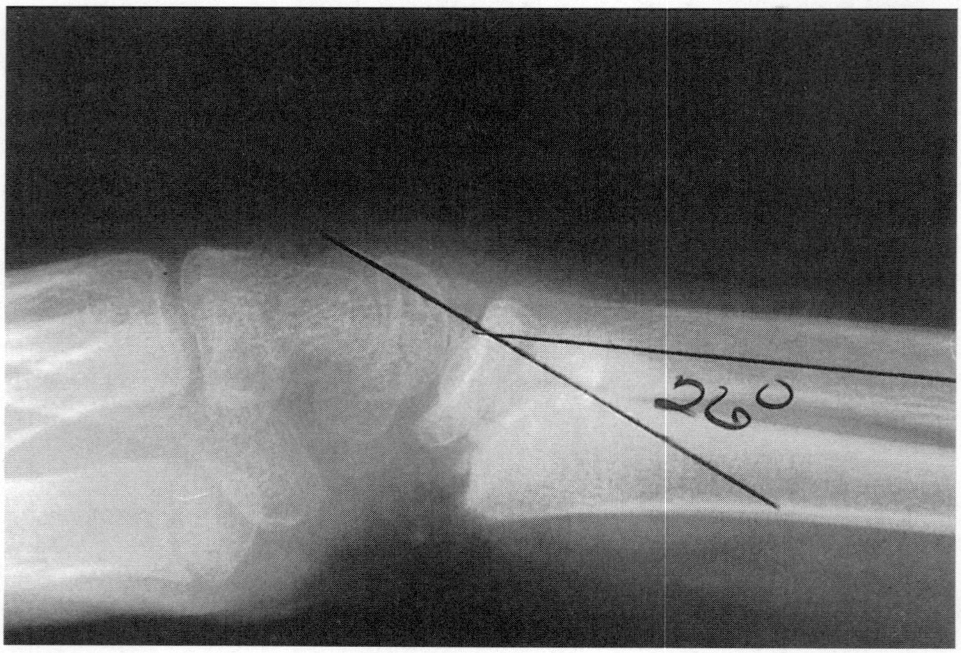
26°

361. On a normal anteroposterior radiograph of the forearm, the bicipital tuberosity is

(A) medial in supination; lateral in pronation
(B) lateral in supination; medial in pronation
(C) medial in supination; not seen in pronation
(D) lateral in supination; not seen in pronation
(E) not seen either in supination or pronation

362. Greenstick fractures differ from complete fractures of the forearm bones in that

(A) both cortices of the involved bone are intact
(B) angular deformity without rational deformity has occurred
(C) reduction is not necessary
(D) recurrent deformity is much more likely in the cast
(E) growth arrest is a more frequent complication

363. Following closed reduction of a type II Monteggia fracture in an 8-year-old child, the arm should be immobilized in a position of

(A) full extension of the elbow; supination
(B) 90° flexion of the elbow; supination
(C) 90° flexion of the elbow; pronation
(D) 100° flexion of the elbow; supination
(E) 100° flexion of the elbow; pronation

364. The age range during which the incidence of supracondylar fractures of the humerus is highest is

(A) 0 to 3 years
(B) 3 to 5 years
(C) 5 to 8 years
(D) 8 to 10 years
(E) 10 to 13 years

365. A 6-month-old patient in a forward-facing car seat had complete quadriplegia after a motor vehicle accident. Radiographs, a CT scan, and a myelogram were normal. Treatment should consist of

(A) observation
(B) a rigid collar
(C) traction with cervical tongs
(D) a Minerva jacket
(E) posterior cervical fusion

366. An absolute indication for operative management of a supracondylar fracture of the humerus in a child is

(A) marked displacement
(B) severe swelling
(C) an open fracture
(D) neurologic compromise
(E) age over 10 years

367. Posterolateral subluxation of the elbow frequently occurs with displaced fractures of the lateral condyle of the humerus because

(A) there is a tear of the medial collateral ligament
(B) there is a fracture of the coronoid process
(C) hemarthrosis distends the elbow joint
(D) the fracture line usually disrupts the lateral crista of the trochlea
(E) there is frequently an associated fracture of the proximal radius

368. All the following deformities may occur following a fracture of the lateral condyle of the humerus in children EXCEPT

(A) cubitus varus
(B) cubitus valgus
(C) lateral condylar spur formation
(D) central growth arrest of the distal humeral physis
(E) avascular necrosis of the lateral part of the medial crista of the trochlea

369. Radiographs of a 4-year-old boy seen 7 days following an elbow injury revealed posterior and medial displacement of the proximal radius and ulna relative to the distal humerus. Optimal treatment is

(A) cast immobilization
(B) closed reduction
(C) closed reduction and percutaneous pinning
(D) open reduction and percutaneous pinning
(E) a sling that allows motion of the elbow

370. All the following statements regarding fractures of the medial epicondyle of the humerus in children are true EXCEPT that

(A) they tend to occur in children older than those with supracondylar fractures
(B) they are frequently associated with elbow dislocations
(C) they rarely cause growth disturbances
(D) the results of late removal of incarcerated fragments are satisfactory
(E) operative stabilization is unnecessary

371. A 5-year-old boy sustained a fracture of the radial neck with 60° of angulation. After closed reduction under general anesthesia, there was 30° of residual angulation. Pronation of the forearm was 70° and supination was 80°. The next step in treatment should be

(A) immobilization in 90° elbow flexion
(B) further closed manipulation and immobilization
(C) closed reduction and percutaneous pinning
(D) open reduction of the radial neck
(E) open reduction and pin fixation of the radial neck

372. Indications for open reduction and internal fixation of fractures of the humeral shaft in children include all the following EXCEPT

(A) open fracture
(B) multiple injuries
(C) associated head injury
(D) associated vascular injury
(E) associated fracture of the ipsilateral forearm

373. A 5-year-old girl sustained a Salter type II fracture of the proximal humerus. Radiographs showed 50 percent apposition of the fracture fragments and 45° of angulation. The most appropriate treatment is

(A) immobilization in a sling and swathe
(B) closed reduction under general anesthesia; immobilization in a sling and swathe
(C) closed reduction under general anesthesia; immobilization in a shoulder spica cast
(D) closed reduction under general anesthesia; percutaneous pinning
(E) open reduction and internal fixation

374. A 7-year-old boy fell from a swing, sustaining no apparent injury. His physical examination was normal, but a lateral radiograph of the cervical spine revealed 3 mm anterior displacement and 10° angulation of C2 on C3. The most appropriate management is

(A) observation
(B) a Minerva cast
(C) cranial tongs and traction
(D) immediate application of a halo ring and vest
(E) closed reduction and posterior spinal fusion

375. All the following statements regarding fractures of the odontoid in children are correct EXCEPT that

(A) the AP radiograph may be normal
(B) nonunion occurs rarely
(C) displacement is usually posterior
(D) the anterior periosteum usually remains intact
(E) a good result can be expected

376. The most common sequela of complete, posttraumatic paraplegia in children is increased susceptibility to

(A) fractures of long bones
(B) dislocations of the hip
(C) spinal deformity
(D) genitourinary complications
(E) decubiti

377. For a 10-year-old boy with a nondisplaced, transcervical fracture of the femoral neck, the most appropriate management is

(A) a hip spica cast
(B) skeletal traction
(C) fixation in situ with pins crossing the physis
(D) fixation in situ with screws short of the physis
(E) open reduction and internal fixation

378. In a child with an injury to the cervical spine, the incidence of injury at another level in the cervical spine is approximately

(A) 5 percent
(B) 10 percent
(C) 15 percent
(D) 25 percent
(E) 50 percent

379. In the treatment of a mid-shaft fracture of the femur in a 7-year-old child in skeletal traction, the traction pin should be inserted in the

(A) proximal tibia with the knee fully extended
(B) proximal tibia with the knee flexed 90°
(C) distal femur with the knee fully extended
(D) distal femur with the knee flexed 90°
(E) distal femur and proximal tibia

380. Pathologic changes on the medial side of the elbow in children who play throwing games, such as pitchers, include all the following EXCEPT

(A) hypertrophy of the medial epicondyle
(B) fragmentation of the epicondylar apophysis
(C) attenuation of the ulnar collateral ligament
(D) microscopic tears of the flexor-pronator group
(E) avulsion fractures of the medial epicondyle

381. A 14-year-old boy sustained the injury in the radiographs below while playing basketball. All the following statements concerning this injury are true EXCEPT

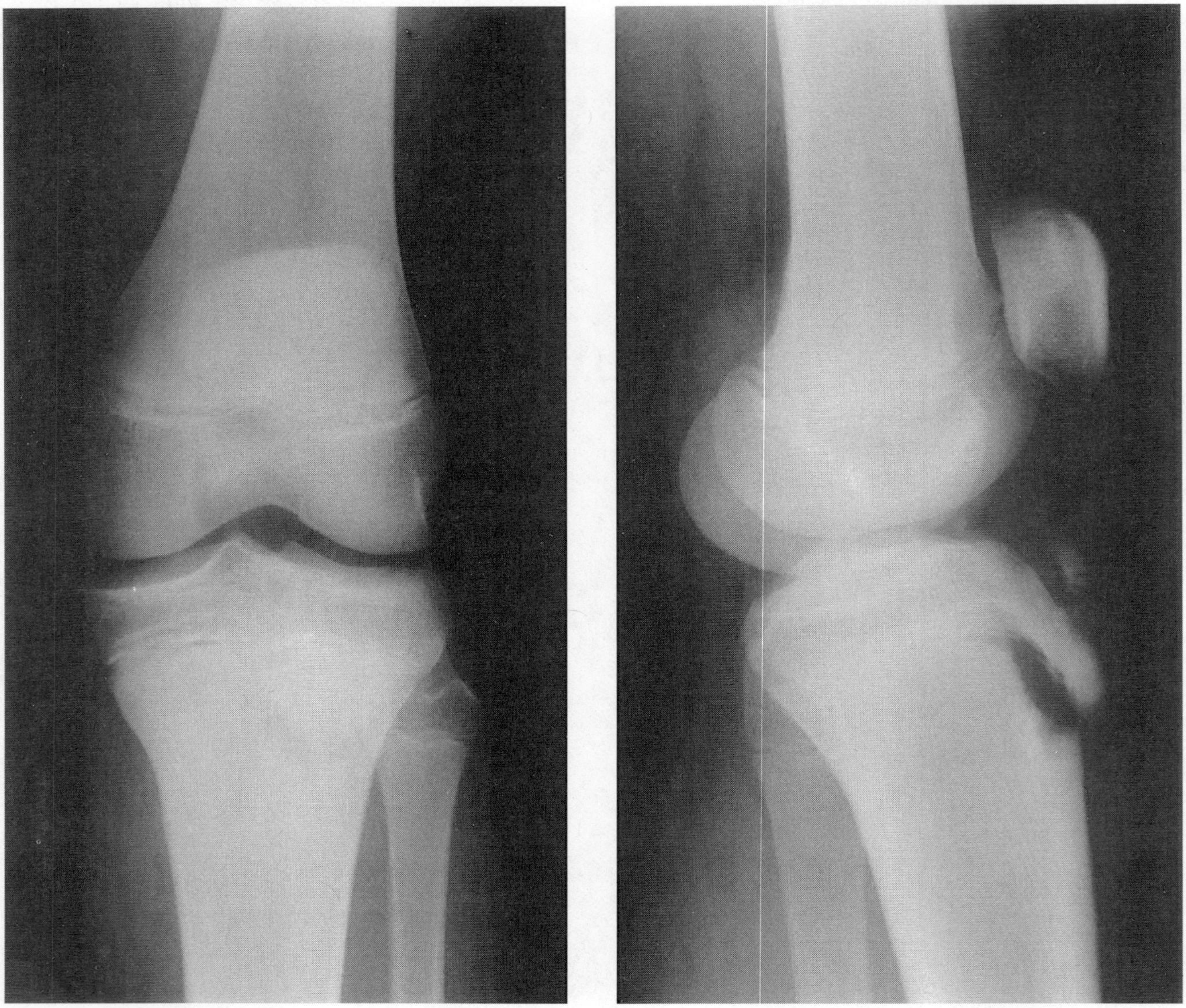

(A) the Osgood-Schlatter lesion often precedes this lesion
(B) closed reduction is often successful
(C) the prognosis for return to full activities is good
(D) the patient is unable to extend the knee fully
(E) growth disturbance is unlikely

382. An 11-year-old girl sustained an isolated, complete rupture of the anterior cruciate ligament (ACL) while playing soccer. A 3-month trial of nonoperative treatment left the patient with marked, symptomatic anterior instability of the knee. The most appropriate treatment for this problem is

(A) extraarticular tenodesis with the iliotibial band
(B) reconstruction with the medial hamstrings
(C) reconstruction with the central third of the patellar tendon
(D) intrasubstance repair
(E) reconstruction with a Gore-Tex allograft

383. Persons less than 20 years of age who sustain a dislocation of the glenohumeral joint will develop recurrent dislocation in approximately what percentage of cases?

(A) 20 percent
(B) 40 percent
(C) 60 percent
(D) 80 percent
(E) 100 percent

384. The most common direction of a traumatic dislocation in a child's knee is

(A) anterior
(B) posterior
(C) medial
(D) lateral
(E) posterolateral

385. In the treatment of a tibial shaft fracture in a 10-year-old boy, what is the maximum amount of shortening that is acceptable?

(A) No shortening is acceptable
(B) 5 mm
(C) 10 mm
(D) 15 mm
(E) 20 mm

386. The sport responsible for the greatest number of spinal cord injuries in children under 18 years of age is

(A) football
(B) ice hockey
(C) diving
(D) gymnastics
(E) trampoline jumping

387. The most common complication following fractures of the tibias in paraplegic children is

(A) nonunion
(B) delayed union
(C) malunion
(D) pressure sores
(E) persistent pain

388. The most common sequela of a fracture of the proximal tibial metaphysis in a child is

(A) nonunion
(B) growth arrest
(C) varus deformity
(D) valgus deformity
(E) rotational malunion

389. Stress fractures of the lower limb in children most commonly occur in the

(A) talus
(B) proximal femur
(C) tibia
(D) fibula
(E) metatarsals

390. An 8-year-old boy injured his right foot in a lawn mower accident. After serial debridements, a clean 10 × 10 cm wound remained on the dorsum of the foot with exposed extensor tendons. The most appropriate management of the soft-tissue injury is

(A) closure by secondary intention
(B) a split thickness skin graft
(C) a soleus flap and split thickness skin graft
(D) a cross-leg pedicle flap
(E) a fasciocutaneous free flap

391. An 11-year-old girl fell and sustained the ankle injury in the figure. The most appropriate next step in the management of this injury is

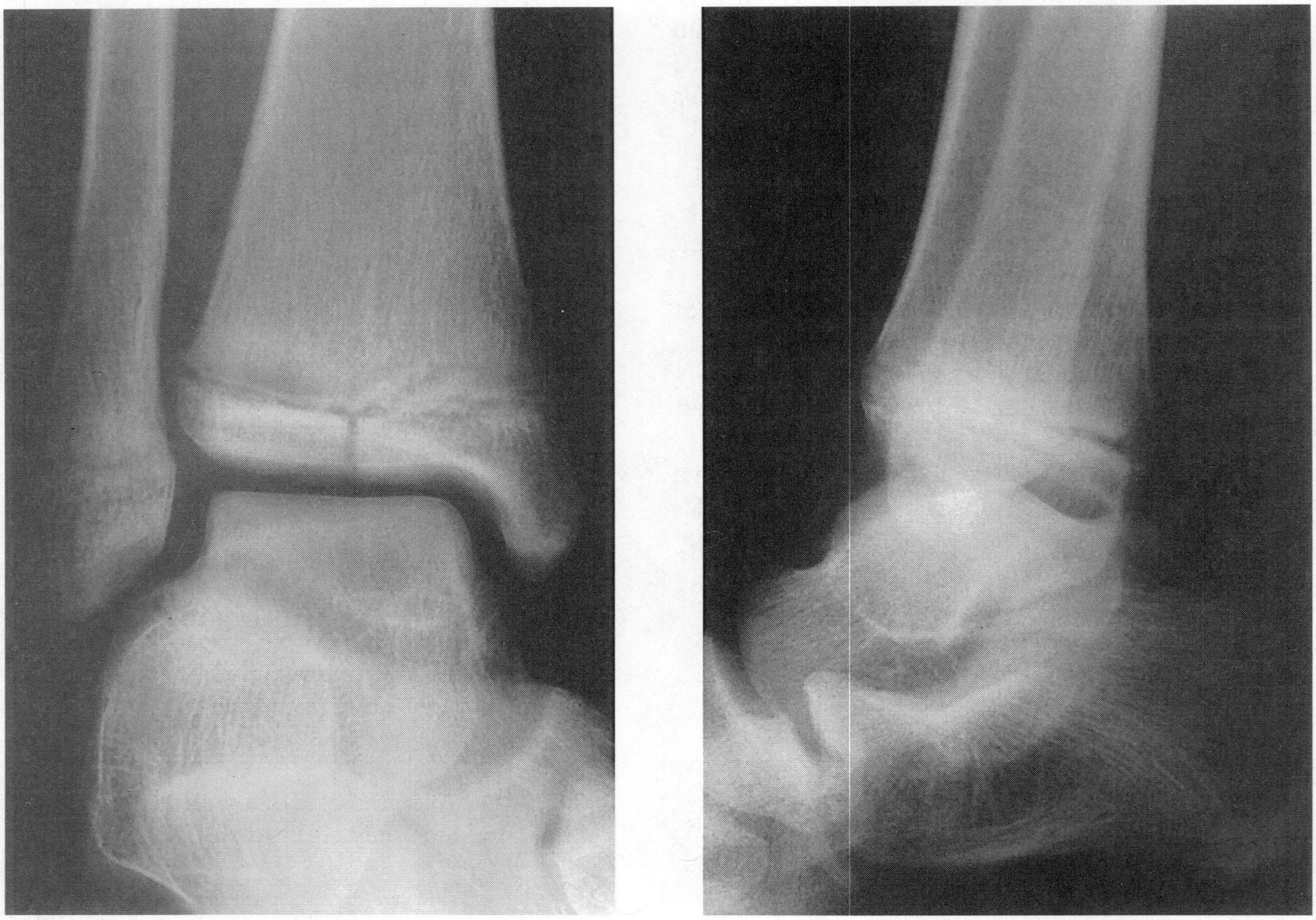

(A) application of a below-knee cast; weight-bearing as tolerated
(B) application of a below-knee cast; non-weight-bearing
(C) application of an above-knee cast; non-weight-bearing
(D) a CT scan to confirm the position of the fragments
(E) open reduction and internal fixation

392. An obese 7-year-old boy sustained an isolated, closed fracture of the femoral shaft in a motor vehicle accident. Skeletal traction was applied through a femoral traction pin. After 5 days of traction and multiple adjustments, the best alignment achieved was that shown below. The most appropriate management now is

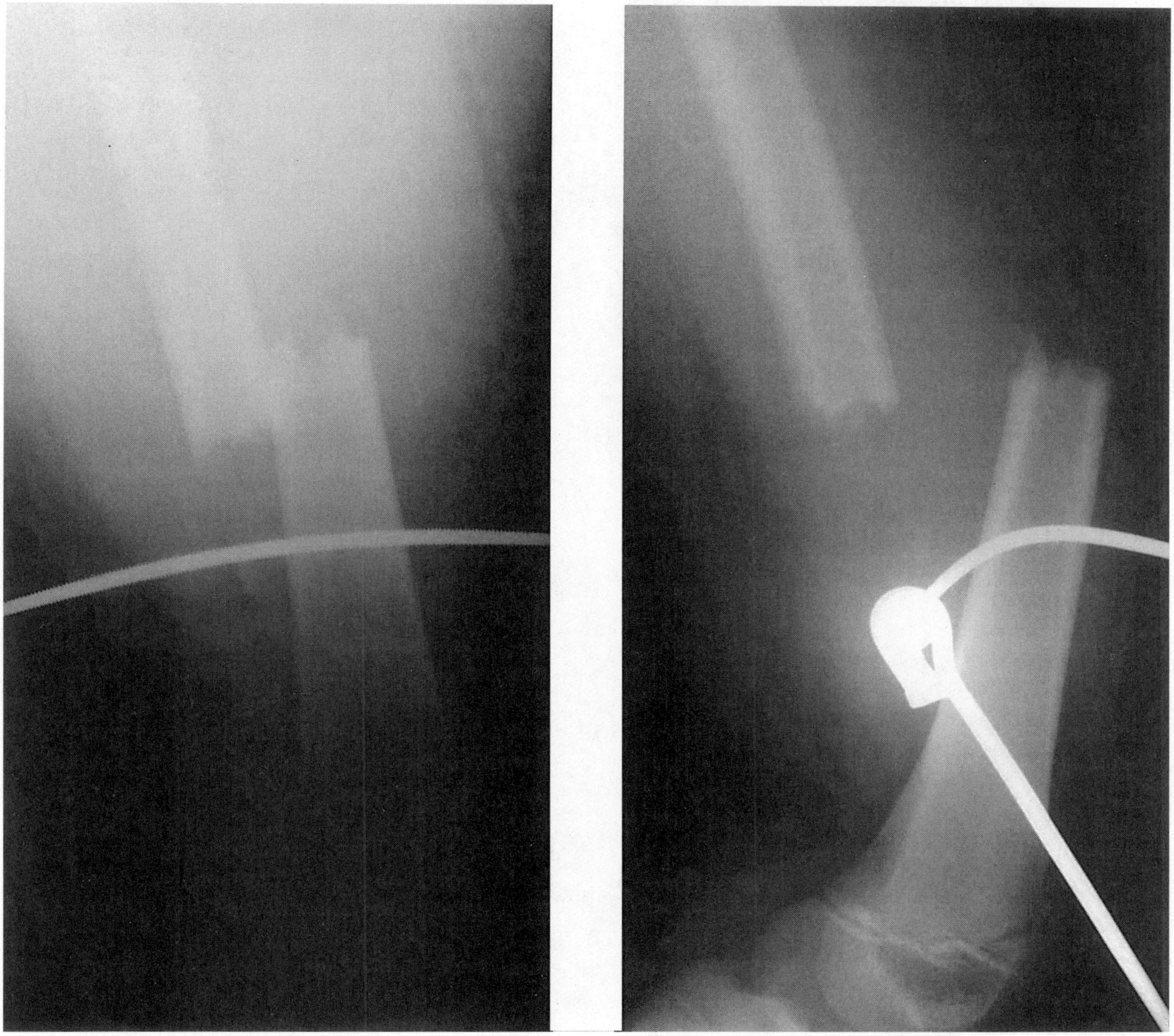

(A) continued skeletal traction
(B) application of a hip spica cast
(C) external skeletal fixation
(D) intramedullary nailing
(E) open reduction and plate fixation

393. A 4-year-old girl who fell on her elbow sustained the injury show below. The most appropriate treatment is

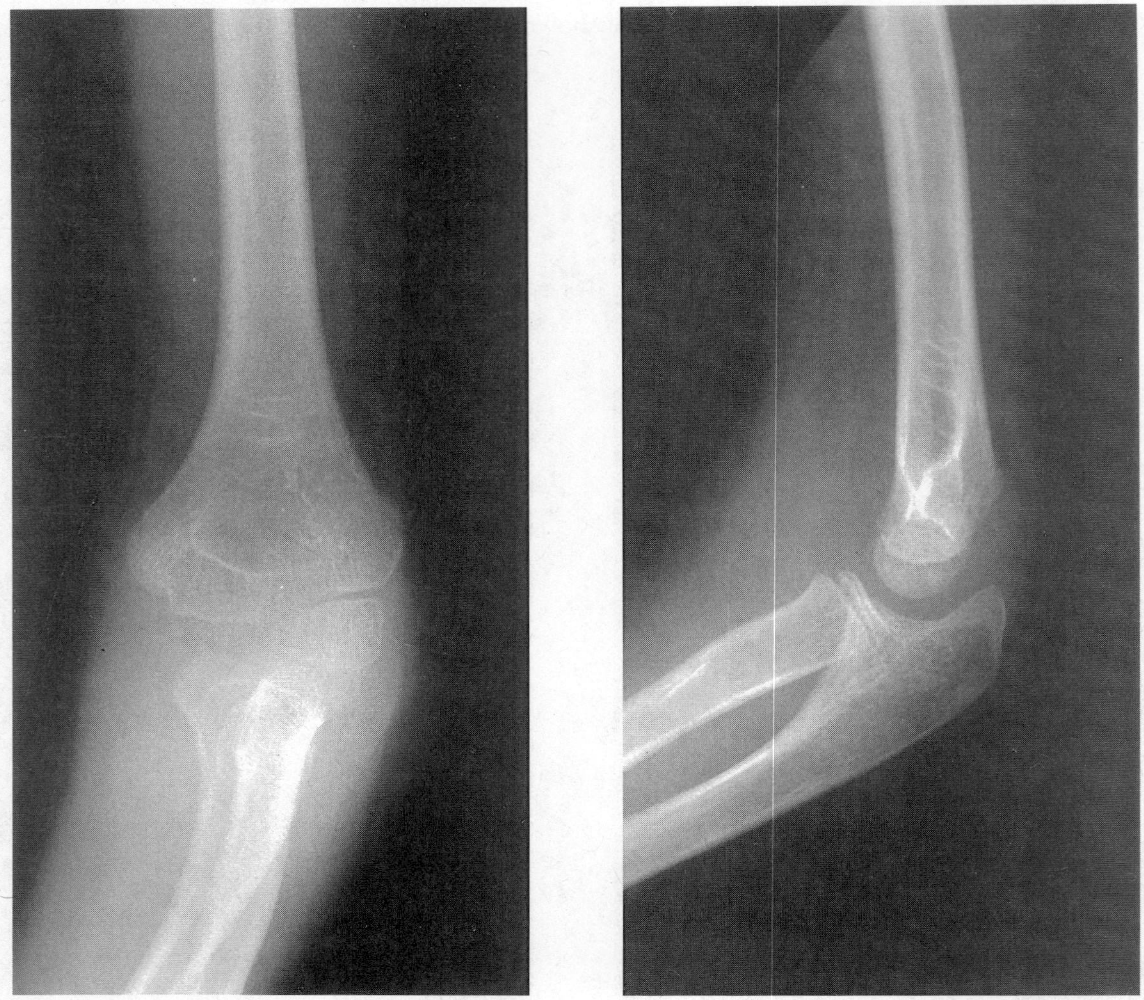

(A) application of an above-elbow cast
(B) closed reduction; application of an above-elbow cast
(C) closed reduction; percutaneous pinning
(D) open reduction; percutaneous pinning
(E) excision of the fracture fragment

394. A 2-year-old boy who fell from a trampoline sustained the injury in the figure. The most appropriate treatment is

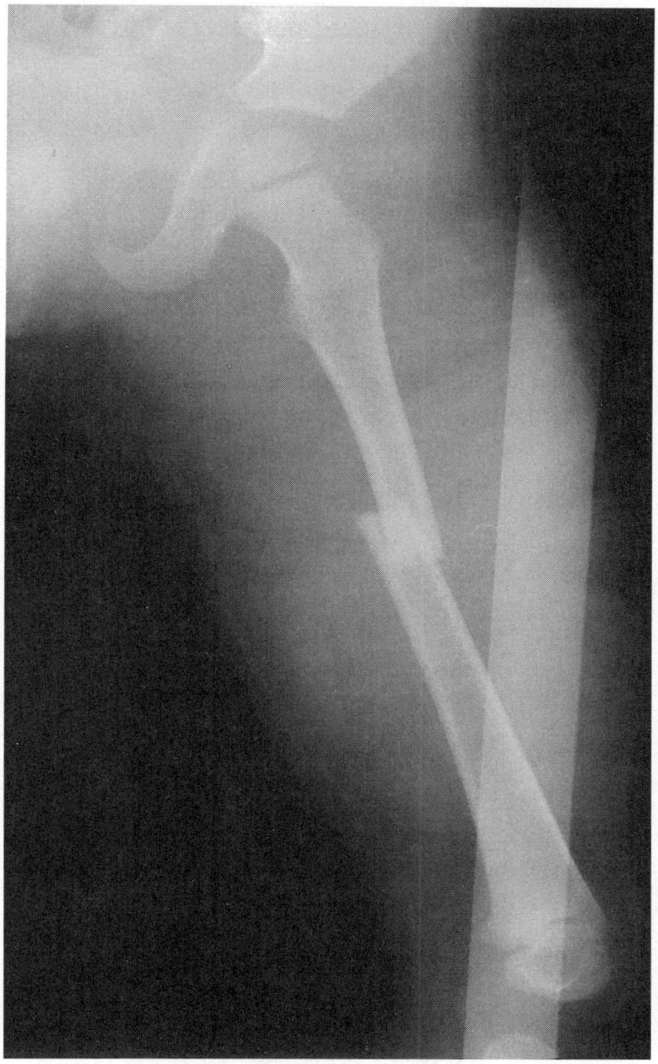

(A) immediate application of a spica cast
(B) skin traction; delayed application of a spica cast
(C) skeletal traction; delayed application of a spica cast
(D) skeletal traction; delayed external fixation
(E) immediate external fixation

395. For a 12-year-old girl with a displaced, closed fracture of the olecranon and no neurovascular deficit, the optimal treatment is

(A) application of an above-elbow cast with the elbow fully extended
(B) application of an above-elbow cast with the elbow flexed 90°
(C) skeletal traction
(D) open reduction and internal fixation
(E) excision of the olecranon fragment

396. A 5-year-old girl fell and sustained the injury in the figure. Her neurovascular status was normal. The optimal treatment is

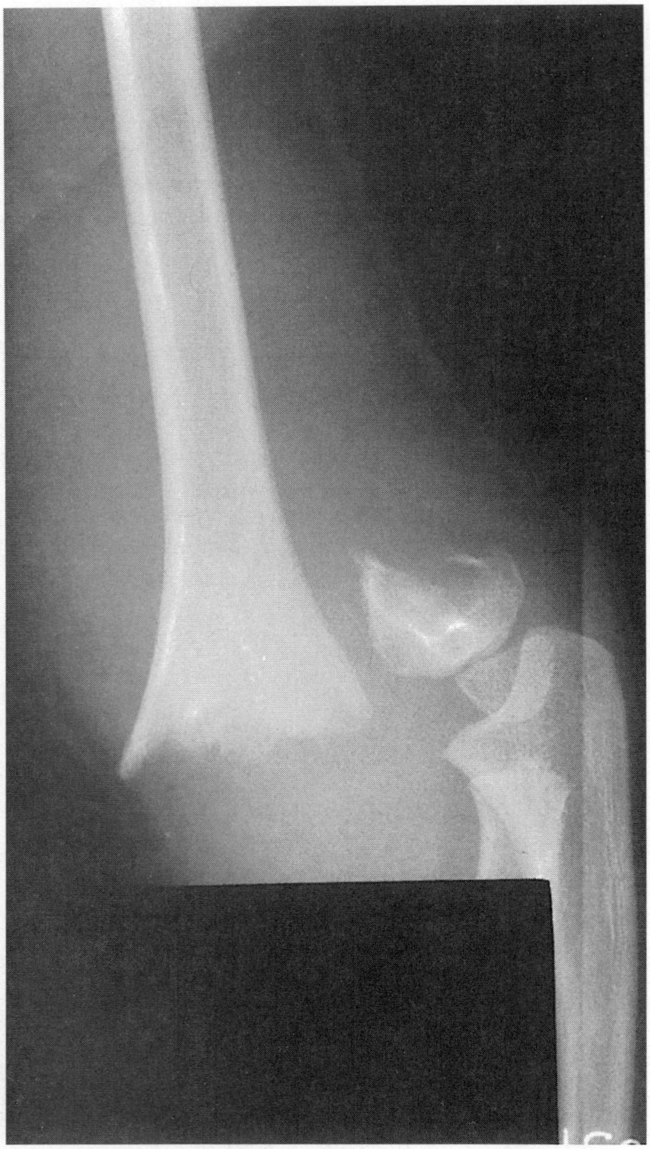

(A) application of an above-elbow cast with the elbow in 90° of flexion
(B) closed reduction; application of an above-elbow cast with the elbow in 110° of flexion
(C) closed reduction and percutaneous pinning
(D) skeletal traction
(E) open reduction and internal fixation

397. An 8-year-old boy struck from behind while running experienced pain in the left proximal thigh, was unable to bear weight, and had limited hip motion. Radiographs of the hip were normal. Six weeks after injury, he still had pain and a limp. Repeat radiographs revealed medial widening of the joint space without fracture. The most likely explanation for these findings is

(A) an early pyarthrosis of the hip
(B) an occult fracture of the femoral neck
(C) an occult injury of the physis
(D) avascular necrosis of the femoral head
(E) an intraarticular cartilaginous loose body

398. A 9-year-old boy sustained a Salter-Harris type IV fracture of the distal tibia with 5 mm of displacement. The most appropriate treatment is

(A) application of an above-knee cast
(B) closed reduction and application of an above-knee cast
(C) open reduction and application of an above-knee cast
(D) open reduction and external fixation
(E) open reduction and internal fixation

399. A 3-year-old girl sustained a greenstick fracture of the proximal tibial metaphysis in a fall. The fibula was intact. Six months following injury, she had 20° of genu valgum, compared with 10° on the contralateral side. Optimal treatment is

(A) observation
(B) a knee-ankle-foot orthosis
(C) serial casting
(D) corrective tibial osteotomy
(E) angular correction with a thin wire external fixator

400. A 13-year-old boy involved in a motor vehicle accident sustained a closed head injury, pulmonary contusion, splenic rupture, and a closed, mid-shaft fracture of the femur. The most appropriate treatment for the femoral fracture is

(A) immediate application of a spica cast
(B) skeletal traction, followed by application of a cast brace
(C) skeletal traction, followed by application of a spica cast
(D) external skeletal fixation
(E) intramedullary nailing

401. The figure is a radiograph of a 1-month-old distal radial fracture in a 6-year-old child who had been treated with a below-elbow cast. There is minimal tenderness at the fracture site. Treatment should consist of

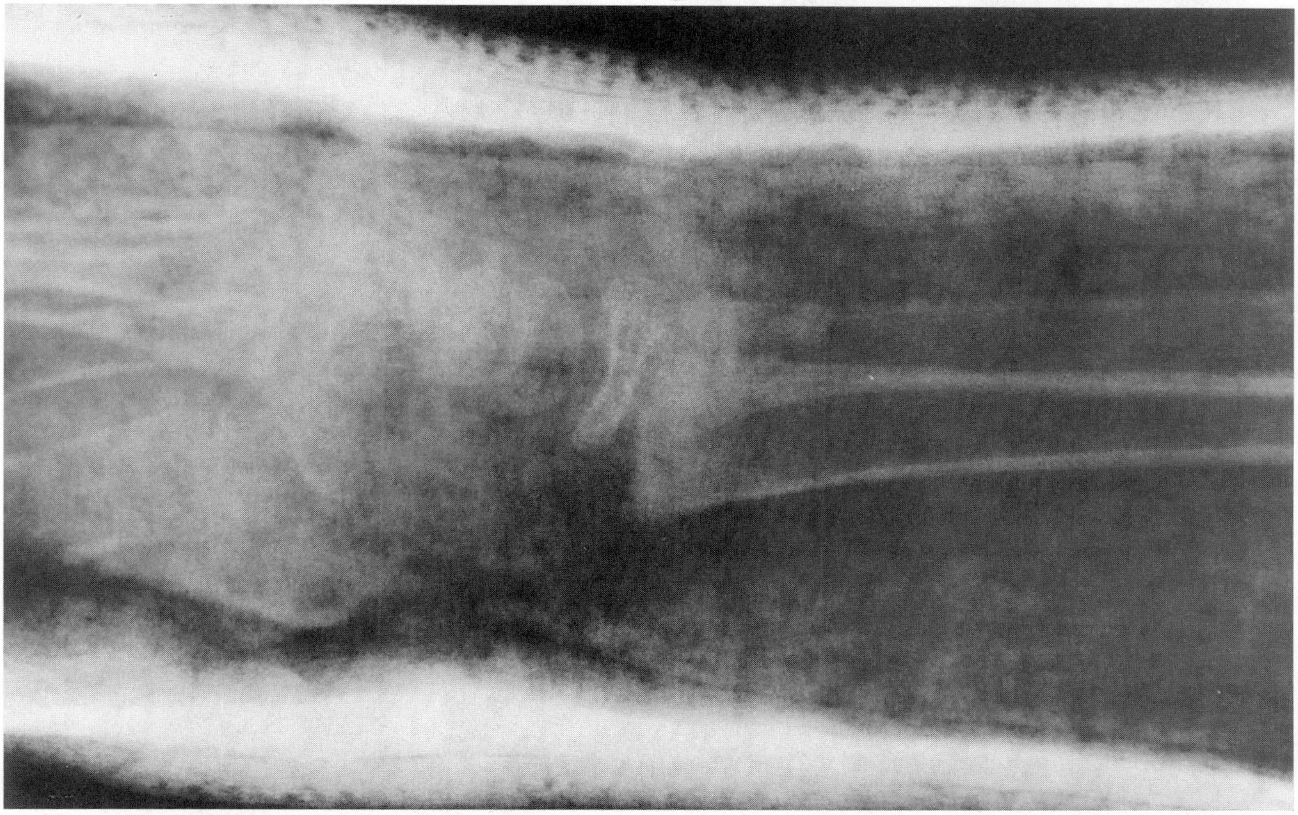

(A) reapplication of a below-elbow cast
(B) closed reduction and an above-elbow cast
(C) closed reduction and percutaneous pinning
(D) open reduction and internal fixation
(E) discontinuation of casting

402. An 11-year-old girl sustained a slipped vertebral apophysis in a fall from a height. She had weakness in great toe extension and decreased sensation over the dorsum of the foot. Recommended treatment is

(A) activity as tolerated
(B) a Jewett brace; activity as tolerated
(C) 2 weeks of bed rest, followed by activity as tolerated
(D) a body cast for 6 weeks
(E) excision of the annulus and vertebral bony margins

403. A 3-year-old girl fell, sustaining a completely displaced fracture of the distal third of the radius with plastic bowing of the ulna measuring 20°. Closed reduction was performed, and postreduction radiographs showed 50 percent apposition of the radial fracture, but the ulna was unchanged. The most appropriate treatment is

(A) immobilization in an above-elbow cast
(B) correction of the bowing of the ulna; immobilization in an above-elbow cast
(C) osteoclasis of the ulna; closed reduction of the radial fracture; immobilization in an above-elbow cast
(D) closed reduction and percutaneous fixation of the radial fracture
(E) open reduction of the radial fracture

404. A 14-year-old boy sustained a traumatic, posterior dislocation of the hip. Closed reduction was performed within 4 h of injury. After reduction, the hip could be flexed to 90° without instability, and the postoperative radiograph showed a concentric reduction without fracture. The most appropriate treatment at this time is

(A) weight-bearing as tolerated
(B) non-weight-bearing on crutches
(C) application of a hip abduction orthosis
(D) skeletal traction
(E) arthrotomy

405. The radiograph is of a 4-year-old girl who fell from a swing, injuring her arm. Her hand was cool and capillary refill time was over 5 s. The next step in the management of this injury is

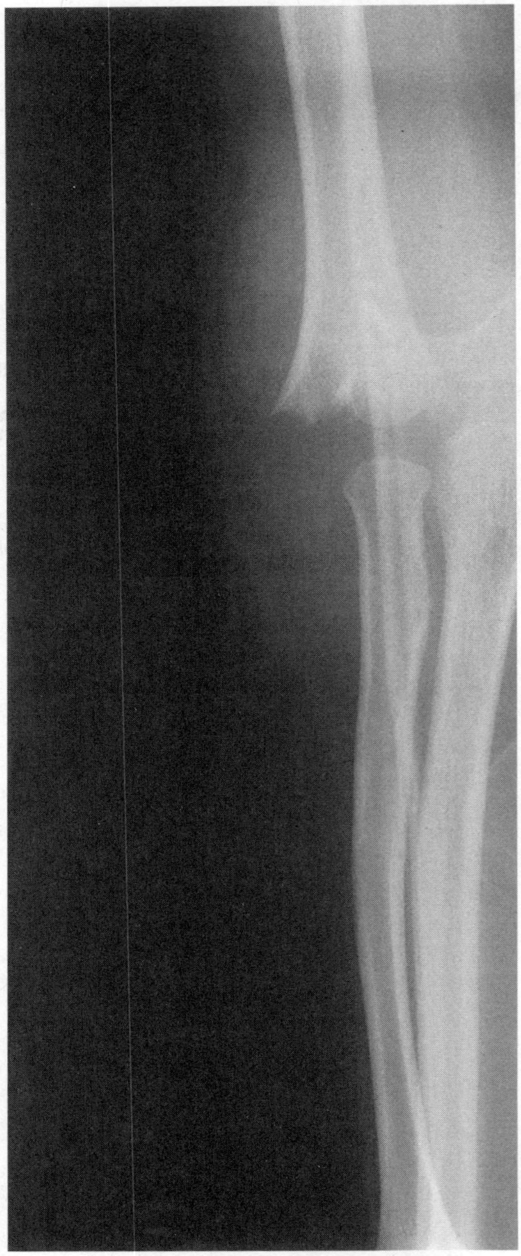

(A) arterial Doppler examination
(B) arteriography
(C) measurement of compartmental pressures
(D) immediate arterial exploration
(E) reduction of the fracture and reexamination

406. An 8-year-old boy sustained a grade II open midshaft fracture of the humerus. Findings in his neurologic examination were within normal limits. Treatment should consist of irrigation, debridement, and

(A) immobilization in a collar and cuff
(B) external skeletal fixation
(C) fixation with Kirschner wires and immobilization in an above-elbow cast
(D) open reduction and plating
(E) flexible intramedullary nailing

407. In a 13-year-old child with an angulated fracture of the tibial shaft, what is the maximum percentage of angulation that can be expected to correct spontaneously?

(A) None
(B) 25 percent
(C) 50 percent
(D) 75 percent
(E) 100 percent

408. A 12-year-old boy sustained a complete, midsubstance rupture of the anterior cruciate ligament (ACL) and an avulsion of the medial collateral ligament (MCL) from its tibial insertion. The knee is grossly unstable to valgus and anteroposterior stresses. The most appropriate treatment is

(A) application of a knee immobilizer; early knee motion
(B) application of an above-knee cast for 6 weeks; vigorous rehabilitation
(C) surgical repair of the MCL; rehabilitation for the ACL
(D) surgical repair of the MCL; intraarticular reconstruction of the ACL
(E) surgical repair of the MCL; extraarticular reconstruction of the ACL

409. The most common problem in the management of fractures of the shaft of the femur in children is

(A) stiffness of the hip and knee joints
(B) angular malunion
(C) rotational malunion
(D) delayed union
(E) anisomelia

410. The incidence of avascular necrosis of the femoral head following fractures of the femoral neck in children is most directly related to the

(A) age of the child
(B) displacement of the fracture
(C) time to treatment
(D) type of treatment
(E) location of the fracture line (physeal, transcervical, cervicotrochanteric)

411. Odontoid fractures in children start to become rare after the age of

(A) 2 years
(B) 4 years
(C) 6 years
(D) 8 years
(E) 10 years

412. The radiologic finding at the base of the fifth metatarsal in the figure is caused by

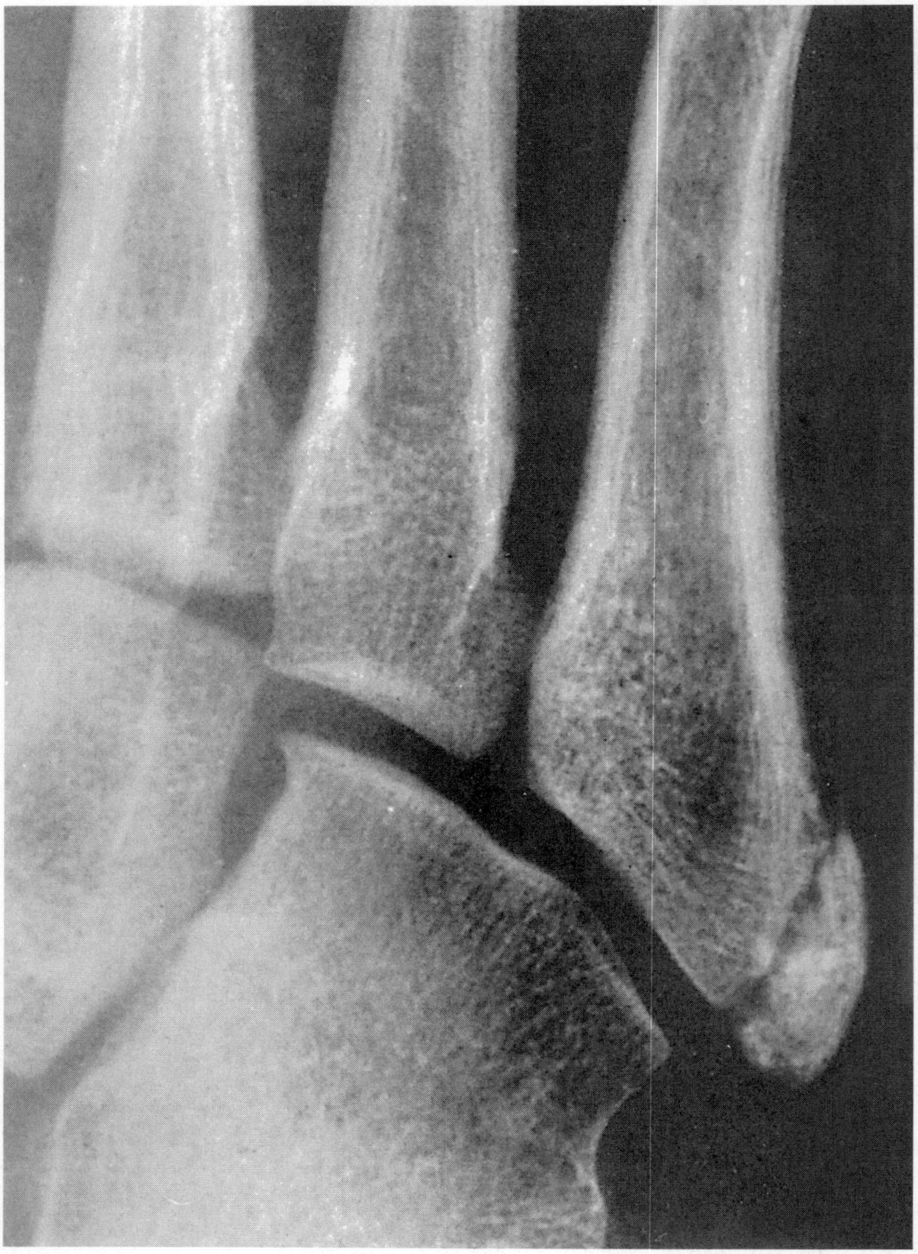

(A) avulsion of bone by the action of the peroneus brevis
(B) avulsion of bone by the action of the abductor digiti minimi
(C) avulsion of bone by the lateral cord of the plantar aponeurosis
(D) failure of bone from repeated stress
(E) normal growth of the fifth metatarsal

413. All the following statements concerning supracondylar fractures of the humerus in children are true EXCEPT that

(A) the incidence is higher in males
(B) they are the most common reason for hospitalization of children with elbow injuries
(C) they are uncommon after age 15
(D) the ulnar nerve is the most frequently injured nerve with this fracture
(E) extension-type fractures are more common than flexion-type fractures

414. Which of the following fractures in a 6-year-old boy is LEAST likely to show significant remodeling?

(A) A dorsally angulated distal radial fracture
(B) A posteriorly angulated supracondylar humeral fracture
(C) An volarly angulated distal radial fracture
(D) A supracondylar humeral fracture in varus
(E) A femoral shaft fracture

Questions 415–416

An 8-year-old girl sustained a displaced supracondylar fracture of the humerus. Her neurovascular status was normal. Closed reduction and percutaneous pinning of the fracture were performed, and the arm was immobilized with the elbow flexed 100°. Two hours later, the patient was unable to actively extend her fingers and complained of pain with passive extension of her fingers.

415. The next step in management is to

(A) remove the splint and extend the elbow
(B) measure compartmental pressure
(C) obtain venous Doppler measurements
(D) obtain an arteriogram
(E) perform fasciotomy of the forearm

416. The above patient's pain decreased and her neurovascular status returned to normal. The next day, however, she complained of the inability to flex the distal phalanges of the thumb and index finger. She had no pain with passive extension of the fingers, capillary refill was normal, and sensation was intact. The most appropriate treatment is to

(A) continue observation of the patient
(B) obtain electromyography and nerve conduction studies
(C) obtain an arteriogram
(D) measure compartmental pressures in the forearm
(E) explore the median nerve

Pediatric Trauma

Answers

342. The answer is E. *(Bernick, Clin Pediatr 9:487–491, 1980.)* To save the tooth, dental care for this patient must be immediate. The tooth should not be allowed to dry out, and ice is not necessary. The best way to preserve the tooth is to replace it promptly in the socket and refer the patient to a dentist immediately.

343. The answer is D. *(Rockwood, pp 629–642.)* Complications of fractures of the lateral condyle of the humerus include malunion, nonunion, avascular necrosis, angular deformity, and neurologic injury. Although a displaced fracture of the lateral condyle may be reduced closed, reduction is very difficult to maintain in a cast. The preferred method of treatment is open reduction and internal fixation with one or two smooth pins.

344. The answer is E. *(Dirschl, Orthop Rev 23:305–312, 1994.)* The incidence of infection following puncture wounds to the foot is 3 to 15 percent. The typical patient is seen 2 to 4 days following injury because of increasing foot pain. Laboratory studies and radiographs are generally normal. *Pseudomonas aeruginosa* is the causative organism in 95 percent of cases. Since antibiotic treatment alone does not eradicate the infection, thorough surgical debridement of necrotic tissue is necessary. Ciprofloxacin is not approved for use in children.

345. The answer is D. *(Rockwood, pp 288–290.)* Up to 1.5 percent of children in the United States are victims of abuse. Most child abuse cases involve children under 3 years of age, with another peak in incidence between 11 and 17 years of age. First-born children, premature babies, stepchildren, and handicapped children are at greater risk. Boyfriends, relatives, siblings, and step-parents are frequent abusers. Nearly half the children abused in one large series were from single-parent homes.

346. The answer is A. *(Rockwood, pp 288–293.)* Recent studies have shown rib fractures to be almost twice as prevalent as fractures of any long bone in abused children. The next most frequently fractured bone is the humerus, followed by the femur and tibia. Skull fractures are slightly less common. Rib fractures occur most often near the transverse process of the vertebrae and may be difficult to diagnose because of the lack of displacement.

347. The answer is B. *(Rockwood, pp 1151–1153.)* Isolated, closed femoral shaft fractures in children under 10 years of age are best managed by immediate closed reduction and application of a spica cast. Exceptions to this rule include fractures with excessive shortening (over 2 cm), patients with multiple injuries, and patients with an unreliable family situation. Skeletal traction is used for older children or for younger children with significant shortening. Surgery is usually reserved for older patients, especially those with multiple injuries.

348. The answer is C. *(Browner, pp 137–139.)* Resuscitation of the trauma patient, pediatric or adult, begins with isotonic crystalloid solution, preferably lactated Ringer's. The initial bolus for a pediatric patient is 30 mL/kg. The patient's response determines further fluid replacement. Continued tachycardia and hypotension following the initial fluid bolus are signs of sufficient hemorrhage to require blood replacement.

349. The answer is D. *(Rockwood, pp 1–5.)* Fractures are more common in children than in adults and more likely to occur after seemingly insignificant trauma. Physeal disruptions constitute approximately 15 percent of all skeletal injuries in children and may result in disturbances of growth. Salter I fractures are more common in infants than in older children. Although the periosteum is thicker and less likely to be completely disrupted in children, it is more easily elevated from the bone in a fracture.

350. The answer is C. *(Rockwood, pp 2–5.)* Fractures heal rapidly in children in part because of thickened, osteogenic periosteum and the abundant blood supply within the developing bone. They heal more rapidly during early childhood than in adolescence. Fractures may stimulate longitudinal growth by increasing blood supply to the physis. Nonunion can occur but is extremely infrequent in children. Injuries to the physis heal in approximately half the time required for union of fractures through the metaphysis or diaphysis.

351. The answer is E. *(Rockwood, pp 61–62.)* Children's fractures do not always remodel, but the remodeling capacity is greater the younger the patient. As the fracture site approaches the physis, the capacity for remodeling increases. The amount of remodeling also varies directly with the degree of angular deformity. There is little remodeling of rotational deformities.

352. The answer is C. *(Cantu, Phys Sports Med 14:76, 1986.)* This patient has a Cantu grade 2 concussion, for which recommended treatment includes withdrawing the athlete from activities for 1 month. Symptoms such as headache, lack of concentration, inability to sleep, or loss of appetite may require further investigation and prolonged restriction from athletic activities.

353. The answer is D. *(Rockwood, pp 153–155.)* There are three types of partial growth arrest: type I, peripheral; type II, central; and type III, combined. Not infrequently, a central lesion becomes apparent after longitudinal growth has resumed because there is tenting of the physis with the apex pointing into the metaphysis. Although hypocycloidal motion tomography at 3-mm intervals has been used for evaluating a suspected partial growth arrest, CT is currently the best imaging modality to confirm a central growth arrest.

354. The answer is B. *(Rockwood, pp 282–285.)* Birth fractures are uncommon, but 75 percent occur in association with breech delivery. Although 92 percent of birth injuries are clavicular fractures, these injuries involve the diaphysis of the bone rather than the epiphysis. The most common sites of epiphyseal injury with birth trauma, in order of decreasing frequency, are the proximal humerus, distal femur, distal humerus, proximal femur, and distal tibia. These fractures may be difficult to identify on plain radiographs, and a week may pass before the fracture can be recognized by the appearance of fracture callus.

355. The answer is C. *(Rockwood, p 321.)* Crushing injury, such as trapping the digit in a door, accounts for the majority of hand fractures in toddlers. Play and sports activities cause most hand fractures and dislocations in slightly older children; in adults, industrial accidents account for the majority. Motor vehicle accidents cause a very small percentage of these fractures in children.

356. The answer is C. *(Rockwood, pp 324–326.)* A hyperflexion force applied to the end of the digit in a preadolescent child is the usual cause of an open Salter type I or II injury. The epiphysis is held in place by the extensor tendon, while the remainder of the phalanx is acutely flexed by the unopposed action of the flexor profundus. Although the open nature of this injury is easily missed, infection is rare. The most common complication of this injury is deformity resulting from tendon imbalance, followed closely by deformity of the nail. Nonunion and growth arrest occur rarely.

357. The answer is D. *(Rockwood, pp 335–341.)* Anatomic reduction of this fracture is important, since the absence of a physis at this end of the phalanx limits remodeling. Closed reduction is usually successful, but maintaining the reduction in a splint is exceedingly difficult. Percutaneous Kirschner wire fixation through the proximal interphalangeal joint is recommended.

358. The answer is C. *(Rockwood, pp 359–361.)* Although dislocations in the hands of children are uncommon because the physes are generally weaker than the capsular and ligamentous structures, the metacarpophalangeal joint is the most commonly dislocated joint. Dislocation of the proximal interphalangeal joint is second in frequency, followed distantly by dislocation of the distal interphalangeal joint.

359. The answer is C. *(Rockwood, pp 372–374.)* The thick cartilage imparts resilience to the carpal bones of the child and makes fractures of the scaphoid uncommon when compared with an adult. Fractures of the proximal pole are almost never seen in the child, and displaced fractures are rare. The distal pole, rather than the waist, is the most common site of fracture in the child.

360. The answer is A. *(Rockwood, pp 378–380.)* Anatomic reduction of acute fractures of the distal radius in children is desirable, but repeated manipulation of physeal fractures is not recommended because of the increased risk of growth disturbance. When more than 10 days have passed since injury, manipulation of the fracture is neither advisable nor, usually, possible. Forceful attempts at reduction are likely to damage the physis and result in growth arrest. Satisfactory remodeling of this fracture may be expected in 5 to 8 months.

361. The answer is A. *(Rockwood, pp 418–420.)* An important goal in the treatment of forearm fractures is restoration of full forearm rotation. Thus, rotational deformity must be corrected, since remodeling will not correct rotational malunions. The bicipital tuberosity is a guide to the rotation of the proximal fragment of the fractured radius. In full supination, the bicipital tuberosity is medial, in full pronation, it is lateral, and in the mid position, it lies posteriorly. This knowledge is critical for obtaining correct rotational alignment of the fracture fragments.

362. The answer is D. *(Rockwood, pp 424–435.)* In a greenstick fracture, one cortex is completely fractured and the other undergoes plastic deformation, which results in angulation or rotation of the bone or both. Angular deformity is more likely to recur following greenstick than complete fractures, but the incidence of growth arrest is no different between the two.

363. The answer is A. *(Rockwood, pp 463–465.)* A type II Monteggia lesion consists of a fracture of the proximal or middle third of the ulna with posterior dislocation of the radial head. After reduction by longitudinal traction with the elbow extended, the arm is immobilized in this position to maintain the reduction.

364. The answer is C. *(Rockwood, pp 527–528.)* Eighty-five percent of supracondylar fractures of the humerus are seen in children below the age of 10. The incidence, which increases during the first 5 years of life, peaks at 5 to 8 years. These fractures are extremely rare after age 15.

365. The answer is B. *(Roge, J Neurosurg 68:25–30, 1988.)* This child has a spinal cord injury without radiographic abnormality, a syndrome unique to children under 8 years of age. The injury occurs most commonly when children are in forward-facing car seats, rather than in rear-facing car seats. Children under 3 rarely recover neurologic function. A rigid collar is used for immobilization.

366. The answer is C. *(Rockwood, pp 575–576.)* The absolute indications for operative intervention for supracondylar fractures of the humerus are (1) an open fracture and (2) vascular compromise that is unrelieved by closed reduction. The presence of a neurologic deficit is not an absolute indication for surgical intervention. Although the inability to obtain an adequate closed reduction is a relative indication for operative management, marked displacement of the fracture is not, by itself, an indication. Massive swelling is a relative contraindication to operative management, and the quality of the reduction rather than the age of the child determines whether or not operative management is indicated.

367. The answer is D. *(Rockwood, pp 623–626.)* The fracture line in this injury commonly extends through the physis medial to the growth center of the lateral condyle and enters the joint, which disrupts the lateral crista of the trochlea and renders the elbow joint unstable. This allows posterolateral subluxation of the proximal radius and ulna on the distal humerus.

368. The answer is D. *(Rockwood, pp 642–647.)* Up to 40 percent of fractures of the lateral condyle heal with cubitus varus angulation, but this deformity is rarely sufficient to require treatment. Cubitus valgus, although seen, is much less common than cubitus varus. Spur formation on the lateral condyle is one of the most common late deformities and may cause apparent cubitus varus. Avascular necrosis of the lateral part of the medial crista of the trochlea is a source of "fishtail" deformity. Central growth arrest of the distal humeral physis has not been reported following fractures of the lateral condyle.

369. The answer is A. *(Rockwood, pp 676–678.)* Fractures involving the entire distal humeral physis are rare and often difficult to diagnose. The only radiographic finding may be posteromedial translation of the proximal radius and ulna relative to the distal humerus. For acute fractures, closed reduction followed by cast immobilization (in the infant) or percutaneous pinning (in the child) may be performed. If the fracture is more than 5 to 6 days old, manipulation increases the risk of avascular necrosis. The arm should be immobilized with the expectation of complete remodeling. Very few children will require an osteotomy at an older age.

370. The answer is D. *(Rockwood, pp 699–703.)* Fractures involving the epicondylar apophyses have a peak incidence at a later age than fractures of the supracondylar region. They are more common in boys than in girls, are associated with an elbow dislocation in up to 50 percent of cases, and rarely cause growth disturbances. If the fractured epicondyle is incarcerated within the joint, it should be removed promptly, since late removal of incarcerated fragments has not been associated with good results. Operative fixation of nondisplaced or minimally displaced fractures is unnecessary; in fact, the outcome may be compromised by internal fixation.

371. The answer is A. *(Rockwood, pp 740–748.)* In uncomplicated fractures of the radial neck with up to 60° of angulation, a satisfactory result can usually be achieved by closed reduction. In the young child, anatomic reduction need not be obtained, as up to 45° of residual angulation is tolerated without significant loss of function. Repeated manipulation is usually no more successful than the initial attempt. One method for testing the adequacy of closed reduction is to test the range of supination and pronation of the forearm. If it is at least 60° in both directions, the reduction is adequate regardless of the radiographic appearance.

372. The answer is A. *(Rockwood, p 837.)* Open reduction and internal fixation (ORIF) of humeral shaft fractures in children carries a higher complication rate than does nonoperative treatment. Indications for ORIF include multiple injuries, head injury, vascular injury, and fractures of the ipsilateral forearm. An open fracture is not an indication for open reduction and internal fixation; it should be treated by aggressive irrigation and debridement, without internal fixation or primary closure of the wound.

373. The answer is A. *(Rockwood, pp 846–851.)* Approximately 80 percent of the longitudinal growth of the humerus occurs at the proximal humeral physis; therefore, there is tremendous potential for remodeling of fractures in this region. With 50 percent apposition and 45° of angulation, an excellent result may be anticipated. This patient's fracture meets these criteria and may be treated in a sling and swathe. Treatment options for more displaced fractures include closed reduction and immobilization or percutaneous pinning. Open reduction is rarely required.

374. The answer is A. *(Rockwood, pp 929–930.)* One of the most frequently overinterpreted findings on radiographs of the cervical spine in children is hypermobility of C2 on C3. Pseudosubluxation of C2 on C3 occurs in 40 percent of children under 8 years of age. A negative history of injury and the absence of neck pain or limited motion are key data to avoid inappropriate treatment of a normal radiographic variant.

375. The answer is C. *(Rockwood, pp 941–944.)* The AP radiograph may be of little value in the diagnosis of a fractured odontoid in a child, as the fracture is often seen only on the lateral view. Anterior displacement with posterior tilting of the odontoid is usually present; however, the odontoid tilts posteriorly in 4 percent of normal children. The rarity of complications and the favorable outcome in young children are in contrast with the results following this fracture in adults.

376. The answer is C. *(Rockwood, pp 969–970.)* The child with spinal cord injury can be expected to have the same problems as the paraplegic adult: increased susceptibility to fractures of long bones, dislocations of the hip, decubiti, and genitourinary complications. In addition, 86 to 100 percent of paraplegic children will develop progressive spinal deformity, which may eventually overshadow the effects of the original injury.

377. The answer is D. *(Rockwood, pp 1057–1063.)* Transcervical fractures account for most fractures of the hip in children. The rate of avascular necrosis is directly related to the amount of fracture displacement, which may increase in traction or a hip spica cast. Closed reduction of displaced fractures, followed by fixation with pins or screws, is recommended. Preferably, the fixation devices should not cross the physis.

378. The answer is D. *(Rockwood, p 921.)* Children under the age of 8 years have a higher incidence of injury to the upper cervical spine than the adolescent or adult. About 25 percent of children with an injury to the cervical spine have multiple-level injury. When the diagnosis of a cervical spine injury is made in a child, careful examination of the remaining cervical spine should be performed.

379. The answer is D. *(Rockwood, pp 1140–1143.)* Tibial pin traction in children in inappropriate because the pin may damage the proximal tibial physis, and traction through the knee may aggravate soft-tissue injury. Femoral pin traction is less likely to damage the physis. The pin should be inserted with the knee in 90° of flexion to allow the iliotibial band to slip behind the lateral femoral condyle. If the pin is inserted with the knee in extension, the iliotibial band lies anterior to the pin, which will limit knee flexion.

380. The answer is C. *(Sullivan, p 149.)* The valgus forces generated during the acceleration phase of pitching result in tension on the medial side of the elbow and compression on the lateral side. Hypertrophy of the medial epicondyle, microscopic tears of the flexor-pronator muscles, fragmentation of the medial epicondylar apophysis, and avulsion fractures of the medial epicondyle have been described in children. Attenuation or tearing of the ulnar collateral ligament occurs in adults but not in children, in whom the medial epicondyle fractures instead.

381. The answer is B. *(Rockwood, pp 1206–1216.)* Avulsion of the tibial tubercle is uncommon, occurs primarily in males between the ages of 14 and 16 years, and may be preceded by the Osgood-Schlatter lesion. The degree of displacement indicates that the extensor mechanism has been completely disrupted. Because successful closed reduction of this lesion is unlikely, open reduction and internal fixation is indicated. The prognosis for return to full athletic activity is excellent.

382. The answer is A. *(Rockwood, pp 1251–1253.)* Operative reconstruction of the ACL in a young child is best avoided unless the knee is extremely unstable after a trial of nonoperative treatment. If operative treatment is necessary in an adolescent with a skeletal age of less than 14 years, an extraarticular tenodesis may be expected to prevent significant pivot shift and protect the menisci during the remaining period of growth. Intraarticular reconstruction may be performed if needed at skeletal maturity.

383. The answer is D. *(Sullivan, p 147.)* Recurrent traumatic dislocation of the shoulder is a problem in young patients, in whom the recurrence rate within 5 years is roughly 80 percent. There is evidence that prolonged immobilization after the initial dislocation reduces the likelihood of recurrence.

384. The answer is A. *(Rockwood, pp 1254–1255.)* Traumatic dislocation of the knee in children is rare because the force necessary to produce dislocation is more likely to produce a fracture of the distal femur or proximal tibia. Dislocations of the knee in children are usually anterior and are commonly associated with multiple trauma. Dislocations of the knee in adults are more commonly posterior.

385. The answer is B. *(Rockwood, pp 1277–1281.)* In the treatment of complete fractures of the tibia and fibula in children, the greatest challenge is often maintaining adequate length. One should strive for anatomic length in boys over 10 and in girls over 8 years of age. The amount of shortening that may be accepted immediately after closed reduction of a tibial fracture is 10 mm in children from 1 to 5 years of age and 5 mm in children between 5 and 10.

386. The answer is C. *(Sullivan, p 145.)* The incidence of major head or spinal cord injury is low in children under 15 years of age but increases significantly in those 15 to 18 years of age. Most injuries of the spinal cord in children result from motor vehicle accidents (38 percent), falls or jumps (16 percent), and gunshot wounds (13 percent). Diving is the only sport responsible for a significant number of spinal cord injuries (9 percent). Football, ice hockey, gymnastics, and trampoline injuries each accounts for approximately 1 percent of all cord injuries.

387. The answer is D. *(Rockwood, pp 1298–1302.)* The only clinical signs of fracture in a paraplegic child may be swelling and warmth in the affected area. Bone formation occurs rapidly in these children, making nonunion and delayed union rare. Most fractures in paraplegic children are nondisplaced, so malunion is also uncommon. The most common complications are pressure sores produced by ill-padded casts or splints. Immobilization should consist of a bulky dressing or a well-padded splint or cast for 2 to 4 weeks.

388. The answer is D. *(Rockwood, pp 1302–1305.)* The most common sequela of a fracture of the proximal tibial metaphysis in a child is a valgus deformity, which usually results from unrecognized valgus angulation at the time of casting combined with compression and slowing of growth in the lateral portion of the physis of the proximal tibia. Because the child holds the injured leg in a flexed position, the valgus deformity may not be apparent initially.

389. The answer is C. *(Rockwood, pp 1436–1438.)* The most common site for stress fractures in children is the tibia, followed by the fibula. Only 2 percent of stress fractures involve the tarsals or metatarsals, and stress fractures of the talus and proximal femur are equally uncommon.

390. The answer is E. *(Rockwood, pp 1440–1441.)* Over 10,000 lawn mower injuries to children are reported annually. Closure by secondary intention and split thickness skin grafting does not provide adequate coverage for exposed extensor tendons, and a soleus muscle flap will not reach the dorsum of the foot. The free flap has replaced the cumbersome cross-leg pedicle flap as the method of choice for treating soft-tissue defects on the dorsum of the foot.

391. The answer is D. *(Rockwood, pp 1358–1363.)* The figure shows a triplane fracture of the distal tibia that appears to be nondisplaced. Since the fracture is intraarticular, anatomic reduction should be obtained. The accuracy of reduction of the articular surface should be assessed with tomograms or a CT scan. If the joint surface is anatomically reduced, immobilization in an above-knee cast is appropriate; otherwise, open reduction and internal fixation is indicated.

392. The answer is C. *(Rockwood, pp 1145–1146, 1150–1151.)* Acceptable alignment of femoral shaft fractures in children can nearly always be achieved through nonoperative means. The amount of angulation that may be accepted is controversial; as a rule, however, angulation exceeding 15° in the frontal plane and 20° in the sagittal plane should be avoided. External skeletal fixation is easily applied, ensures good fracture alignment, and allows mobilization of the patient. Intramedullary fixation may cause avascular necrosis, and plate fixation involves extensive dissection.

393. The answer is A. *(Rockwood, pp 630–635.)* The figure shows a nondisplaced fracture of the lateral humeral condyle. When displaced less than 2 mm, lateral condylar fractures can be treated by immobilization alone, provided rotational deformity is not present. Displacement of the fracture can occur in the cast, so serial radiographs should be obtained early in the treatment period.

394. The answer is A. *(Rockwood, pp 1151–1153.)* In children 2 to 5 years of age, fractures of the femoral shaft are best treated by immediate application of a spica cast. Contraindications to immediate casting include fractures having a propensity for excessive shortening and patients with multiple injuries or a poor family situation.

395. The answer is D. *(Rockwood, pp 766–772.)* Displaced fractures of the olecranon require anatomic reduction of the articular surface, which is best achieved by open reduction and internal fixation. Cast immobilization alone will not restore articular alignment, and skeletal traction will usually not maintain anatomic alignment. Excision of the olecranon is rarely indicated in the growing child.

396. The answer is C. *(Pirone, J Bone Joint Surg 70-A:641–650, 1988.)* Displaced extension-type supracondylar fractures of the humerus in children are best managed by closed reduction and percutaneous Kirschner wire fixation. Skeletal traction is preferred in the presence of a compromised or extremely swollen soft-tissue envelope. Open reduction and internal fixation are indicated if acceptable alignment is not achieved by closed means or if there is an associated vascular injury requiring surgical repair.

397. The answer is E. *(Caudle, J Bone Joint Surg 70-A:1568–1570, 1988.)* Traumatic dislocation of the hip with spontaneous relocation occurs in children 10 years of age and younger. Portions of the articular cartilage or the secondary ossification centers of the acetabulum, which do not begin to ossify until after 8 years of age, may be entrapped in the joint, causing widening of the medial joint space.

398. The answer is E. *(Rockwood, p 1366.)* A Salter-Harris type IV fracture of the distal tibia usually results from inversion of the ankle. The incidence of premature closure of the medial portion of the distal tibial physis is high following this injury. Anatomic alignment of the articular surface is desirable, and open reduction and fixation with smooth Kirschner wires or cancellous screws is the most appropriate treatment for this injury. Care should be taken that fixation devices do not cross the physis.

399. The answer is A. *(Rockwood, pp 1302–1308.)* Greenstick fractures of the proximal tibial metaphysis frequently result in overgrowth of the medial portion of the proximal tibial physis, causing genu valgum. The genu valgum usually resolves with further growth; only deformities greater than 20° should be considered for surgical correction.

400. The answer is E. *(Rockwood, pp 1150–1153.)* The amount of growth remaining in the greater trochanter is negligible in the child over 12 years of age. Therefore, intramedullary nailing of the femoral shaft fracture in this patient is appropriate. Early stabilization of long-bone fractures in multiply-injured patients is highly desirable.

401. The answer is A. *(Rockwood, pp 396–399.)* One month following a distal radial fracture, significant healing will have taken place, and closed manipulation will not be possible. The distal radial and ulnar physes contribute up to 80 percent of the growth of the forearm, and the excellent potential for remodeling makes surgical correction unnecessary. Because the fracture site is still tender, continued immobilization is recommended.

402. The answer is E. *(Rockwood, pp 961–962.)* Neurologic symptoms resulting from a slipped vertebral apophysis usually do not respond to conservative therapy. Because the disk is not degenerated or herniated, simple disk excision will not decompress the nerve roots. Excision of the annulus and any bone protruding into the spinal canal is necessary.

403. The answer is A. *(Rockwood, pp 451–453.)* Correction of ulnar bowing is not necessary in a child under 4 years of age because remodeling will correct the deformity within 6 to 12 months. Older children may have a loss of forearm rotation if the bowing is not reduced. An above-elbow cast is necessary to prevent recurrent displacement of the radial fracture.

404. The answer is B. *(Rockwood, pp 1111–1116.)* If a congruent and stable reduction of a simple posterior dislocation of the hip is achieved, arthrotomy, skeletal traction, and bracing are unnecessary. Controversy exists as to whether patients should be allowed immediate motion or kept in traction for a short period following reduction. The majority view, however, is that patients should be kept non-weight-bearing on crutches for 3 to 4 weeks.

405. The answer is E. *(Rockwood, pp 591–594.)* Vascular compromise following supracondylar fractures of the humerus in children occurs in about 5 percent of cases. Fractures with posterolateral displacement are particularly susceptible to vascular injury. If the circulation to the hand is not restored by closed reduction of the fracture, arterial exploration is indicated. Arteriography and arterial Doppler studies only delay the restoration of blood flow to the limb.

406. The answer is A. *(Rockwood, p 837.)* Open fractures of the humerus in children require early aggressive irrigation and debridement, appropriate antibiotic coverage, and delayed wound closure. An open humeral fracture in a child is not, in itself, an indication for open reduction and internal fixation. A collar and cuff supplemented with a swathe is the most appropriate treatment.

407. The answer is B. *(Rockwood, pp 1286–1288.)* Spontaneous correction of axial malalignment following diaphyseal fractures of the tibia in children does not occur as readily as following fractures of the forearm or femur. In children 9 to 12 years old, up to 50 percent of the angulation will remodel, but in children over 12, 25 percent or less will correct spontaneously.

408. The answer is C. *(Rockwood, pp 1252–1253.)* The combination of MCL and ACL injuries is fairly common in the older adolescent. If the MCL is torn in its midsubstance or avulsed from its tibial insertion, operative repair is indicated. If the MCL is avulsed from its femoral origin, 6 weeks in a cast brace followed by vigorous rehabilitation is usually adequate treatment. Reconstruction of the ACL is performed only if symptomatic instability follows rehabilitation.

409. The answer is E. *(Rockwood, pp 1155–1158.)* Goals in the treatment of fractures of the femoral shaft in children are union with adequate alignment and femoral lengths within 1 cm of each other. Inequality of leg length (anisomelia) is the most common complication of femoral shaft fractures in children; discrepancies of over 2 cm are noticeable to both the family and the child. Angular malunion occurs frequently, but remodeling lessens this deformity. Rotational malunion, delayed union, and joint stiffness are uncommon.

410. The answer is B. *(Rockwood, pp 1073–1079.)* Avascular necrosis is the most common and most devastating complication following hip fractures in children. Although avascular necrosis may occur following nondisplaced fractures, 26 of the 27 patients who developed avascular necrosis in one series had displaced fractures. The incidence of avascular necrosis is more directly related to the initial displacement of the fracture than to the age of the child, type of treatment, delay until treatment, or location of the fracture line.

411. The answer is C. *(Rockwood, p 941.)* Fractures of the odontoid are the most common cervical injuries in children, occurring at an average age of 4 years. These fractures are, in reality, growth plate injuries at the base of the odontoid process. The cartilage line at the base of the odontoid has the histologic appearance of a synchondrosis rather than a physis; and it closes much earlier than a physis, fusing to the body of the axis by 6 years of age. Fractures of the odontoid in children are rare after the age of 6.

412. The answer is E. *(Rockwood, pp 1428–1432.)* Avulsion fractures of the base of the fifth metatarsal are common in children and must be differentiated from the apophyseal growth center at the base of the fifth metatarsal. The long axis of the apophysis is parallel to the shaft of the metatarsal, is not present before age 8, and is usually united to the shaft by age 12 to 15. Avulsion fractures of the base of the fifth metatarsal are perpendicular to the shaft of the metatarsal.

413. The answer is D. *(Rockwood, pp 527–530.)* Males sustain almost twice as many supracondylar fractures as females. Two-thirds of children hospitalized with elbow injuries have supracondylar fractures, yet these injuries are rare after age 15. Ninety-eight percent of supracondylar fractures are caused by extension injuries. The radial nerve is the most frequently injured nerve, accounting for 41 percent of all nerve palsies with this fracture, followed by the median nerve (36 percent) and the ulnar nerve (22 percent).

414. The answer is D. *(Rockwood, p 61.)* Remodeling is greatest when a fracture is near the physis, and when the deformity is in the plane of motion of the joint. It is minimal when the angulation is at right angles to the plane of motion of the joint, as in varus angulation of a supracondylar fracture. Remodeling in the diaphysis is largely a process of rounding off the angularity of the bone, so significant remodeling potential exists for a femoral shaft fracture in a 6-year-old patient.

415. The answer is A. *(Perone, J Bone Joint Surg 70-A:641–650, 1988.)* Supracondylar fractures of the humerus can be associated with extensive soft-tissue swelling that compromises circulation. Flexion of the elbow beyond 90° increases circulatory compromise. The next step in the management of this patient is to remove the splint, extend the elbow, and reevaluate the vascular status with the elbow extended.

416. The answer is A. *(Perone, J Bone Joint Surg 70-A:641–650, 1988.)* Injury to the anterior interosseous nerve is one of the most common neural injuries seen with supracondylar fractures of the humerus. It results in paralysis of the flexor digitorum profundus to the index finger and the flexor pollicis longus. No sensory deficit is detectable. This injury is usually a neuropraxia that will recover spontaneously.

Adult Diseases and Disorders: Upper Limb

Frank C. Wilson, M.D., and
Donald K. Bynum, M.D.

DIRECTIONS: Each question below contains five suggested responses. Select the **one best** response to each question.

417. Rupture of the extensor digiti quinti proprius (extensor digiti minimi) occurs most often as a result of

(A) DeQuervain's tenosynovitis
(B) carpal bossing
(C) osteoarthritic carpal spurring
(D) prominence of the ulnar styloid
(E) rheumatoid arthritis

418. In an intrinsic minus deformity, or clawhand, all the following are present EXCEPT

(A) decreased grip strength
(B) negative Froment's sign
(C) weakness of abduction and adduction of the fingers
(D) flattening of the metacarpal arch
(E) hyperextension of the metacarpophalangeal joints

419. A positive Bunnell test is seen most often in association with which of the following finger deformities?

(A) Intrinsic minus
(B) Intrinsic plus
(C) Lumbrical plus
(D) Swan-neck
(E) Boutonnière

420. Which of the following findings is most characteristic of the anterior interosseous syndrome?

(A) Weakness of the palmaris longus
(B) Weakness of the flexor carpi radialis longus
(C) Loss of precise pinch
(D) Sensory deficit over the base of the palm
(E) Sensory deficit in the volar forearm

421. Scapholunate advanced collapse (SLAC) typically involves all the following areas EXCEPT the

(A) radiolunate joint
(B) radial styloid
(C) radioscaphoid joint
(D) capitolunate joint
(E) scaphocapitate joint

422. For a middle-aged, right-handed man with rheumatoid arthritis, a disabling boutonnière deformity of the right index finger, and an extension contracture of the DIP joint, optimal treatment would be

(A) release of the lateral bands distal to the DIP joint
(B) silicone arthroplasty of the PIP joint
(C) reconstruction of the lateral bands distal to the DIP joint
(D) reconstruction of the lateral bands proximal to the PIP joint
(E) arthrodesis of the PIP joint in 25 to 30° of flexion

423. A 46-year-old man with mild diabetes mellitus developed Dupuytren's disease in his dominant right hand. There were 30° fixed flexion deformities of the MCP joints in the long, ring, and little fingers and 10° flexion contractures of the PIP joints in the same digits. The optimal treatment would be

(A) injection of painful, prominent nodules with corticosteroids
(B) subcutaneous fasciotomy of the involved digits
(C) excision of palmar nodules with Z-plasty closure
(D) subtotal palmar fasciectomy
(E) total palmar fasciectomy

424. In a patient suspected of having suppurative flexor tenosynovitis of the thumb, which of the following signs is LEAST likely to be present?

(A) Pain on passive extension of the thumb
(B) Slight flexion of the interphalangeal joint
(C) Marked tenderness over the volar aspect of the thumb and thenar area
(D) Symmetric swelling of the thumb
(E) "Pointing" of the infection at the insertion of the flexor pollicis longus

425. Dupuytren's disease commonly involves all the following structures in the hand EXCEPT

(A) the palmar aponeurosis
(B) Cleland's ligament
(C) Grayson's ligament
(D) the pretendinous bands
(E) the natatory ligaments

426. A 42-year-old woman with rheumatoid arthritis (RA) had persistent elbow pain and motion limited to 20 to 115°. The radiographic appearance of the joint is shown below. The most appropriate treatment is

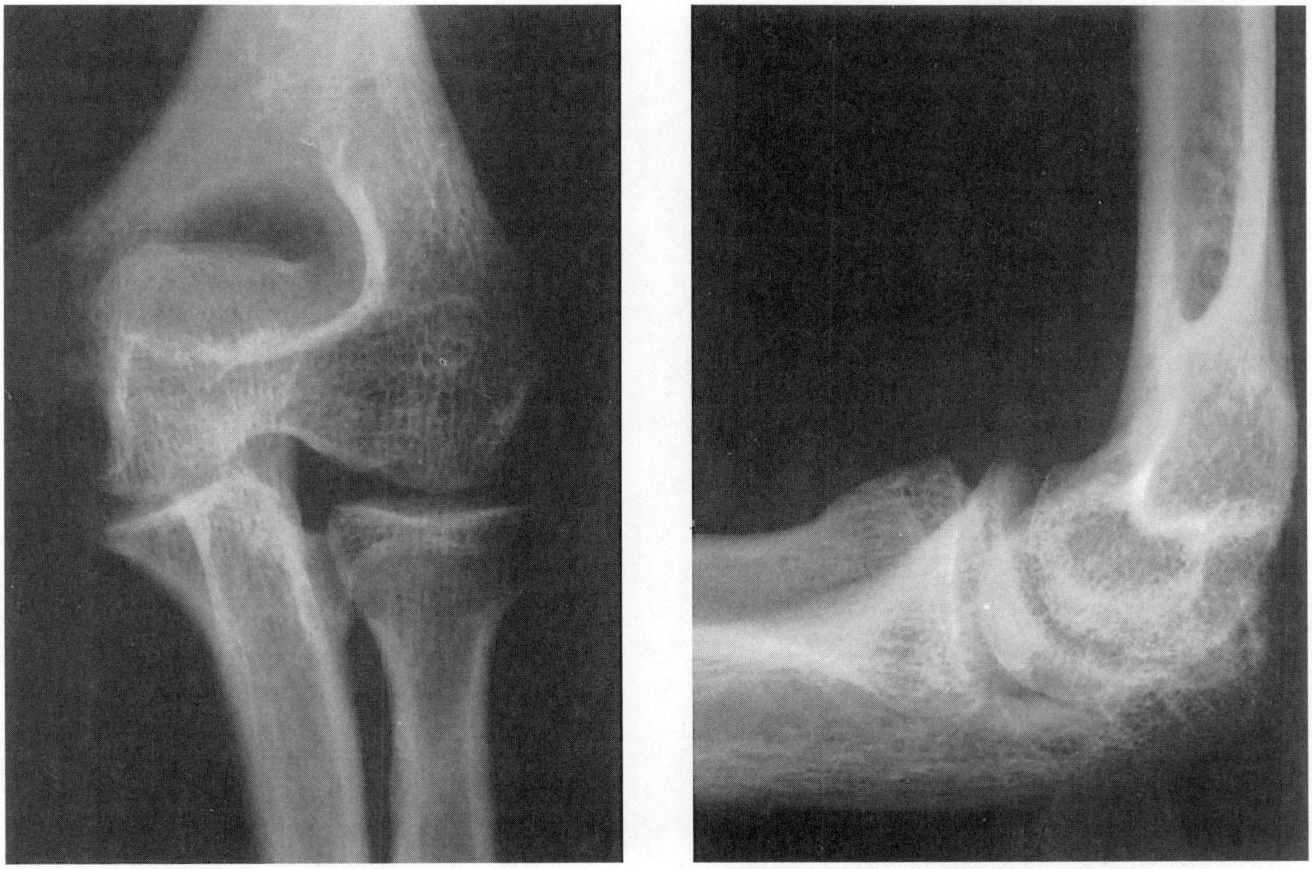

(A) synovectomy
(B) synovectomy with radial head excision
(C) semiconstrained total elbow arthroplasty
(D) excisional arthroplasty with silastic interposition
(E) arthrodesis of the humeroulnar joint

427. Which of the following is a risk factor for the development of adhesive capsulitis of the glenohumeral joint?

(A) Advanced age (over 65)
(B) Male sex
(C) Hyperthyroidism
(D) Ipsilateral Colles' fracture
(E) Ipsilateral rotator cuff tear

428. The most frequent late complication of non-constrained total shoulder arthroplasty is

(A) loosening of the humeral component
(B) fracture of the humerus at the tip of the humeral stem
(C) loosening of the glenoidal component
(D) deep infection
(E) dislocation of the prosthetic joint

429. Glenohumeral replacement is most successful in patients with

(A) rheumatoid arthritis
(B) posttraumatic arthritis
(C) osteoarthritis
(D) postinfectious arthritis
(E) cuff-tear arthropathy

430. A 34-year-old lawyer had 3 months of activity-related pain in the anterolateral aspect of her dominant shoulder. There was no history of trauma. The pain was increased by flexion of the internally rotated shoulder. The next step in management should be

(A) instillation of a local anesthetic into the subacromial area
(B) a short period of immobilization
(C) ultrasonography of the shoulder
(D) arthroscopy of the glenohumeral joint
(E) MRI of the shoulder

431. Three months following a fall on her outstretched, nondominant hand, a 55-year-old clerk complained of slowly decreasing pain in the ipsilateral shoulder. Examination revealed tenderness over the bicipital groove and soft-tissue crepitus in the same area with passive movement of the shoulder. Following normal routine radiographs, the study in the figure was performed. Management at this time should consist of

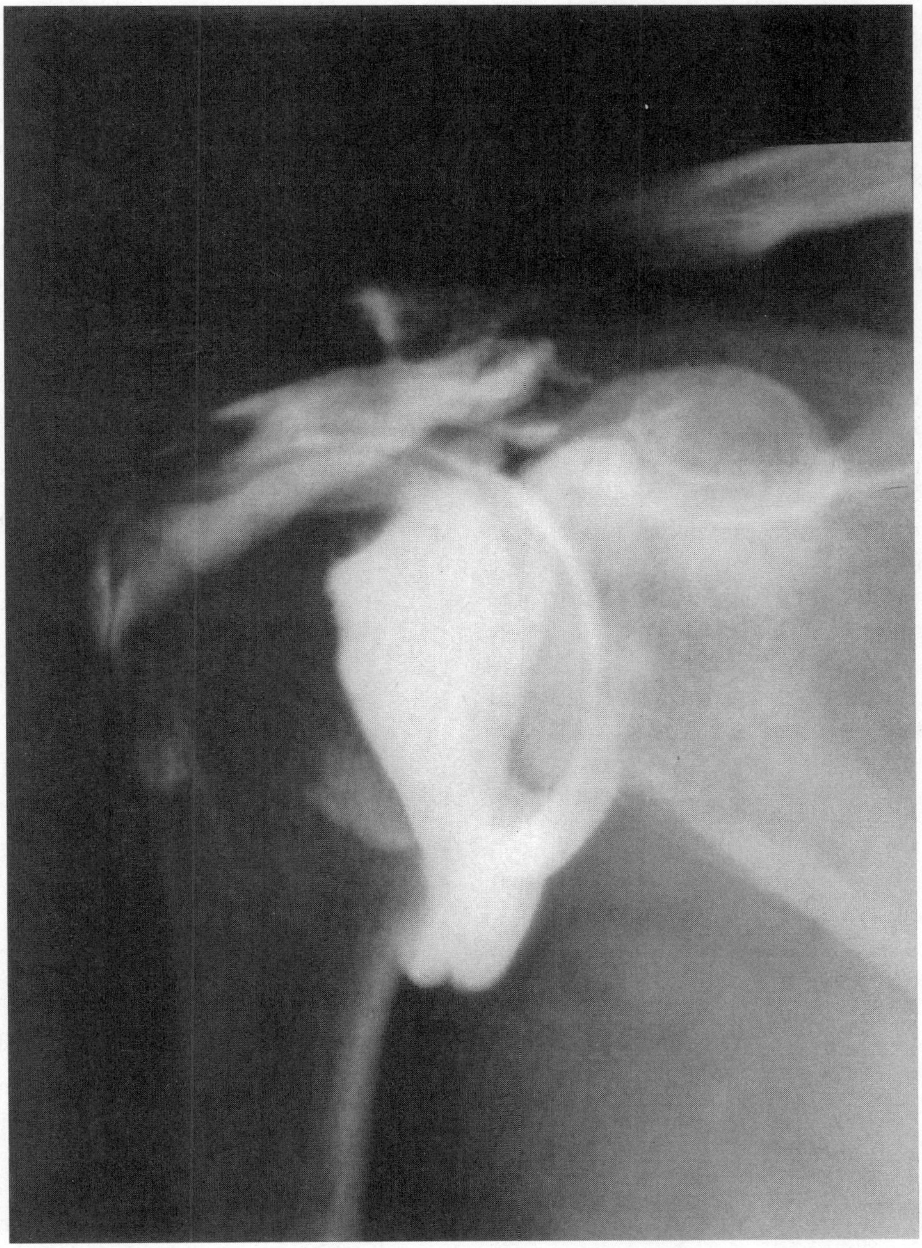

(A) an MRI of the affected shoulder
(B) nonsteroidal anti-inflammatory drugs (NSAIDs) and immobilization of the shoulder
(C) NSAIDs and range-of-motion exercises within pain limits
(D) arthroscopic subacromial decompression
(E) open arthrotomy and repair

432. To prevent injury to the musculocutaneous nerve during an anterior approach to the shoulder, the surgeon should avoid

(A) the deltopectoral interval
(B) division of the inferior fibers of the subscapularis
(C) lengthening of the subscapularis and anterior capsule more than 2 cm
(D) release of the conjoint tendon
(E) dissection medial to the coracobrachialis

433. The posterior approach to the shoulder is most safely and easily accomplished by dissection

(A) along the inferior border of the teres major
(B) between the teres major and the teres minor
(C) between the teres minor and the infraspinatus
(D) between the infraspinatus and the supraspinatus
(E) between the long and lateral heads of the triceps

434. The optimal prosthesis following a transradial amputation in the dominant arm of a 33-year-old farmer is

(A) a VO hook, quick change wrist unit, saddle harness
(B) a VC hook flexion wrist unit, self-suspended socket
(C) a mechanical hand, friction wrist unit, saddle harness
(D) a mechanical hand, wrist flexion unit, strap harness
(E) an APRL hook, friction wrist unit, back harness

435. In patients with carpal tunnel syndrome, electrodiagnostic studies typically show

(A) increased distal motor and sensory latencies, decreased median nerve conduction velocity, and decreased muscular insertional activity
(B) decreased distal motor and sensory latencies, decreased median nerve conduction velocity, and increased muscular insertional activity
(C) decreased distal motor and sensory latencies, increased median nerve conduction velocity, and increased muscular insertional activity
(D) increased distal motor and sensory latencies, decreased median nerve conduction velocity, and increased muscular insertional activity
(E) decreased distal motor and sensory latencies, decreased median nerve conduction velocity, and decreased muscular insertional activity

436. The most sensitive and specific procedure for the early detection of avascular necrosis (AVN) of the proximal humerus is

(A) routine x-rays taken in multiple oblique projections
(B) MRI
(C) arthrography
(D) CT arthrography
(E) scintigraphy and CT

437. All the following factors play a role in the etiology of tears of the rotator cuff EXCEPT

(A) degenerative changes in the rotator cuff
(B) hypovascularity of the supraspinatus tendon
(C) acute bursitis
(D) abnormalities of the acromion
(E) acute trauma

438. Anterior tenderness over the proximal humerus associated with a rupture of the rotator cuff most likely results from

(A) bicipital tendinitis
(B) inflammatory changes at the torn margins of the cuff
(C) associated calcific tendinitis
(D) subluxation of the biceps tendon
(E) deltoid myalgia

439. Findings on examination of a patient with an old, massive tear of the rotator cuff are LEAST likely to include

(A) tenderness over the bicipital groove
(B) atrophy of the deltoid
(C) atrophy of the spinati
(D) superior translation of the humeral head with attempted abduction
(E) a positive impingement sign

440. The natural history of calcium deposits in the rotator cuff is

(A) progressive enlargement of the deposit with increasing symptoms
(B) rupture of the cuff subsequent to degenerative changes associated with the calcium deposit
(C) spontaneous resolution within 48 h of peak symptoms
(D) subsidence of symptoms, followed by recurrent episodes of pain
(E) spontaneous resolution of symptoms in 7 to 10 days

441. Pathologic findings encountered in the frozen shoulder commonly include all the following EXCEPT

(A) osteopenia of the underlying bone
(B) acute inflammatory changes in the capsule
(C) fibrosis between the capsule and rotator cuff
(D) fibrosis between the rotator cuff and deltoid
(E) calcium deposits in the rotator cuff

442. The most important physical sign for the diagnosis of anterior instability of the glenohumeral joint is a positive

(A) apprehension sign
(B) impingement sign
(C) resisted straight arm raising sign
(D) resisted forearm supination sign
(E) drop arm sign

443. The pathology of recurrent posterior subluxation of the shoulder is most often a

(A) reverse Bankart lesion
(B) Hill-Sachs lesion
(C) fracture of the posterior lip of the glenoid
(D) generalized ligamentous laxity
(E) redundancy of the posterior capsule

444. Operative correction of multidirectional instability of the glenohumeral joint is based on

(A) capsular plication of the most symptomatic side
(B) tenodesis of the long head of the biceps
(C) reefing of the subscapularis tendon
(D) obliteration of the inferior capsular pouch
(E) restoration of the normal slope of the glenoid

445. The most useful diagnostic information for distinguishing an old posterior dislocation of the shoulder from a frozen shoulder is

(A) an AP radiograph of the shoulder
(B) a transthoracic lateral radiograph of the shoulder
(C) palpation of the dislocated head in the subclavicular area
(D) marked internal rotation deformity of the arm
(E) increased prominence of the scapular spine seen with dislocation

446. A 34-year-old laborer sustained an injury to his dominant shoulder 3 weeks ago. Based on the findings in the figure, the most appropriate management is

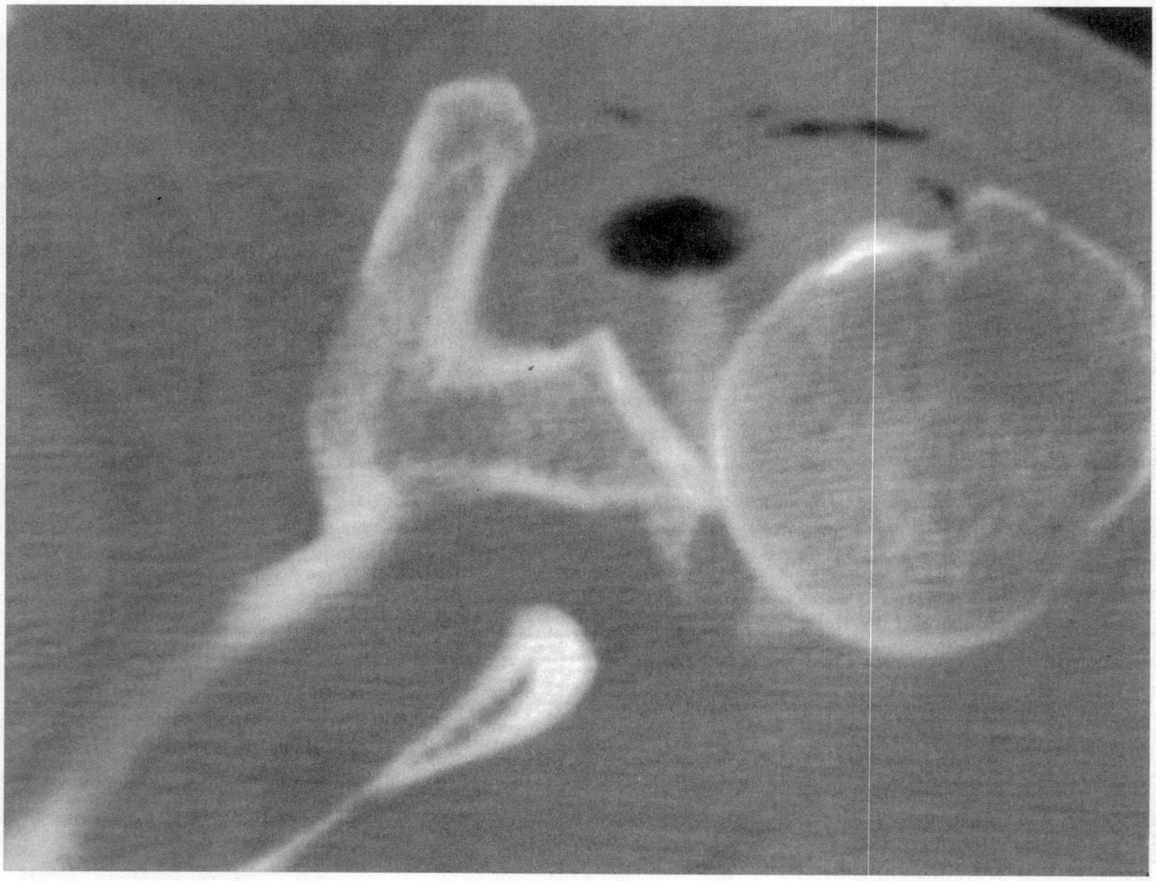

(A) closed reduction under general anesthesia
(B) observation for 3 months to determine final functional level
(C) open reduction and subscapularis transfer through an anterior approach
(D) open reduction and infraspinatus transfer through a posterior approach
(E) open reduction through combined anterior and posterior approaches

447. A 62-year-old housewife had long-standing rheumatoid arthritis and disabling pain in her dominant left shoulder. Her bone stock was well preserved, but she had a large tear of the rotator cuff. The optimal management is

(A) nonoperative
(B) synovectomy and debridement
(C) humeral head replacement, synovectomy, and debridement
(D) total shoulder arthroplasty using oversized humeral and glenoidal components
(E) total shoulder arthroplasty with reconstruction of the rotator cuff and acromioplasty

448. According to Neer, the incidence of disruption of the rotator cuff in patients with rheumatoid arthritis of the shoulder is approximately

(A) 5 percent
(B) 20 percent
(C) 35 percent
(D) 50 percent
(E) 65 percent

449. In patients with rheumatoid arthritis, rupture of the tendon of the long head of the biceps in the intertubercular groove is usually best treated by

(A) a brief period of rest in a sling, followed by gradual resumption of full activities
(B) immobilization of the arm in a splint that maintains the shoulder and elbow flexed for 6 weeks
(C) excision of the intraarticular portion of the biceps and tenodesis of the distal end in the bicipital groove
(D) primary repair of the biceps tendon
(E) free tendon grafting of the biceps tendon

450. Satisfactory or better results following total shoulder arthroplasty for osteoarthritis may be expected in approximately what percentage of patients?

(A) 50 percent
(B) 60 percent
(C) 70 percent
(D) 80 percent
(E) 90 percent

451. In a 42-year-old patient with a painful shoulder and the radiograph shown in the figure, which of the following findings would best confirm the radiographic diagnosis?

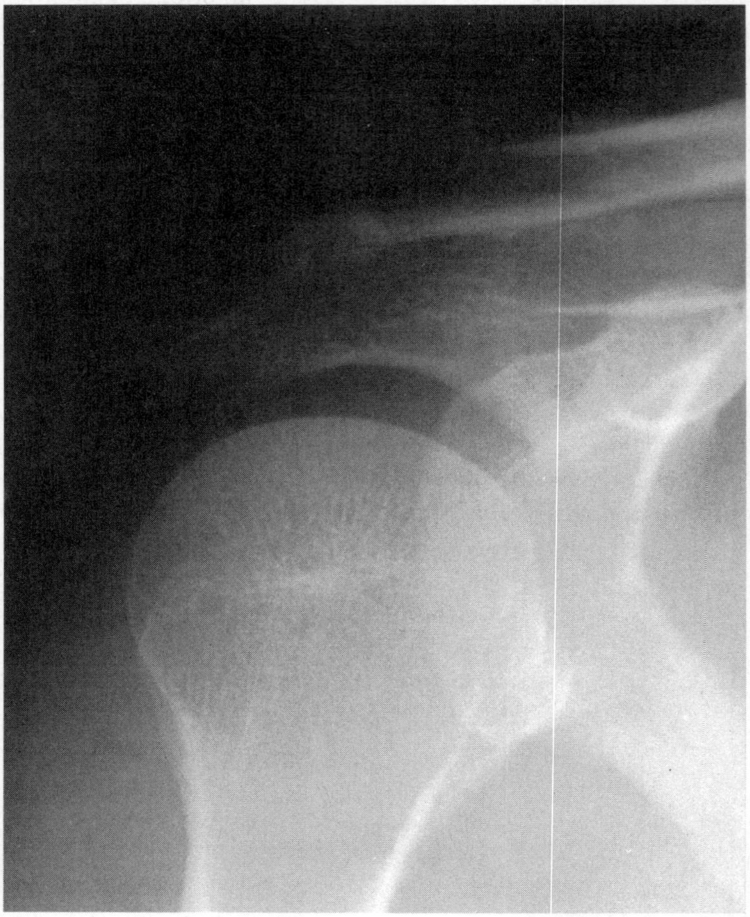

(A) Pain with forced horizontal adduction of the arm across the chest
(B) Superior localization of the pain
(C) Abolition of pain by injection of the acromioclavicular joint with local anesthetic
(D) Abolition of pain by injection of the subacromial space with a local anesthetic
(E) A subacromial spur on a supraspinatus outlet radiograph

452. Osteolysis of the outer clavicle has been observed in association with all the following EXCEPT

(A) hypothyroidism
(B) scleroderma
(C) rheumatoid arthritis
(D) trauma
(E) weight lifting

453. Entrapment of the suprascapular nerve is typically characterized by

(A) winging of the scapula, atrophy of the rhomboid muscles, and hypesthesia in the infraspinous region
(B) weakness of abduction and external rotation, atrophy of the spinati muscles, and normal sensation
(C) weakness of abduction, atrophy of the supraspinatus muscle, and hypesthesia in the supraspinous region
(D) weakness of scapular elevation, atrophy of the trapezius, and normal sensation
(E) inferior subluxation of the humerus, weakness of the deltoid, and hypesthesia over the lateral shoulder

454. The provocative position for reproducing the pain of lateral epicondylitis is

(A) elbow extension, forearm pronation, wrist flexion
(B) elbow flexion, forearm pronation, wrist flexion
(C) elbow flexion, forearm supination, wrist extension
(D) elbow extension, forearm pronation, wrist extension
(E) elbow flexion, forearm supination, wrist extension

455. The preferred treatment for acute, nonpyogenic olecranon bursitis is

(A) rest and avoidance of mechanical irritation
(B) administration of NSAIDs
(C) aspiration followed by a compressive dressing
(D) injection of corticosteroids
(E) bursectomy

456. All the following conditions have been associated with the development of myositis ossificans about the elbow joint EXCEPT

(A) thermal trauma
(B) surgical procedures about the elbow
(C) physical trauma
(D) paraplegia
(E) immobilization of the elbow

457. The optimal management of a clean digital tip amputation of the ring finger without bone loss in the dominant hand of a 32-year-old male laborer is

(A) shortening of the bone as needed, followed by primary closure
(B) amputation through the DIP joint and primary closure
(C) split-thickness skin grafting
(D) full-thickness skin grafting
(E) nonoperative, with healing by secondary intention

458. A 51-year-old right-handed carpenter sustained a clean amputation through the base of the distal phalanx of his right index finger. The most appropriate management is

(A) nonoperative, with healing by secondary intention
(B) a cross-finger pedicle flap
(C) Kutler lateral V-Y flaps
(D) a volar advancement flap
(E) a thenar flap

459. A major contraindication to fusion of the basal (trapeziometacarpal) joint of the thumb is

(A) stiffness of the first metacarpophalangeal joint
(B) stiffness of the scaphotrapezial joint
(C) stiffness of the thumb interphalangeal joint
(D) an occupation requiring heavy labor
(E) posttraumatic arthritis

460. Triscaphe arthrodesis is indicated for all the following EXCEPT

(A) nonunion of the scaphoid
(B) instability of the midcarpal joints
(C) arthritis of the radiocarpal joint
(D) dorsal intercalated segment instability (DISI)
(E) Kienböck's disease

461. The most common pattern of degenerative arthritis encountered in the wrist is

(A) triscaphe arthritis
(B) scapholunate advanced collapse (SLAC)
(C) scapholunate arthritis
(D) triquetrolunate arthritis
(E) capitolunate arthritis

462. Degenerative arthritis in the wrist develops most often as a result of pathology affecting the

(A) lunate
(B) scaphoid
(C) capitate
(D) radiolunate joint
(E) scapholunate joint

463. The most reliable and accepted technique for arthroplasty of the metacarpophalangeal joints is

(A) insertion of a double-stemmed Vitallium-hinged replacement
(B) insertion of a silicone elastomer spacer
(C) insertion of a silicone prosthesis with in-growth fixation
(D) resection of the joint surfaces
(E) resection of the joint surfaces with soft-tissue interposition

464. All the following are important considerations for a successful metacarpophalangeal (MCP) arthroplasty EXCEPT

(A) the functional status of the proximal and distal interphalangeal joints
(B) the functional status of the wrist joints
(C) release of MCP capsular contracture
(D) release of intrinsic contracture
(E) amount of osteopenia in the hand

465. A 36-year-old man with rheumatoid arthritis had long-standing, disabling pain at the base of the thumb in his dominant hand. A radiograph is shown below. The optimal surgical management of the first carpometacarpal (CMC) joint is

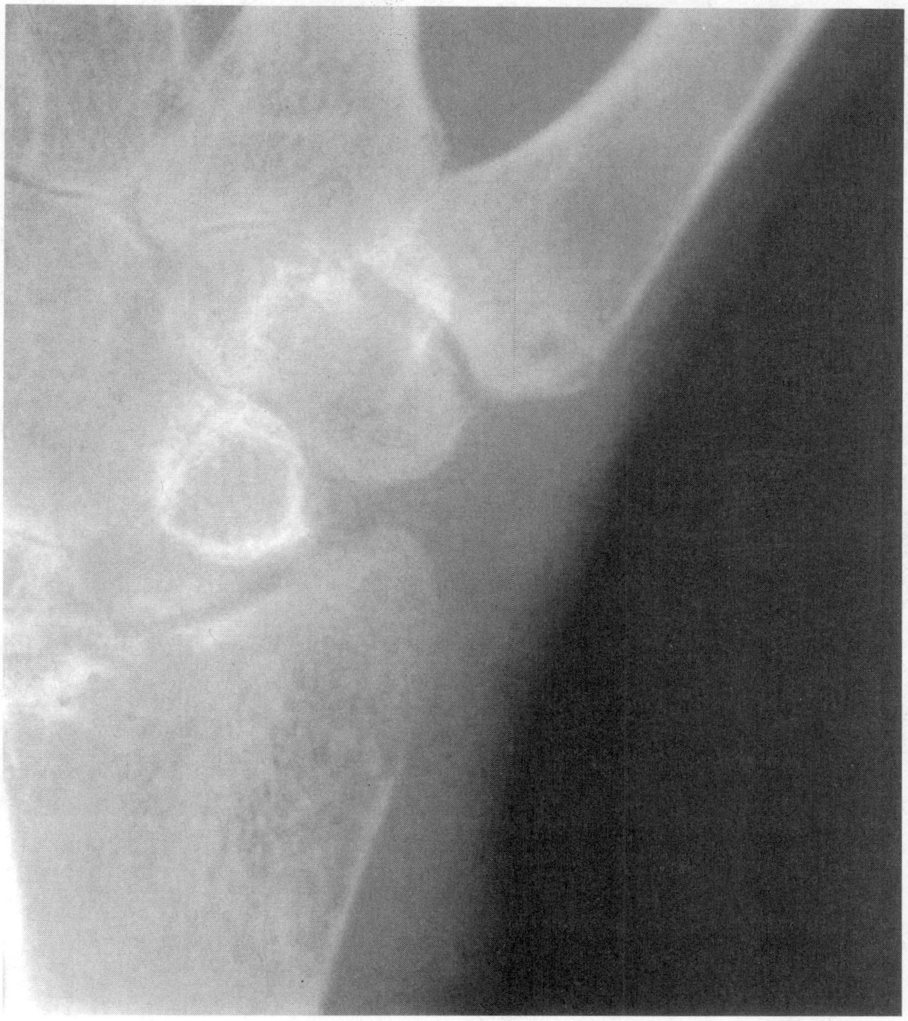

(A) arthrodesis of the CMC joint
(B) excision of the trapezium
(C) capsular arthroplasty of the CMC joint
(D) titanium condylar arthroplasty
(E) silicone replacement of the trapezium

466. A 62-year-old woman had a painful nondominant wrist 8 weeks after a motor vehicle accident. A lateral radiograph is shown below. The most appropriate management is

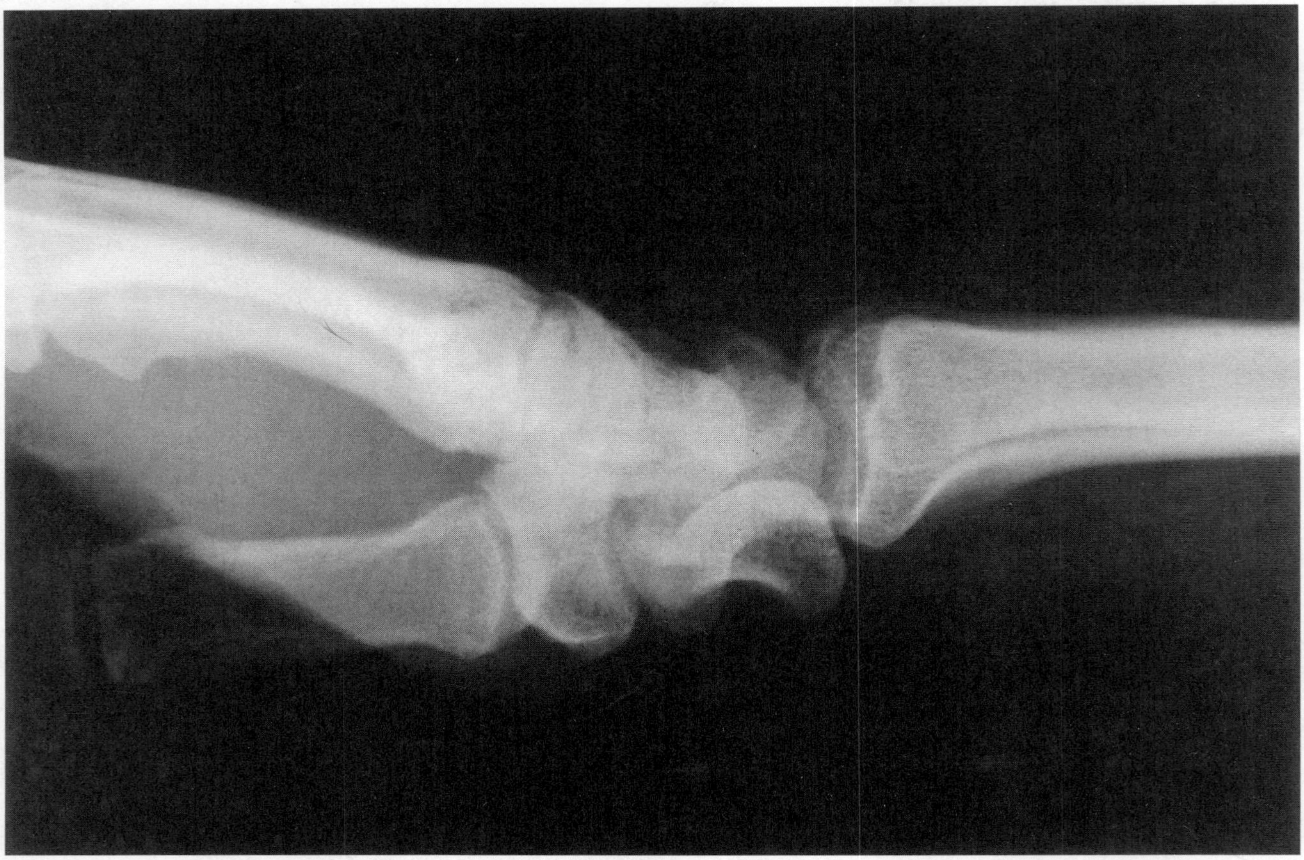

(A) arthroplasty of the radiocarpal joint with a silicone prosthesis
(B) proximal row carpectomy
(C) arthrodesis of the radiocarpal joint
(D) excision of the lunate, with insertion of a tendon spacer
(E) open reduction and arthrodesis of the scapholunate joint

467. The use of a double-stemmed, hinged, silicone elastomer prosthesis for arthroplasty of the radiocarpal joint is contraindicated in patients with

(A) osteoarthritis, good bone stock, and limited wrist motion
(B) rheumatoid arthritis and minimal deformity
(C) rheumatoid arthritis and "loose" wrist motion
(D) posttraumatic arthritis following scapholunate dissociation
(E) osteoarthritis and minimal deformity

468. The best indication for total wrist arthroplasty is a patient

(A) over age 50, with rheumatoid arthritis involving only one wrist
(B) under age 50, with rheumatoid arthritis involving both wrists
(C) over age 50, with old septic arthritis of the wrist
(D) under age 50, with posttraumatic arthritis following scapholunate dissociation
(E) under age 50, with posttraumatic arthritis following an intraarticular fracture of the distal radius

469. A 55-year-old executive had a painful flexion deformity of her nondominant wrist following a stroke and was unable to extend her fingers when she reached for an object. Active grasp was present. When the wrist was held in neutral, the metacarpophalangeal joints rested in 70 to 80° of flexion. The most appropriate management is

(A) injection of phenol into the median nerve at the elbow
(B) an intensive program of splinting and physical therapy to stretch contracted muscles, joint capsules, and ligaments
(C) neurectomy of the motor branches of the median nerve in the forearm
(D) superficialis to profundus (STP) release
(E) flexor origin release (flexor "slide")

470. Without prompt, effective splinting, a hand that has sustained a crushing injury is most likely to develop which of the following patterns of contracture?

(A) Finger interphalangeal (IP) extension, metacarpophalangeal (MCP) flexion, thumb flexion, wrist extension
(B) Finger IP flexion, MCP extension, thumb adduction, wrist flexion
(C) Finger IP extension and MCP extension, thumb flexion, wrist flexion
(D) Finger IP flexion and MCP flexion, thumb abduction, wrist extension
(E) Finger IP flexion and MCP flexion, thumb adduction, wrist flexion

471. Posttraumatic stiffness following a crushing injury to the hand is best avoided by positioning the fingers in

(A) full metacarpophalangeal (MCP) flexion and full interphalangeal (IP) extension
(B) full MCP flexion and 30 to 45° IP flexion
(C) 30 to 45° MCP flexion and full IP extension
(D) 30 to 45° MCP flexion and 30 to 45° IP flexion
(E) full MCP extension and full IP flexion

472. The optimal management of long-standing extension contractures of the metacarpophalangeal joints is

(A) the use of a nonelastic, three-point fixation splint
(B) a rigorous and closely supervised rehabilitation program to strengthen all finger flexors
(C) manipulation under anesthesia, followed by instillation of hydrocortisone
(D) volar plate capsulodesis (Zancolli)
(E) dorsal capsulotomy and release of the lateral bands from the metacarpal heads

473. The muscles most severely affected in Volkmann's ischemic contracture are the

(A) flexor digitorum superficialis and flexor carpi radialis
(B) flexor digitorum superficialis and flexor pollicis longus
(C) flexor carpi ulnaris and pronator teres
(D) flexor digitorum profundus and flexor pollicis longus
(E) flexor digitorum profundus and flexor carpi ulnaris

474. The preferred surgical procedure for correction of swan-neck deformities caused by intrinsic contractures in patients with rheumatoid arthritis is

(A) crossed intrinsic transfer
(B) tenodesis of the intrinsic muscles
(C) transection of the lateral band proximal to the metacarpophalangeal joint
(D) silastic arthroplasty of the proximal interphalangeal joint
(E) release of the ulnar distal intrinsic muscles

475. Which of the following clinical pictures best describes the shoulder-hand syndrome?

(A) Younger females; distal to proximal spread of symptoms; frozen shoulder; damp, pale skin; extension deformity of fingers; osteoporosis
(B) Older males; proximal to distal spread of symptoms; decreased elbow motion; clawing of fingers; normal bone radiographs
(C) Older females; proximal to distal spread of symptoms; frozen shoulder; pale, dry skin; extension deformity of fingers; osteoporosis
(D) Younger females; distal to proximal spread of symptoms; decreased forearm rotation; damp, red skin; flexion deformities of the PIP joints; osteoporosis
(E) Older males; proximal to distal spread of symptoms; decreased elbow and wrist motion; dry, red skin; extension deformity of the fingers; normal bone radiographs

476. A 61-year-old patient with rheumatoid arthritis had pain and subluxation of the metacarpophalangeal (MCP) joints caused by ulnar deviation and flexion deformities. All flexor tendons were intact. A radiograph of the patient's hand is shown below. The most appropriate treatment is

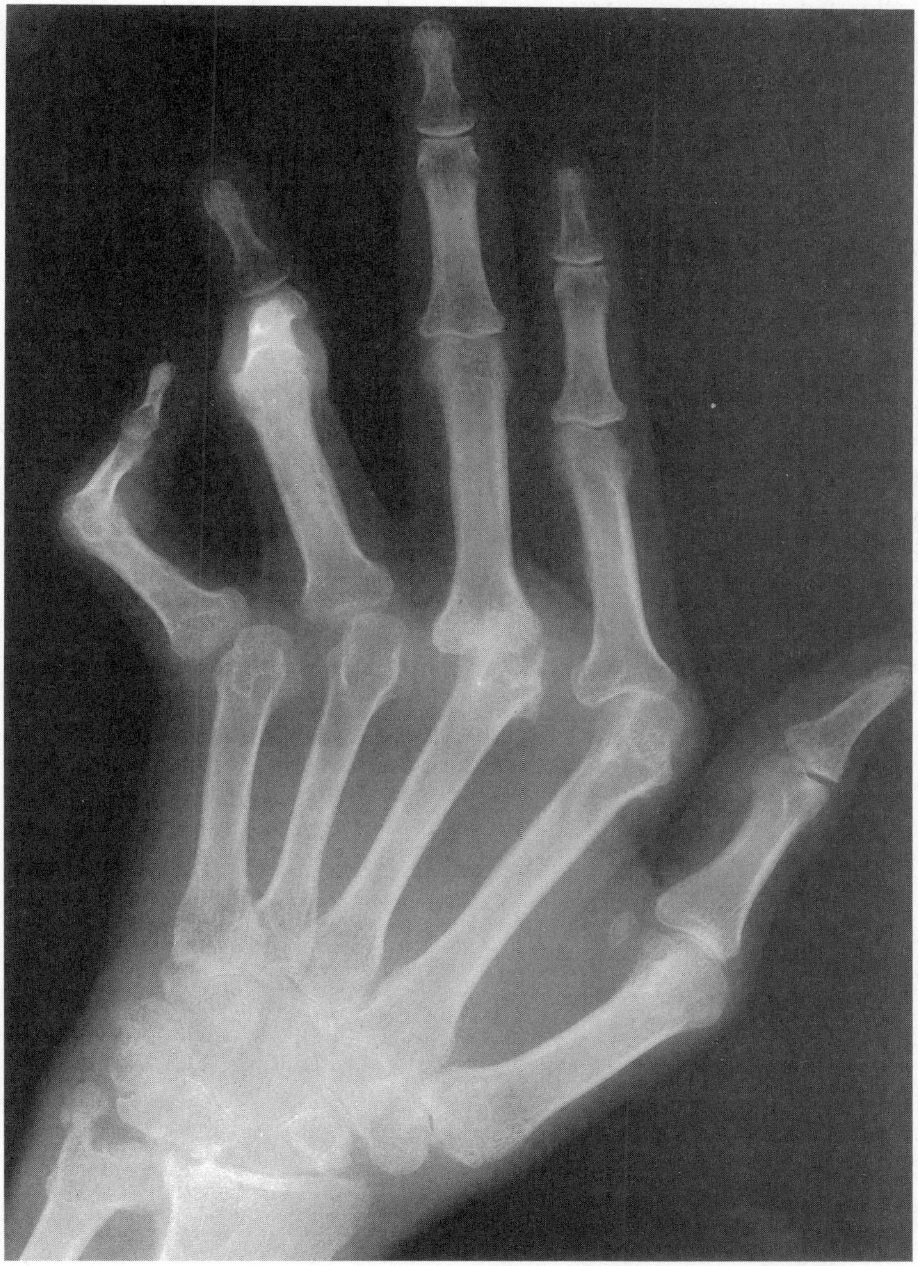

(A) a carefully designed physical therapy program to stretch contracted structures and strengthen weak muscles
(B) splinting and intraarticular injection of corticosteroids
(C) arthrodesis of the MCP joints
(D) soft-tissue reconstruction of the MCP joints
(E) arthroplasty with silicone implants

477. Compartmental syndrome of the forearm is most often characterized by which of the following clinical patterns?

(A) Distal pallor and pulselessness, pain, decreased distal sensation, and weakness of muscles in the involved compartment
(B) Normal distal color and pulses, increase of pain by passive stretch of the involved muscles, normal sensation and strength
(C) Distal pallor, skin coolness and pulselessness, decreased distal sensation, and weakness of the involved muscles
(D) Normal distal color and skin temperature, increase of pain by passive stretch of involved muscles, decreased distal sensation, and weakness of the involved muscles
(E) Distal pallor and skin coolness, pain, diminished pulses, normal distal sensation, and weakness of muscles in the involved compartment

Adult Diseases and Disorders: Upper Limb

Answers

417. The answer is E. *(Miller, p 121.)* Rheumatoid arthritis is frequently associated with doral tenosynovitis and dorsal subluxation of the ulnar head, which lies beneath the extensor digiti quinti proprius (EDQP) tendon. DeQuervain's tenosynovitis affects the tendons in the first dorsal compartment (extensor pollicis brevis [EPB] and abductor pollicis longus [APL]). Carpal bossing typically involves the tendons in the second dorsal compartment (extensor carpi radialis longus and brevis [ECRL/B]). Osteoarthritis (with dorsal spurring) is unusual in the wrist. Impingement by the ulnar styloid most commonly affects the tendon in the sixth dorsal compartment (extensor carpi ulnaris [ECU]).

418. The answer is B. *(Miller, p 121.)* The intrinsic minus, or clawhand, deformity results from a lesion of the median and ulnar nerves in the distal forearm or wrist. Loss of ulnar nerve function results in paralysis of the adductor pollicis, which leads to instability of the thumb MCP joint and weakness of pinch (*positive* Froment's sign). With paralysis of the interossei and lumbricals, abduction and adduction of the fingers are lost and grip strength reduced. Unopposed action of the long extensor tendons in the fingers results in hyperextension of the MCP joints, and unopposed action of the long finger flexors causes flexion of the IP joints.

419. The answer is B. *(Miller, p 121.)* A positive Bunnell test (more passive flexion of the PIP joint when the MCP joint is flexed than when it is extended) is seen most often in conditions causing spasm or contracture of the intrinsic muscles, such as cerebral palsy or rheumatoid arthritis, which produces MCP flexion and extension of both IP joints. This picture is the opposite of that seen in an intrinsic minus hand. In a lumbrical plus deformity, active flexion of the MCP joint causes extension of the PIP joint. MCP flexion is not a significant component of the swan neck deformity (PIP hyperextension and DIP flexion); nor is the MCP joint affected in the boutonnière deformity (PIP flexion and DIP hyperextension).

420. The answer is C. *(Miller, pp 122–124.)* In the anterior interosseous syndrome, there is weakness of the radial half of the flexor digitorum profundus (FDP), the flexor pollicis longus (FPL), and the pronator quadratus. Weakness in the FPL causes loss of precise pinch. Typically, patients with this disorder are unable to make an "OK" sign. There are no sensory branches of the anterior interosseous branch of the median nerve, which is most often entrapped at the origin of the deep head of the pronator teres.

421. The answer is A. *(Miller, p 132.)* Scapholunate advanced collapse commonly follows scaphoid fracture or scapholunate dissociation and is manifested by degeneration of the radial styloid-scaphoid area, radioscaphoid joint, capitolunate joint, and sometimes the scaphocapitate joint. Classically, the radiolunate joint is spared.

422. The answer is E. *(Miller, p 134.)* The PIP flexion and DIP hyperextension seen in boutonnière deformities result from volar subluxation of the lateral bands following rupture or attenuation of the insertion of the central slip into the base of the middle phalanx. Fixed hyperextension of the DIP joint indicates long-standing deformity. Soft-tissue procedures usually fail if the DIP joint is fixed in extension. Arthroplasties, especially if extensor balance is not restored, also commonly fail. Arthrodesis is the preferred procedure for such cases.

423. The answer is D. *(Miller, p 136.)* Dupuytren's contracture typically involves the palmar aponeurosis and its digital prolongations in the palm. It also involves Grayson's ligament, the pretendinous bands, the natatory ligaments, and the spiral bands in the digits. Characteristically, it does not involve the superficial transverse ligament or Cleland's ligament. Surgery is indicated for significant MCP involvement and *any* PIP involvement. Subcutaneous release risks injury to the neurovascular structures and is associated with a high rate of recurrence. Total fasciectomy is associated with more frequent postoperative palmar hematomas and skin sloughs. Subtotal palmar fasciectomy is usually curative, with fewer postoperative complications. In diabetics, the open-palm technique of McCash is preferred.

424. The answer is E. *(Miller, p 126.)* The classic presentation of suppurative flexor tenosynovitis (Kanavel's four cardinal signs) is represented by choices A through D. Localization, or "pointing," of the infection is uncommon.

425. The answer is B. *(Miller, pp 135–136.)* All the choices are involved except Cleland's ligament, which lies *dorsal* to the digital neurovascular bundle. Grayson's ligament provides the volar cover and is therefore likely to be involved, as are the other volar structures mentioned. Associating Cleland with "ceiling" and Grayson with "ground" helps in remembering the location of these ligaments.

426. The answer is B. *(Miller, p 143.)* Excision of the radial head facilitates synovectomy and is an especially useful procedure before extensive destruction of the joint occurs. There is insufficient joint destruction to warrant total elbow replacement. Interpositional arthroplasty often results in satisfactory motion but can result in instability, especially in patients with RA. Arthrodesis of the elbow causes unacceptable functional disability.

427. The answer is D. *(Miller, p 98.)* Adhesive capsulitis of the glenohumeral joint (frozen shoulder) may be precipitated by any condition leading to prolonged immobilization of the shoulder. Predisposing factors include female sex, middle age, diabetes mellitus, hypothyroidism, and injury. Tears of the rotator cuff and frozen shoulders are rarely associated.

428. The answer is C. *(Miller, p 99.)* Radiolucency at the bone-cement interface is noted in approximately 30 percent of glenoidal components following total shoulder arthroplasty, although radiographic loosening is not necessarily symptomatic. Loosening of the humeral component is rare, with or without the use of cement. Because the humerus is not a weight-bearing bone, fractures are less common after shoulder than after hip replacement. Dislocation, which is infrequent, usually occurs early rather than late in the postoperative course.

429. The answer is C. *(Miller, p 99.)* Osteoarthritic joints have the most favorable prognosis, due in large part to the integrity of the rotator cuff, which is usually intact in this disorder. Patients with rheumatoid arthritis frequently have thinned or torn rotator cuffs, and cuff-tear arthropathy is associated with massive, retracted tears of the rotator cuff. More scarring is present in patients with postinfectious arthritis, and the risk of postoperative infection is greater.

430. The answer is A. *(Miller, p 97.)* Abolition of the patient's pain following subacromial injection of a local anesthetic (positive impingement test) suggest an early stage of the impingement syndrome. In such conditions, MRI is rarely necessary. Ultrasonographic findings in cases of early impingement syndrome have not been clearly defined. Since the pathology is primarily extraarticular, arthroscopy would be of little value, and treatment should not be undertaken until the diagnosis is established.

431. The answer is C. *(Miller, p 98.)* The arthrogram is diagnostic for a tear of the rotator cuff; hence, MRI is unnecessary. Many patients with tears of the rotator cuff who place limited demands on their shoulder will become asymptomatic with time, although there are no data to suggest that this outcome is more likely when shoulder motion is interdicted. Since the optimal period (3 weeks) for repair of a cuff tear has been passed, there is no need for surgery—arthroscopic or open—at this time, especially since the patient is continuing to improve.

432. The answer is E. *(Miller, p 308.)* The musculocutaneous nerve is best protected by avoiding dissection on the medial aspect of the coracobrachialis. Normally, the nerve enters this muscle 5 to 8 cm below the coracoid process; however, in almost 30 percent of cases, the nerve enters the muscle above the 5-cm zone of safety. It is preferable to release the conjoint tendon rather than retract it vigorously.

433. The answer is C. *(Miller, p 308.)* After detaching or splitting the deltoid, the posterior capsule of the shoulder should be approached in the internervous plane between the infraspinatus and the teres minor. The infraspinatus is supplied by the suprascapular nerve and the teres minor by the axillary nerve. Since the axillary nerve and posterior humeral circumflex artery lie just below the teres minor, it is important to stay superior to this muscle.

434. The answer is A. *(Miller, p 224.)* Depending upon the specific needs of the farmer, a VO or VC terminal unit could be used. Mechanical hands are more cosmetic but less functional and heavier than hooks. The APRL hook has many positive features, but expense precludes routine use. A quick change wrist unit is preferred because of its adaptability and reliability. Friction units tend to slip with heavy load, and flexion units are used primarily for bilateral amputees. The saddle harness is especially suited to heavy use. The strap harness is used for short above-elbow amputations or disarticulations.

435. The answer is D. *(Miller, pp 74–75.)* In patients with carpal tunnel syndrome, distal motor and sensory latencies are typically increased to over 3.5 ms, median nerve conduction velocity is reduced to under 50 m/s, and insertional activity of the muscles innervated by the median nerve is increased.

436. The answer is B. *(Miller, p 73.)* MRI is the most sensitive technique for early detection of AVN, and it is 98 percent reliable in determining the age of the disease. MRI also allows direct assessment of overlying cartilage. Scintigraphy and CT is a newer technique, the reliability of which has not been fully determined.

437. The answer is C. *(Cruess, p 962.)* All the choices except acute bursitis play roles in the causation of tears of the rotator cuff. Degenerative changes, which result from daily use, grind the rotator cuff between the coracoacromial "mortise" and the "pestle" of the humeral head. Because of the hypovascularity of the supraspinatus tendon adjacent to its insertion tissue, repair cannot keep pace with degeneration. Impingement on the cuff is increased by inferior projections of the acromion, and the precipitating event in cuff tears is often acute trauma, although it may be trivial in nature.

438. The answer is A. *(Cruess, pp 963–964.)* Tears of the rotator cuff commonly uncover the biceps tendon, subjecting it to impingement, with secondary inflammatory changes. Little or no inflammation is seen at the margins of the tear, and calcific tendinitis is rarely seen in combination with tears of the rotator cuff. The incidence of recurrent subluxation of the biceps tendon is not known to be increased by tears of the rotator cuff, and deltoid pain is not a characteristic feature of tears of the rotator cuff.

439. The answer is B. *(Cruess, pp 969–970.)* Selective myopathy is common with massive, retracted tears of the rotator cuff; compensatory hypertrophy of the deltoid results from chronically impaired function of the spinati muscles. Associated bicipital tendinitis is common, and the impingement sign is often strikingly positive. With large defects, the rotator cuff is unable to stabilize the humeral head against the glenoid, so that with attempted abduction the humeral head pistons superiorly.

440. The answer is E. *(Cruess, p 984.)* As a result of surrounding inflammatory hyperemia, all but very large calcium deposits are spontaneously resorbed; symptoms usually subside within 7 to 10 days. There are no data to support calcific tendinitis as predisposing to tears of the rotator cuff. Recurrence is infrequent.

441. The answer is E. *(Cruess, p 987.)* Osteopenia is frequently encountered in patients with frozen shoulders, perhaps related to disuse. Capsular fibrosis and scarring is a hallmark of frozen shoulders, with the fibrosis often involving the cuff and deltoid as well. The association of adhesive capsulitis and calcific tendinitis is rare.

442. The answer is A. *(Cruess, p 992.)* Classically, a patient with recurrent anterior instability or subluxation exhibits marked apprehension when the relaxed shoulder is stressed in abduction and external rotation. The impingement sign and the drop arm sign indicate disease of the rotator cuff. A positive resisted straight arm raising test (Speed's test) and a positive resisted forearm supination test (Yergason's sign) suggest pathology in the biceps tendon.

443. The answer is E. *(Cruess, p 998.)* Recurrent posterior subluxation follows capsular redundancy caused by the initial displacement. The posterior labrum offers minimal support to the humeral head. Since the lesion is a subluxation rather than a dislocation, there is little impaction of the humeral head on the posterior glenoidal rim and hence no Hill-Sachs lesion. Erosion of the posterior lip of the glenoid and generalized ligamentous laxity are rarely encountered.

444. The answer is D. *(Cruess, p 1004.)* Elimination of the inferior capsular pouch provides anterior, inferior, and posterior stability. Capsular plication on only one side (as well as subscapularis reefing) will increase the displacement forces on the opposite side of the joint. Any Bankart lesion should be repaired, since the inferior pouch attaches to the labrum.

445. The answer is D. *(Cruess, p 1006.)* In posterior dislocation of the shoulder, AP radiographs are frequently read as normal. Transthoracic lateral radiographs are difficult to interpret. The humeral head is palpable not in the subclavicular area, but posteriorly, which reduces, rather than increases, prominence of the scapular spine. Patients with an old posterior dislocation of the shoulder usually have marked internal rotation deformities of the arm, often 50° or more.

446. The answer is C. *(Cruess, p 1006.)* Given the duration of this locked posterior dislocation of the glenohumeral joint, closed reduction is not likely to be successful. Continued observation will lead to further degeneration of the humeral head, which predisposes to posttraumatic arthritis. An anterior approach provides adequate exposure in most cases, although occasionally a combined approach is necessary to achieve reduction. Since over 50 percent of the articular surface of the humeral head is intact, reduction is worthwhile; however, the size of the defect in the humeral head suggests the need for subscapularis transfer as recommended by McLaughlin or Neer.

447. The answer is E. *(Cruess, p 1013.)* When the shoulder is the major source of disability in patients with rheumatoid arthritis, a surgical approach is indicated. Synovectomy and debridement do not generally improve function or significantly reduce pain. Since both sides of the joints are involved, replacement of both the humeral and glenoidal surfaces should be undertaken, if glenoidal bone stock is adequate. Repair of the rotator cuff would be made more difficult by the use of large components. It is often possible to mobilize and repair large cuff defects in rheumatoid patients, and repairs should be protected by an acromioplasty.

448. The answer is C. *(Cruess, p 1012.)* In Neer's experience with rheumatoid shoulders, the rotator cuff was disrupted in one-third of patients. Rupture occurs primarily from the effects of prolonged synovitis on the rotator cuff. With progressive thinning and attrition of the cuff, the humeral head displaces cephalad, leading to impingement and further degenerative changes, which increases the likelihood of rupture.

449. The answer is A. *(Cruess, p 1016.)* Rupture of the long head of the biceps is not usually a disabling feature of rheumatoid arthritis. Prolonged immobilization, especially in nonfunctional positions, is contraindicated in patients with rheumatoid arthritis. If this condition is encountered as part of total shoulder arthroplasty, excision of the intraarticular portion and tenodesis of the distal tendon should be carried out, but this procedure is rarely justified as an isolated procedure. Primary repair is usually impossible and results of free tendon grafting do not justify the additional surgical complexity.

450. The answer is E. *(Neer, J Bone Joint Surg 64-A:331–337, 1982.)* In Neer's series of 40 patients with osteoarthritis who underwent total shoulder arthroplasty, 36 had excellent and 3 had satisfactory results. Other authors have reported similar results. Functional improvement is better in osteoarthritis than in rheumatoid arthritis because the rotator cuff is less functional in rheumatoid patients.

451. The answer is C. *(Cruess, p 1027.)* The radiograph shown is negative except for the presence of arthritic changes in the acromioclavicluar (AC) joint. While pain with horizontal adduction and superior localization of pain are common findings in this disorder, the most specific diagnostic test is abolition of the pain by installation of a local anesthetic into the AC joint. Subacromial injection and radiographs of the supraspinatus outlet would be more useful in the evaluation of suspected impingement syndrome.

452. The answer is A. *(Cruess, p 1028.)* Resorption of the distal clavicle (and often of the adjacent acromion) is seen in patients with rheumatoid arthritis and scleroderma, and occasionally in weight lifters and after minor trauma. The specific cause of this resorption is unclear. Osteolysis of the distal clavicle has not been associated with hypothyroidism.

453. The answer is B. *(Cruess, p 1037.)* Entrapment of the suprascapular nerve usually occurs in the scapular notch as the nerve passes over the superior border of the scapula and beneath the superior transverse scapular ligament. Both spinati muscles are involved, producing weakness of abduction and external rotation. Since the suprascapular nerve is purely a motor nerve, there are no sensory findings.

454. The answer is A. *(Cruess, p 1058.)* Lateral epicondylitis is produced by small disruptions in the conjoined aponeurosis of the extensor carpi radialis brevis and extensor communis muscles near their origin from the lateral epicondyle. Pain results from the inflammatory response, which also initiates healing. The pain is reproduced by positioning the elbow, forearm, and wrist in those positions that exert greatest tension on the forearm extensor muscles, i.e., elbow extension, forearm pronation, and wrist flexion.

455. The answer is A. *(Cruess, p 1070.)* Acute olecranon bursitis most frequently results from acute or repetitive trauma. With avoidance of further trauma, the swelling will usually subside spontaneously. Corticosteroid injections do not facilitate this process, and bursectomy is reserved for chronic bursitis in which the bursal sac is thickened and fibrotic. Aspiration, with or without compression, is usually followed by prompt recurrence.

456. The answer is E. *(Cruess, p 1070.)* The development of myositis ossificans about the elbow is most often related to trauma, which may be thermal, physical, or surgical. It has also been reported to occur in 20 percent of patients with paraplegia or quadriplegia. Immobilization of the elbow in the absence of trauma, while leading to stiffness, has not been associated with the development of myositis ossificans.

457. The answer is E. *(Green, p 54.)* Allowing the fingertip to heal by secondary intention results in fewer complications than does any surgical treatment. In addition, the patient is generally able to return to work sooner following nonoperative treatment. Tenderness, cold intolerance, and hypesthesia are also more common after skin grafting than after secondary healing.

458. The answer is B. *(Green, pp 56–60.)* In laborers, as much length of the digits as possible should be preserved, especially in the thumb and index finger. All the surgical techniques listed provide full-thickness coverage, which is desirable in laborers. Almost two-thirds of patients undergoing V-Y flap repairs have hypersensitivity or numbness, and over 40 percent complain of difficulty in grasping small objects. Volar flap advancement, which requires more extensive surgery, is more appropriate for thumb than for finger amputations. The use of a thenar flap in a patient this age carries the unnecessary risk of joint stiffness. The return of sensibility to cross-finger flaps is excellent in most cases.

459. The answer is A. *(Green, p 99.)* Studies have shown that 75 percent of the compensation for fusion of the basal joint of the thumb comes from compensatory motion in the first MCP joint, while 25 percent is derived from the scaphotrapezial joint. Fusion of the basal joint of the thumb is generally preferred over arthroplasty in heavy laborers. Posttraumatic arthritis, since it is usually confined to one joint with preservation of motion in the joints needed for compensation, is an ideal indication for fusion.

460. The answer is C. *(Green, p 113.)* Triscaphe arthrodesis involves fusion of the scaphoid, trapezium, and trapezoid to one another. It provides excellent load transference to the radius and therefore should not be used in the presence of radiocarpal arthritis. In addition to the remaining choices, the procedure is used for rotary subluxation of the scaphoid, triscaphe degenerative disease, and radial dislocations of the wrist. No studies to date have shown subsequent degenerative changes in other joints of the wrist.

461. The answer is B. *(Green, p 124.)* The SLAC pattern of degenerative arthritis accounts for over one-half of all arthritic problems of the wrist. The radioscaphoid joint is involved initially and, with increasing lack of radial support, the capitate slides off the radial side of the lunate, leading to degenerative changes first in the capitolunate joint and later the hamatolunate joint.

462. The answer is B. *(Green, pp 125–127.)* Scapholunate advanced collapse (SLAC), which is the most common pattern of degenerative arthritis of the wrist, is most frequently caused by rotary subluxation of the scaphoid, followed by nonunion of the scaphoid, midcarpal instability, and intraarticular fractures of the radioscaphoid joint. Each of these conditions involves injury, deformity, or instability of the scaphoid. Any injury to the scaphoid can produce a pattern that predisposes to full SLAC destruction; however, the radiolunate joint is highly resistant to degenerative change, even with significant displacement of the lunate.

463. The answer is B. *(Green, p 143.)* Resection arthroplasties of the metacarpophalangeal joints, with or without soft-tissue interposition, do not afford sufficient stability for good function. Loosening, stem protrusion, and breakage have caused significant problems with metallic devices, whether or not cement was used. Silicone implants with ingrowth fixation also have a high rate of failure due to breakage. The state of the art for MCP arthroplasty is the silicone elastomer spacer, originally designed by Swanson to improve stability following resectional arthroplasty.

464. The answer is E. *(Green, p 151.)* Each of the choices listed in A through D is important for a successful outcome following MCP arthroplasty. With significant PIP and DIP deformity or contracture, function following MCP arthroplasty can be significantly limited. If contracted, as is usually the case in rheumatoid arthritis, the ulnar collateral ligament and capsule must be released for a successful arthroplasty. After the arthroplasty, if the test for intrinsic tightness is positive, the intrinsics should be lengthened or released. Arthroplasty of the MCP joints is most successful in patients with rheumatoid arthritis, most of whom have marked osteopenia.

465. The answer is E. *(Green, pp 161–162.)* The radiograph shows rheumatoid changes in both the carpometacarpal (CMC) and trapezioscaphoid articulations. Thus, neither arthrodesis nor arthroplasty of the carpometacarpal joint alone would adequately address the problem. The titanium condylar implant for the

CMC joint was developed for degenerative or posttraumatic changes localized to that joint. Optimal management for this patient would therefore be removal of the entire trapezium and replacement by either an implant or soft tissue.

466. The answer is D. *(Green, pp 167–169.)* The radiograph shows volar dislocation of the lunate. While one might consider excisional arthroplasty alone, the best choice among those listed is excision with interposition of a tendon spacer. Given the liklihood of avascular necrosis (Kienböck's disease), with subsequent radiocarpal collapse if the lunate is openly reduced, this alternative is not attractive, even when combined with scapholunate arthrodesis. Radiocarpal arthroplasty or arthrodesis and proximal row carpectomy entail more surgery and longer convalescence than necessary in this elderly patient.

467. The answer is C. *(Green, p 167.)* Hinged silicone elastomer prostheses function primarily to occupy the space left following proximal row carpectomy. This prosthesis is most useful in patients with rheumatoid arthritis who do not have severe deformity or rupture of the wrist extensors. The implant, especially when reinforced by grommets, is indicated for young persons with good bone stock and limited, painful motion. If normal or excessive motion is present as a result of soft-tissue instability, as seen in "loose" rheumatoid arthritis, the incidence of postoperative implant fracture is high.

468. The answer is A. *(Green, pp 172–173.)* Elderly patients with rheumatoid arthritis involving only one wrist are the preferred candidates for total wrist arthroplasty. The less radical procedure of silicone elastomer arthroplasty is favored when the rheumatoid process involves both wrists. For the younger patient with posttraumatic arthritis or any patient with old septic arthritis, both of which typically involve only one wrist, arthrodesis is the preferred procedure.

469. The answer is E. *(Green, pp 227–230.)* Flexor origin release usually provides 4 to 5 cm of lengthening, which would allow adequate extension of the fingers with the wrist in a dorsiflexed position. Possession of the intelligence and motivation necessary for an optimal result is suggested by the patient's occupation as an executive. Where more length is required (for more severe deformities), an STP tendon lengthening in the distal forearm would be necessary. The presence of active grasp is required for success following either of these procedures. As a general rule, patients with painful limbs are unable to cooperate in rehabilitation programs. Chemical neurectomy with phenol is often useful early; however, only the motor branches should be injected, not the entire nerve. Operative neurectomy is a more permanent procedure that should be reserved for patients with painful severe deformity and no hope of functional recovery.

470. The answer is B. *(Green, p 550.)* After a crushing injury of the hand, accumulating edema fluid forces the MCP joints into extension, which increases tension in the long flexors, resulting in flexion of the IP joints and wrist. Edema and fibrosis of the intrinsic muscles of the thumb pull the thumb into adduction. Thus, the "negative hand" seen after a neglected crushing injury is one of IP flexion, MCP extension, thumb adduction, and wrist flexion.

471. The answer is A. *(Green, pp 550–551.)* Early management of crush injuries of the hand is critical to the prevention of stiffness and deformity. A grossly edematous hand should be splinted as close to the intrinsic plus position (full MCP flexion and full IP extension) as possible. The MCP joints can be maintained in full flexion because their volar plates, unlike those of the IP joints, are collapsible and therefore do not migrate to the same degree as those of the IP joint. Also, since "checkreins" do not develop in the MCP joints, their optimal position is full flexion, which places the capsule and collateral ligaments on full stretch.

472. The answer is E. *(Green, p 558.)* Surgical treatment is usually required for long-standing extension contractures of the MCP joints. The anatomy of the MCP volar plate is such that even surgically induced volar plate capsulodesis will stretch out, with recurrence of deformity. Thus, dorsal capsulotomy and release of the lateral bands is necessary.

473. The answer is D. *(Green, p 593.)* Volkmann's contracture is the result of arterial and venous circulatory disturbances in closed osseofascial compartments resulting from buildup of tissue fluid pressure within the compartments. In the forearm, the greatest circulatory impairment is seen in the middle third of the muscle bellies and in those muscles closest to the bone. The pathology is centered around the anterior interosseous artery; therefore, the muscles most severely affected are the flexor digitorum profundus and flexor pollicis longus, followed by the flexor digitorum superficialis and pronator teres. Involvement of the wrist flexors is relatively mild.

474. The answer is B. *(Green, pp 612–619.)* Intrinsic tenodesis achieves the treatment goals of releasing the PIP extension contracture and improving extension of the DIP joint. Crossed intrinsic transfers are indicated for the correction of ulnar drift with secondary tightness of the ulnar intrinsic muscles. Transection of the lateral band is used for correction of swan-neck deformities following posttraumatic contracture of necrotic interosseous muscles. Silastic arthroplasty would not be indicated unless joint destruction was also present and would not, in itself, correct intrinsic tightness. Distal intrinsic release is an acceptable alternative; however, it must be performed on both sides of the finger for optimal effectiveness.

475. The answer is C. *(Green, p 631.)* The shoulder-hand type of reflex sympathetic dystrophy (RSD) is caused by an injury in the region of the neck or shoulder girdle or a painful visceral lesion, such as a myocardial infarct or a peptic ulcer. The syndrome favors older females, and symptoms (painful paresthesias) typically spread from proximal to distal. A frozen shoulder is a constant feature, forearm rotation is often limited, and the finger joints are usually stiff in extension, as opposed to the flexion posture seen in other forms of RSD. The skin is typically drier and less red in the shoulder-hand syndrome than in other forms of RSD, and osteoporosis is frequent.

476. The answer is E. *(Kelley, pp 713–714.)* Were this a young patient with well-preserved joints, soft-tissue reconstruction might be considered. Given the articular destruction, however, arthrodeses or arthroplasties are the preferred treatment modalities. In general, arthroplasty is preferred for the MCP joints, while fusion is often favored for the PIP joints. Neither bracing nor physical therapy is likely to offer significant benefit in the correction of established deformity.

477. The answer is D. *(Rockwood, p 663.)* The classic picture of compartmental ischemia is persistent and increasing pain that is accentuated by passive stretch of the involved muscles, diminished distal sensation (which indicates ischemia of nerves in the involved compartment), weakness of compartmental muscles, and palpable tenderness and tenseness over the involved compartment. Even with severe ischemia, distal color and skin temperature are often normal, and distal pulses are rarely obliterated by increased compartmental pressure.

Adult Diseases and Disorders: Spine and Pelvis

Frank C. Wilson, M.D., and
Joe T. Minchew, M.D.

DIRECTIONS: Each question below contains five suggested responses. Select the **one best** response to each question.

478. The primary clinical effect of decreased disk height resulting from degenerative disk disease is

(A) nerve root compression
(B) increased stress on adjacent soft-tissue structures
(C) increased loading of facet joints
(D) loss of spinal motion
(E) radicular pain

479. A 56-year-old man has had 1 month of persistent lower back pain and radiculopathy. The most appropriate treatment is

(A) activity as tolerated, with strengthening and flexibility exercises
(B) laminectomy and disk excision
(C) appropriate imaging studies and chemonucleolysis if the disk is not sequestrated
(D) appropriate imaging studies and percutaneous aspiration of the disk if it is not sequestrated
(E) appropriate imaging studies and microdiskectomy

480. In most cases, the cause of low back pain is

(A) nerve root irritation
(B) overloading of the facet joints
(C) instability
(D) muscle strain
(E) unknown factors

481. The LEAST common cause of spinal instability is

(A) spinal surgery
(B) acute injury
(C) degenerative disk disease
(D) unilateral spondylolysis
(E) muscular insufficiency

482. When a vertical force of 1000 newtons is applied to the top of the sacrum, the force borne by the sacroiliac joints is approximately

(A) 100 newtons
(B) 250 newtons
(C) 500 newtons
(D) 750 newtons
(E) 1000 newtons

483. The figures show AP and lateral myelograms of a 68-year-old woman. Examination would most likely reveal

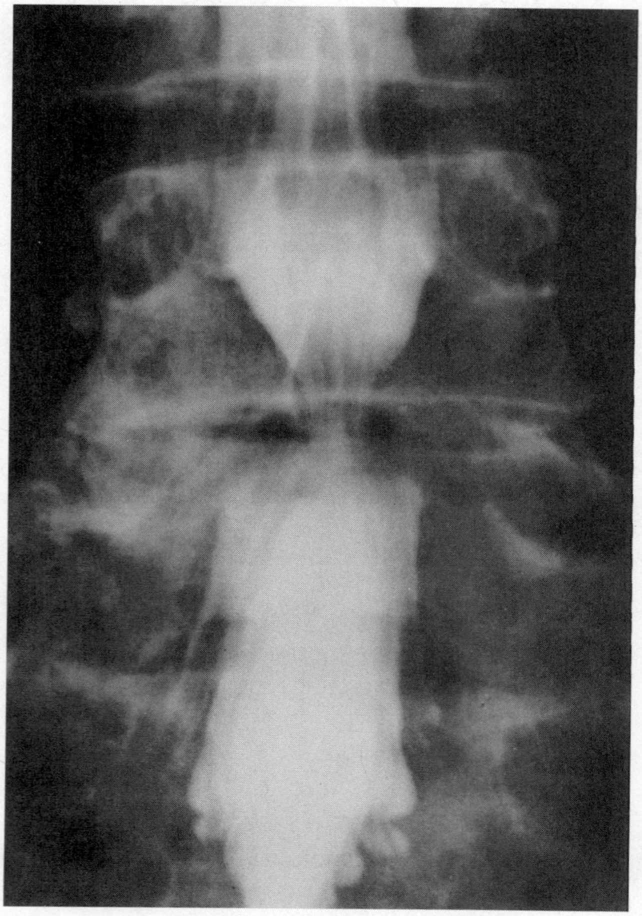

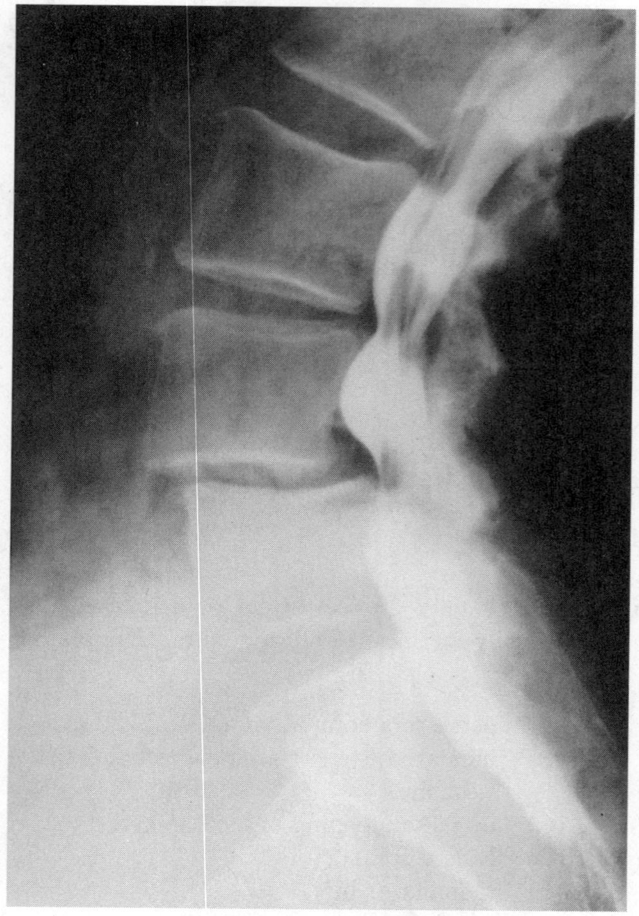

(A) weakness of the left extensor hallucis longus (EHL) and tibialis posterior muscles; decreased sensation on the dorsum of the foot; absent ankle jerk
(B) normal motor, sensory, and reflex findings in the lower limbs
(C) weakness of the right EHL and tibialis posterior muscles; decreased sensation on the dorsum of the foot; absent ankle jerk
(D) bilateral footdrop; decreased sensation in a stocking distribution below the knees with saddle anesthesia; absent knee and ankle jerks
(E) weakness of the left tibialis anterior muscle; decreased sensation on the medial calf and ankle; absent knee jerk

484. The primary biochemical changes in the pathogenesis of degenerative disk disease are

(A) a decrease in the proteoglycan content of the disk and annulus and calcification of the vertebral end plates
(B) a change in the proteoglycans of the disk with disproportionate loss of keratan sulfate, an increase in collagenization of the annulus, and softening of the vertebral end plates
(C) decreased collagenization of the disk and thinning of the vertebral end plates
(D) increased water content of the nucleus, changes in the collagenous architecture of the annulus, and thinning of the vertebral end plates
(E) increased proteoglycan and collagenous content of the nucleus, decreased collagenization of the annulus, and thickening of the vertebral end plates

485. Acute lumbar disk herniation occurs most commonly in patients in the age group

(A) under 20 years
(B) 20 to 30 years
(C) 31 to 50 years
(D) 51 to 70 years
(E) over 70 years

486. The most common direction for symptomatic herniation of a lumbar intervertebral disk is

(A) posteriorly
(B) posterolaterally
(C) anteriorly
(D) anterolaterally
(E) intraforaminally

487. The most common direction for symptomatic herniation of a cervical intervertebral disk is

(A) posteriorly
(B) posterolaterally
(C) anteriorly
(D) anterolaterally
(E) intraforaminally

488. The incidence of myelopathy in patients with spondylosis of the cervical spine is approximately

(A) 5 percent
(B) 15 percent
(C) 25 percent
(D) 50 percent
(E) 75 percent

489. The most frequent predictor of acute myelopathy in patients with spondylosis of the cervical spine is the presence of

(A) an unstable segment
(B) a central soft disk herniation
(C) a vascular malformation of the cord
(D) a midcervical canal diameter of 17 to 20 mm
(E) a congenital vertebral anomaly

490. In adults, cervical instability most commonly results from

(A) degenerative disk disease
(B) a flexion-extension injury
(C) a rotational injury
(D) increased ligamentous laxity
(E) hypoplastic facet joints

491. The pathogenesis of the lesion seen in the figure is most likely

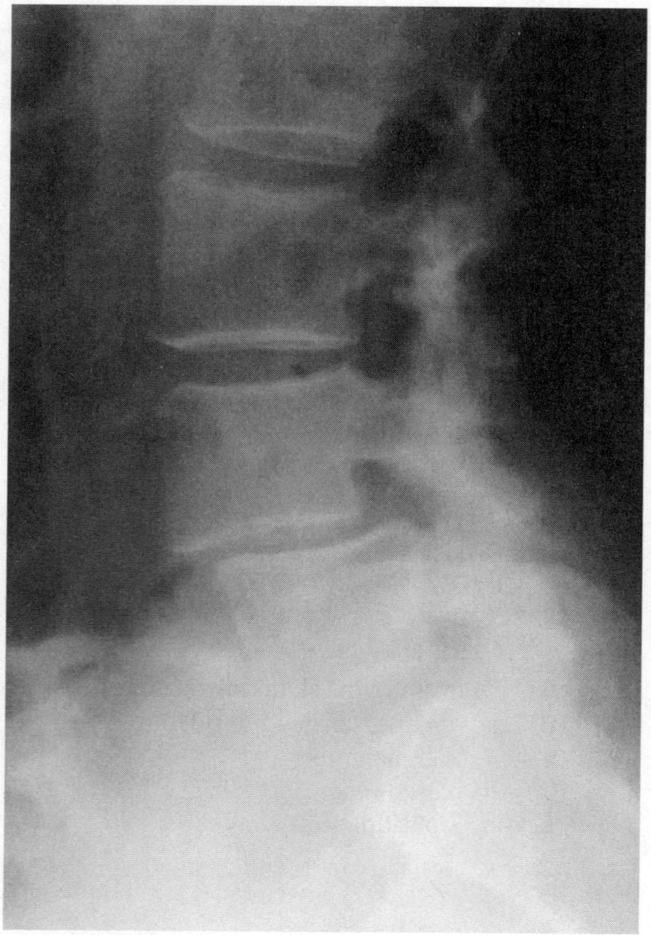

(A) degenerative
(B) congenital
(C) metastatic
(D) traumatic
(E) iatrogenic

492. In degenerative spondylolisthesis of the lumbar spine, the maximum vertebral slippage is

(A) 10 percent
(B) 20 percent
(C) 30 percent
(D) 40 percent
(E) 50 percent

493. The sensory changes expected with an acute disk herniation at the C7–T1 level are at the

(A) back of the neck and anterior chest
(B) deltoid area
(C) index and middle fingers
(D) thumb and index finger
(E) ring and little fingers

494. The motor changes most commonly encountered with an acute disk herniation at the C5–6 level are primarily in the

(A) extensor digitorum communis
(B) interossei
(C) biceps and extensor carpi radialis
(D) biceps and deltoid
(E) triceps

495. Cervical traction and compression tests are most useful in the diagnosis of

(A) vascular insufficiency of the cervical cord
(B) cervical radiculopathy
(C) cervical myelopathy
(D) arthritis of the facet joints
(E) intraspinal tumors of the cervical region

496. In asymptomatic persons between 30 and 70 years of age, radiographic evidence of spondylosis of the cervical spine is present in approximately

(A) 10 percent
(B) 20 percent
(C) 35 percent
(D) 50 percent
(E) 75 percent

497. The major advantage of contrast CT over routine myelography in the evaluation of cervical radiculopathy is the

(A) visualization of areas distal to myelographic blockade
(B) assessment of foraminal encroachment
(C) more accurate assessment of spinal canal diameter
(D) differentiation of disk compression from compression by other soft-tissue lesions
(E) safety and simplicity of the technique

498. The primary advantage of contrast CT over MRI in the evaluation of cervical spondylosis is

(A) more accurate identification of the cause of neurologic compression
(B) better localization of the disease level
(C) greater sensitivity for inflammatory processes
(D) greater specificity for inflammatory processes
(E) more accurate depiction of marrow changes

499. In the study of patients with cervical spondylosis, the greatest value of electromyography (EMG) is to

(A) exclude compressive neuropathies in the upper limb
(B) distinguish anterior horn cell degeneration from upper motor neuron disease
(C) identify cervical radiculopathies that affect only the sensory nerve root
(D) detect cervical radiculopathy early after the onset of symptoms
(E) localize the level of neural compression

500. Which of the following is most important in the early management of cervical radiculopathy?

(A) Immobilization
(B) Traction
(C) Nonsteroidal anti-inflammatory drugs (NSAIDs)
(D) Exercises to strengthen the paravertebral musculature
(E) Trigger-point injections

501. In cervical spondylosis, the plain radiographic changes most likely to be associated with clinical symptoms are in the

(A) disk spaces
(B) apophyseal joints
(C) foramina
(D) posterior articular processes
(E) soft tissues

502. The physical findings most likely to be associated with herniation of the C6–7 disk are

(A) hypesthesia of the thumb; weakness of elbow extension
(B) hypesthesia of the long finger; weakness of wrist flexion
(C) hypesthesia of the index finger; weakness of shoulder abduction
(D) hypesthesia of the lateral forearm; weakness of elbow flexion
(E) hypesthesia of the ring and little fingers; weakness of the hand intrinsics

503. The most common neurologic complication of surgery on the cervical spine is injury to the

(A) spinal cord
(B) nerve roots
(C) sympathetic chain
(D) recurrent laryngeal nerve
(E) ansa cervicalis

504. In an otherwise healthy patient with mild spastic paraparesis and the CT/myelogram shown in the figure, the most appropriate treatment is

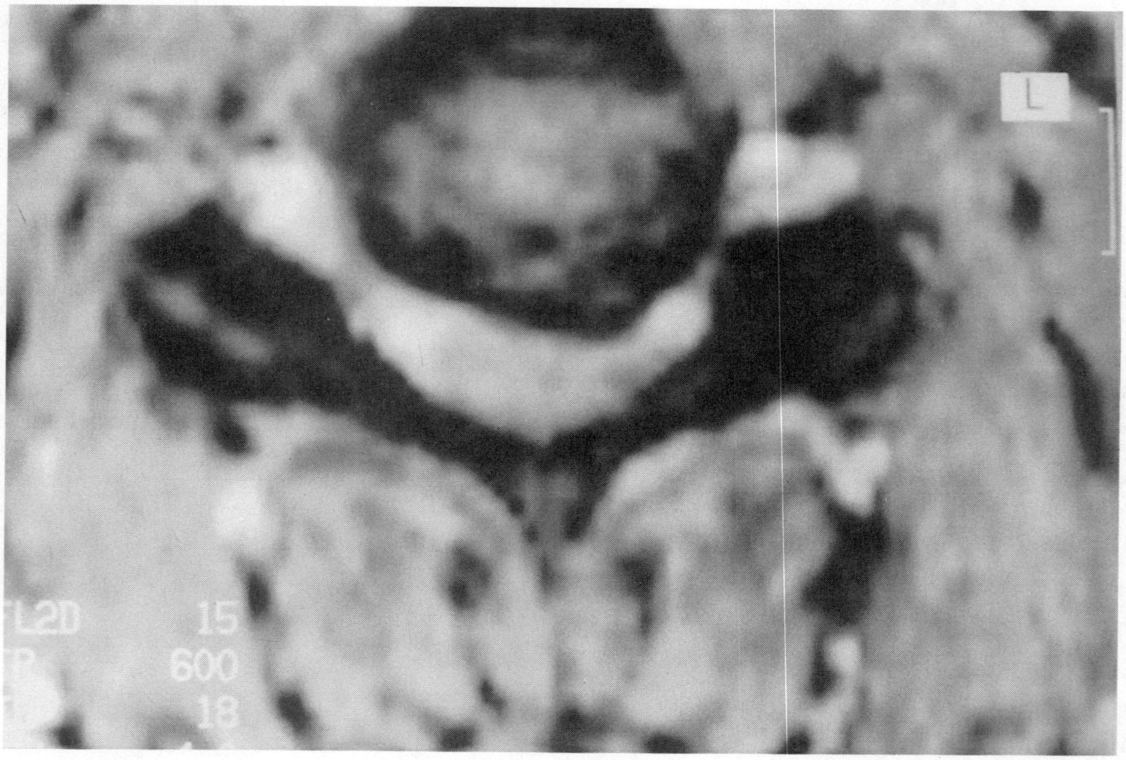

(A) immobilization in a soft cervical collar and careful observation for progression of the neurologic deficit
(B) immobilization in a soft cervical collar, cervical traction, and an isometric exercise program
(C) foraminal decompression
(D) decompressive laminectomy with reconstruction of the spinal canal
(E) anterior decompression and fusion

505. The preferred management of a symptomatic patient with the CT/myelogram of the thoracic spine shown in the figure is

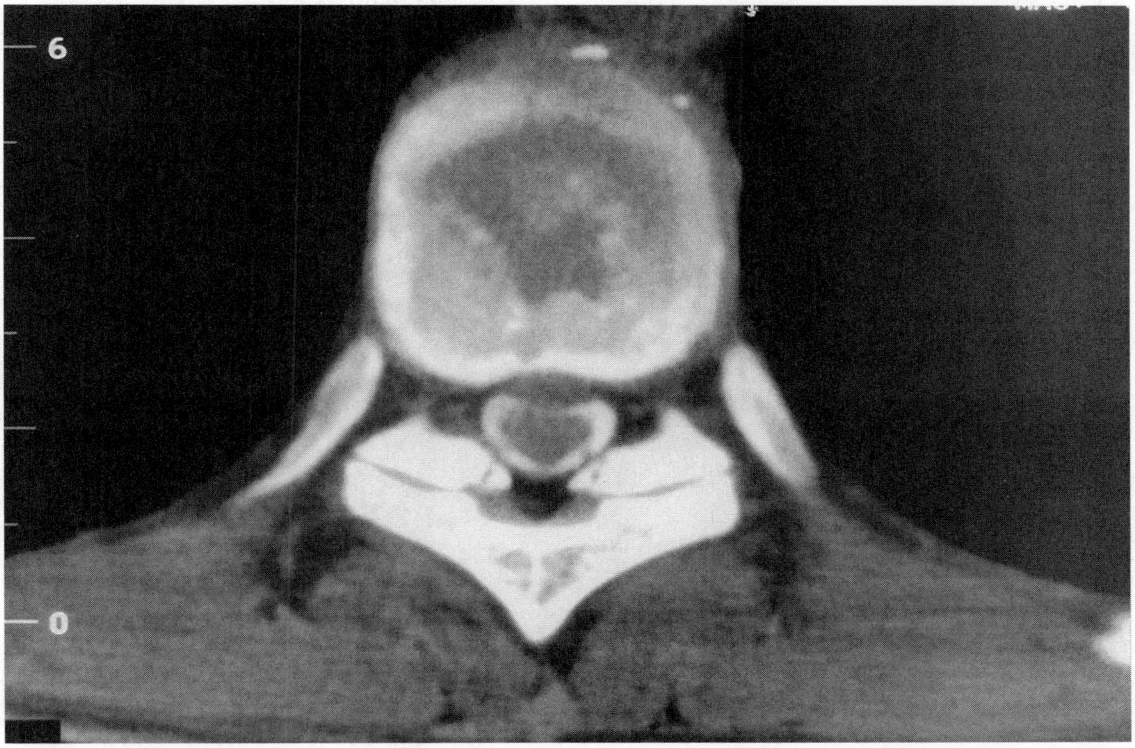

(A) bed rest
(B) physical therapy
(C) oral anti-inflammatory agents
(D) epidural steroids
(E) surgical intervention

---

506. The posture associated with the greatest lumbar intradiskal pressure is

(A) sitting, trunk flexed
(B) sitting, trunk erect
(C) standing, trunk flexed
(D) standing, trunk erect
(E) lying, lateral decubitus

507. In a patient with radiographic evidence of degenerative disk disease in the lumbar spine, pain referred to the sacroiliac joint and upper buttocks most likely results from

(A) compression of the L3 nerve root
(B) compression of the L4 nerve root
(C) compression of the L5 nerve root
(D) compression of the S1 nerve root
(E) abnormal stimulation of the annulus or facet joint capsule

508. The factor most frequently associated with an increased risk of lumbar disk herniation is

(A) pregnancy
(B) obesity
(C) height over 6′2″
(D) repetitive lifting and twisting
(E) increased lumbar lordosis

509. The most reliable finding to distinguish neurogenic claudication from vascular claudication is

(A) reduction of the neurologic deficit by rapid ambulation
(B) changes in limb coloration with elevation and dependency
(C) lack of symptom production by the bicycle test
(D) confinement of pain to the posterior thigh
(E) production of pain by walking uphill

510. The single most valuable confirmatory radiographic test for the diagnosis of acute herniation of a lumbar disk is

(A) metrizamide myelography
(B) diskography
(C) epidural venography
(D) MRI
(E) CT

511. The most likely location of a sensory deficit resulting from the myelographic lesion shown in the figure is the

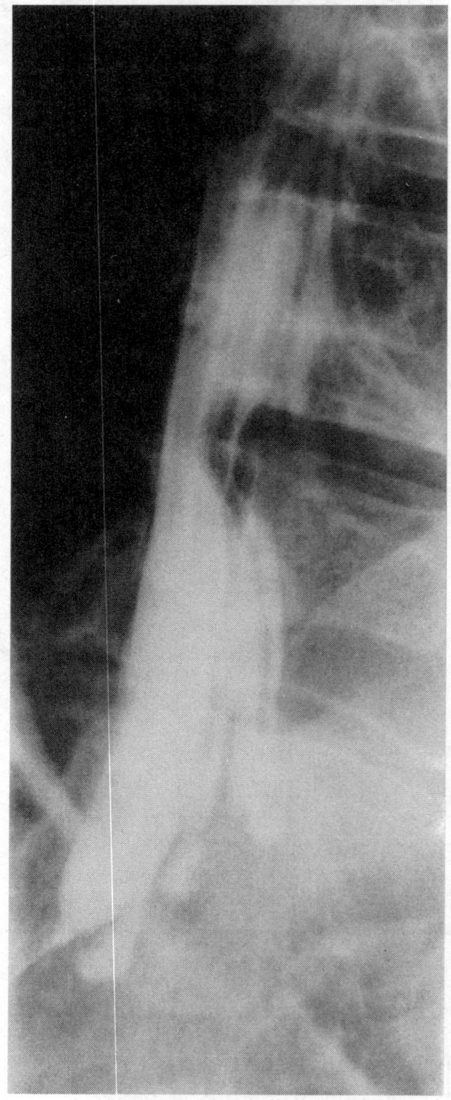

(A) anterior knee
(B) posterior calf
(C) dorsal foot
(D) lateral foot
(E) medial leg

512. Electromyography (EMG) is most helpful in evaluating disorders of the lower back in the

(A) differentiation of disk disease from diabetic neuropathy
(B) differentiation of disk disease from peripheral nerve injury
(C) early evaluation of nerve root compression
(D) confirmation of clinical and imaging findings
(E) detection of secondary nerve root involvement

513. The structural abnormality most likely to be associated with significant low back pain is

(A) spondylolysis
(B) facet hypoplasia
(C) lumbarization of S1
(D) sacralization of L5
(E) spina bifida occulta

514. A 56-year-old man had constant, nonradiating low back pain that was unaffected by posture or rest and had not responded to appropriate conservative care. Plain radiographs were normal. The most valuable screening procedure would be a

(A) facet block with lidocaine and corticosteroids
(B) bone scan
(C) GI series
(D) CT scan
(E) gadolinium-enhanced MRI scan

515. A 36-year-old man with sciatica, no neurologic deficit, and a negative straight leg raising test had not responded to 6 weeks of activity modification. Plain radiographs were normal, and an MRI is shown in the figure. The next diagnostic or therapeutic procedure should be

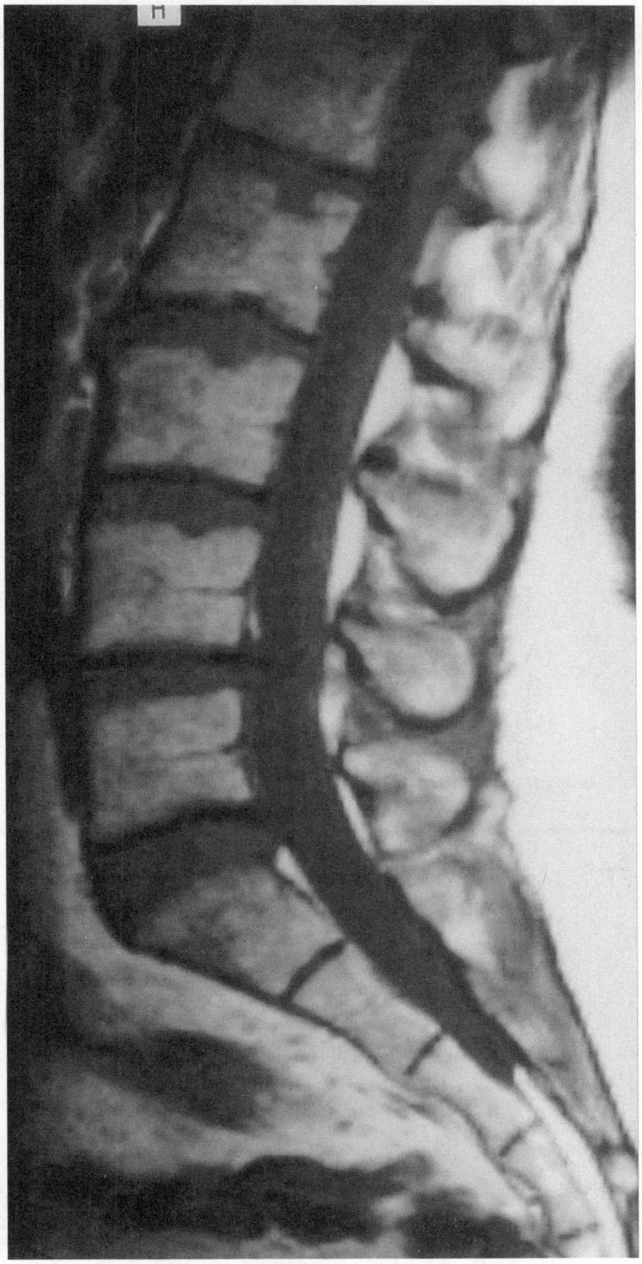

(A) microdiskectomy
(B) psychosocial evaluation
(C) chymopapain injection
(D) continued nonoperative care
(E) percutaneous automated nucleotomy

516. A 42-year-old woman had sciatica and an absent ankle jerk. The CT scan in the figure had not improved after 3 months of nonoperative treatment. The next diagnostic or therapeutic procedure should be

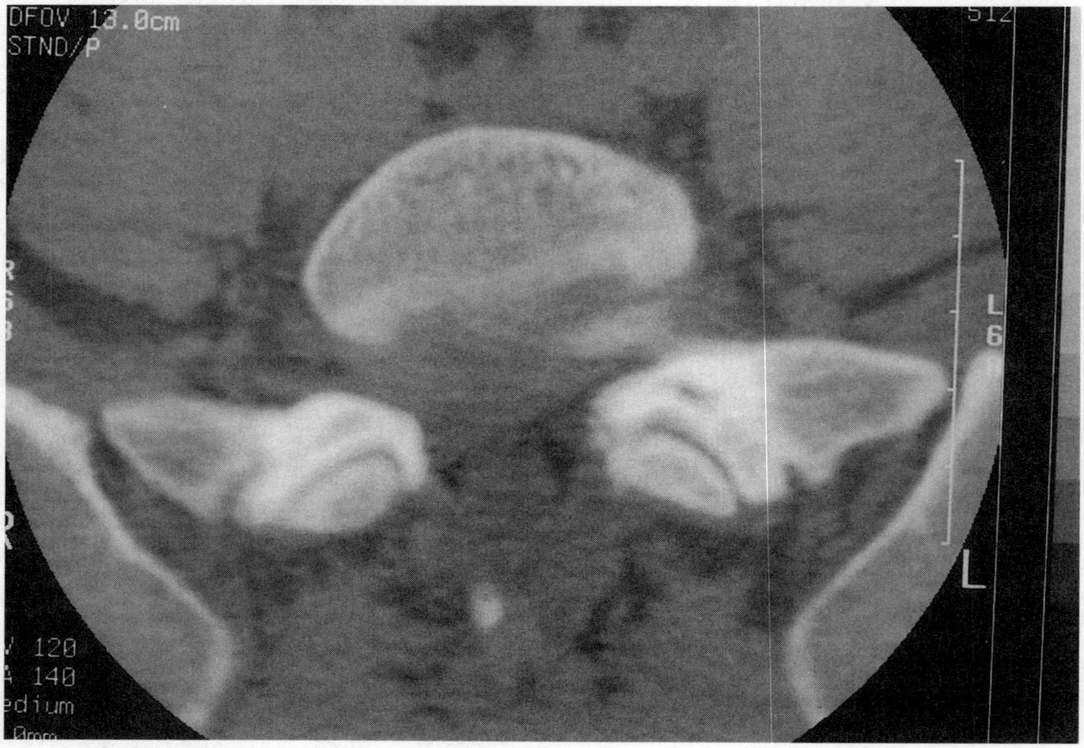

(A) EMG studies
(B) a psychosocial evaluation
(C) an MRI scan
(D) a CT myelogram
(E) a surgical procedure

---

517. A 37-year-old man had low back pain radiating to the leg and paresthesias 3 days after a lifting-twisting injury. The remainder of the history was unremarkable. Examination revealed decreased sensation on the lateral border of the foot and an absent ankle jerk. The next diagnostic or therapeutic procedure should be

(A) MRI
(B) AP and lateral radiography of the lumbar spine
(C) AP, lateral, and oblique radiography of the lumbar spine
(D) CT myelography
(E) activity modification and medications

518. In patients with rheumatoid arthritis, the most common abnormality in the cervical spine is

(A) anterior atlantoaxial subluxation
(B) posterior atlantoaxial subluxation
(C) subaxial subluxation
(D) atlantoaxial rotatory subluxation
(E) basilar invagination

519. A 50-year-old man had an acute onset of back and radiating lower limb pain. The figure is an axial T1-weighted MRI image at the L4–5 level. The most likely findings on examination would be

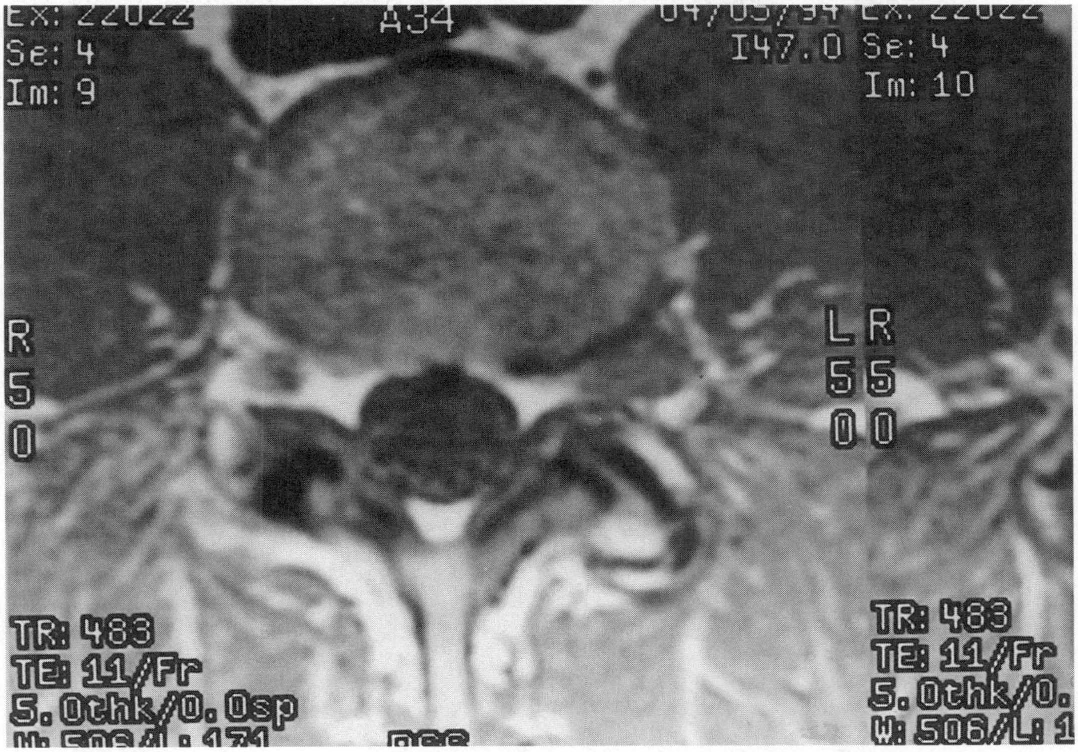

(A) decreased sensation on the right lateral calf and dorsum of the foot; weakness of the right extensor hallucis longus and tibialis posterior muscles
(B) decreased sensation on the left medial calf; weakness of the left tibialis anterior muscle; absent left quadriceps reflex
(C) decreased sensation on the left lateral calf and dorsum of the foot; weakness of the left extensor hallucis longus and tibialis posterior muscles
(D) numbness and tingling of both lower extremities, saddle anesthesia, weakness of anterior tibial and extensor hallucis longus muscles, absent ankle jerks bilaterally
(E) decreased sensation on the right posterior calf and lateral foot; weakness of the left peroneal musculature, absent left ankle jerk

520. A 49-year-old patient complained of low back pain radiating to both legs and paresthesias in both legs and feet. Examination revealed decreased perineal sensibility and bilateral weakness of the extensor hallucis longus and peroneal muscles. An MRI scan is shown below. The most appropriate treatment is

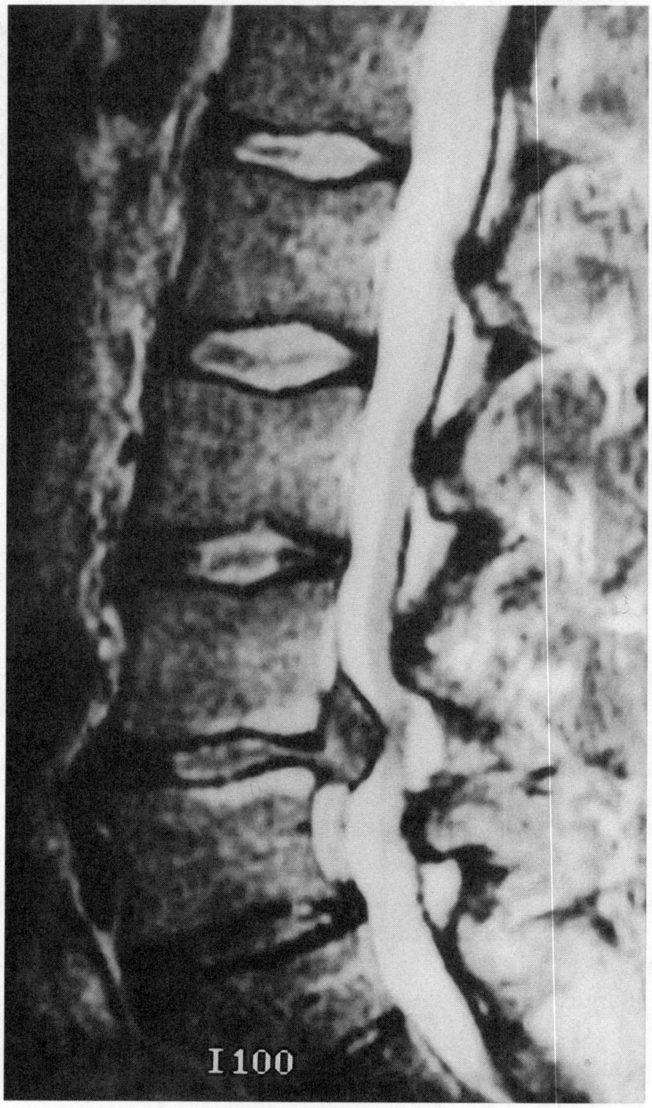

(A) oral anti-inflammatory medications and activity modification
(B) epidural steroid injections
(C) emergent diskectomy
(D) oral steroids
(E) physical therapy

521. A 47-year-old man had low back pain and severe, burning pain radiating to both lateral calves 1 year after having undergone laminectomy, diskectomy, and spinal arthrodesis at L4–5. A CT myelogram is shown below. The most likely explanation of this patient's leg pain is

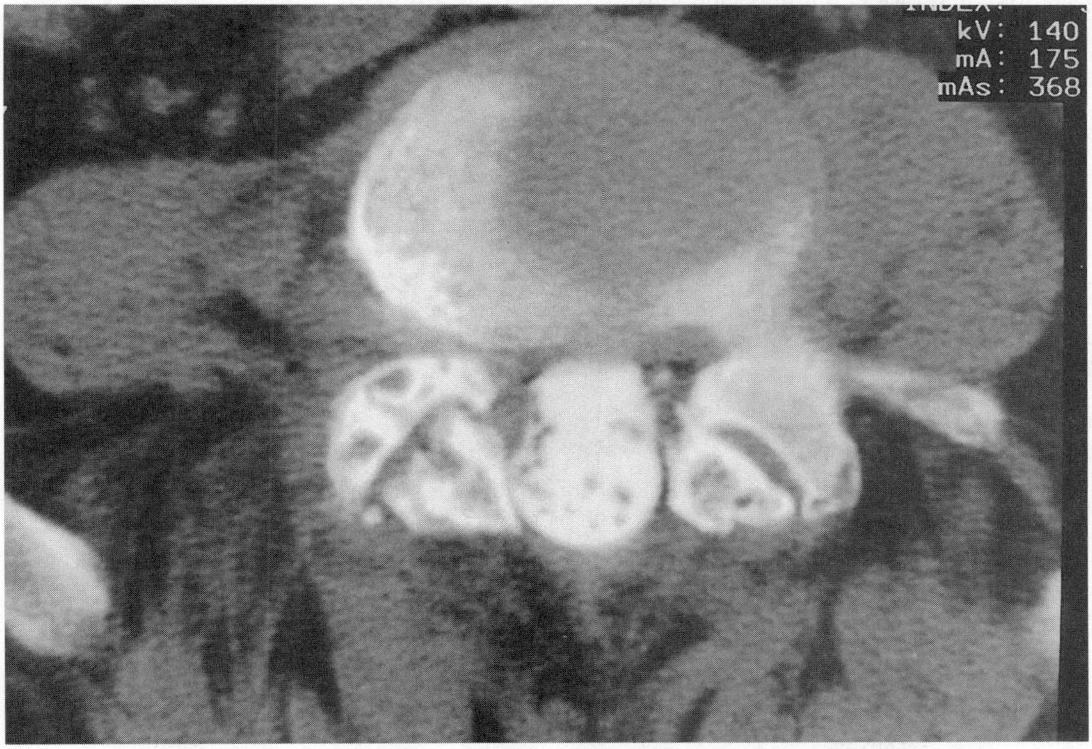

(A) stenosis of the lateral recess
(B) recurrent or residual herniated nucleus pulposus
(C) adhesive arachnoiditis
(D) pseudarthrosis of the fusion
(E) functional pain syndrome

522. The figures below are precontrast (*left*) and postcontrast (*right*) sagittal MRI images of a 33-year-old man who underwent L4–5 diskectomy 3 months previously for recalcitrant L5 radiculopathy. The patient had complete relief of pain for 2 months. Over the last 4 weeks, however, he has had the return of severe pain, preoperative neurologic findings, and tension signs. The most likely cause of the pain is

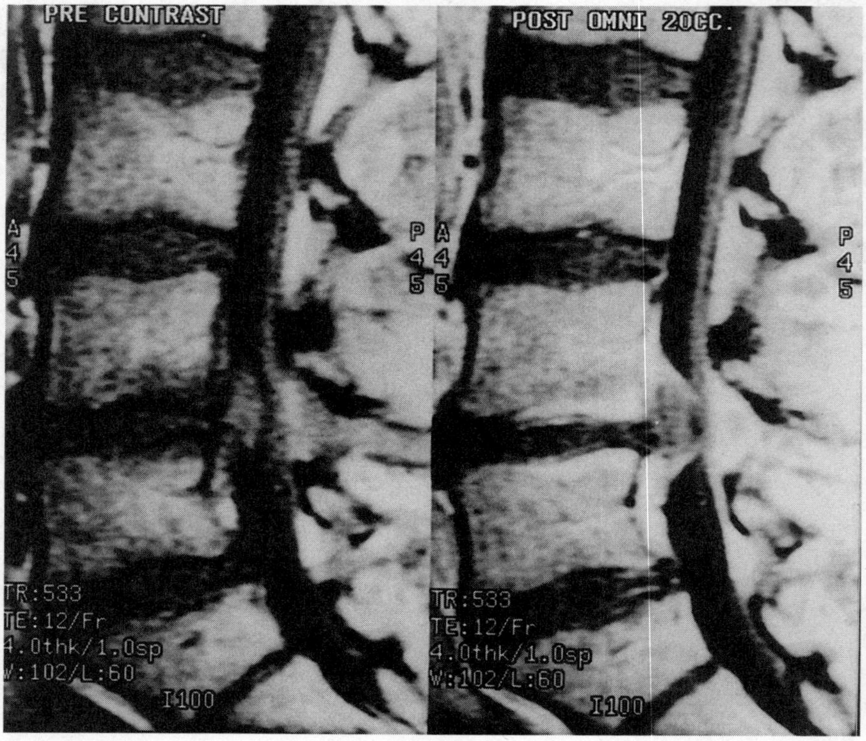

(A) lateral recess stenosis
(B) recurrent or residual herniated nucleus pulposus
(C) adhesive arachnoiditis
(D) epidural or perineural scar formation
(E) functional pain syndrome

523. A 51-year-old Asian man complained of mild neck pain, bilateral hand numbness, and clumsiness. Examination revealed hyperreflexia and extensor plantar responses bilaterally. A CT myelogram is shown below. The most likely diagnosis is

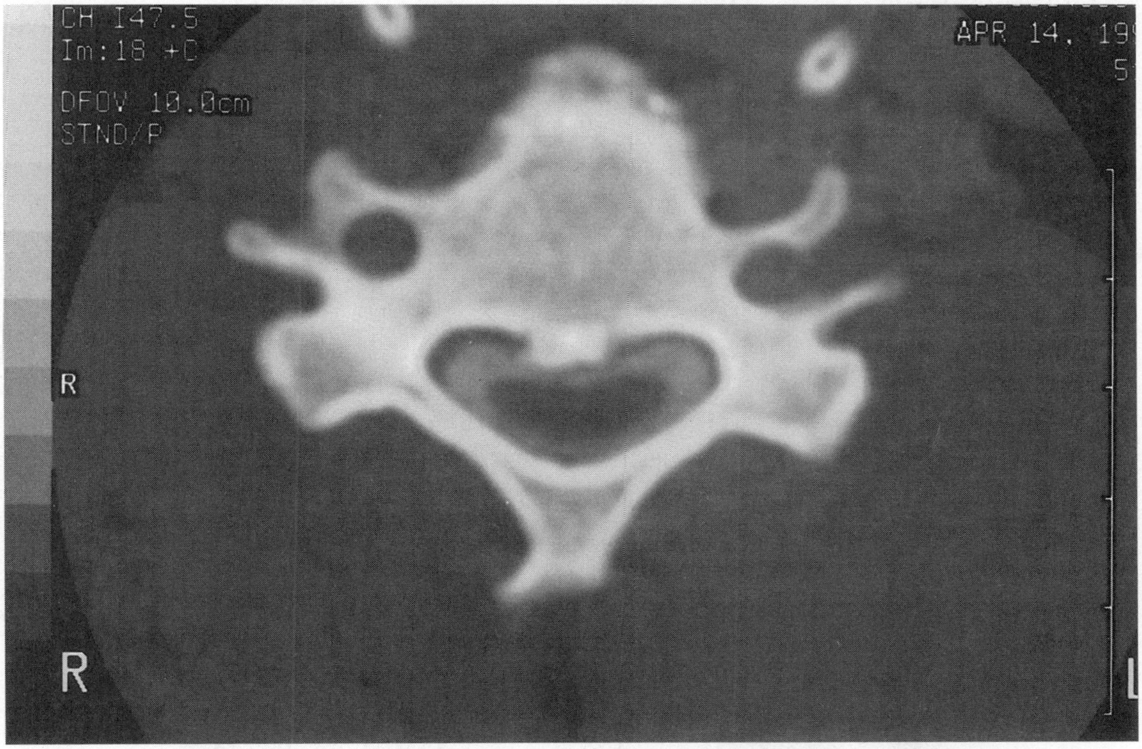

(A) a large, central "soft" disk herniation
(B) a large, central "hard" disk herniation
(C) cervical spondylosis
(D) ossification of the posterior longitudinal ligament
(E) uncovertebral spondylosis

524. A 27-year-old man has had 4 months of gradually worsening low back and lumbosacral pain, worse in the morning, associated with significant stiffness, and improved by exercise and NSAIDs. Examination revealed decreased lumbar mobility in all directions, normal sensation, and no weakness. An AP radiograph is shown below. The most useful physical finding for confirming the diagnosis is

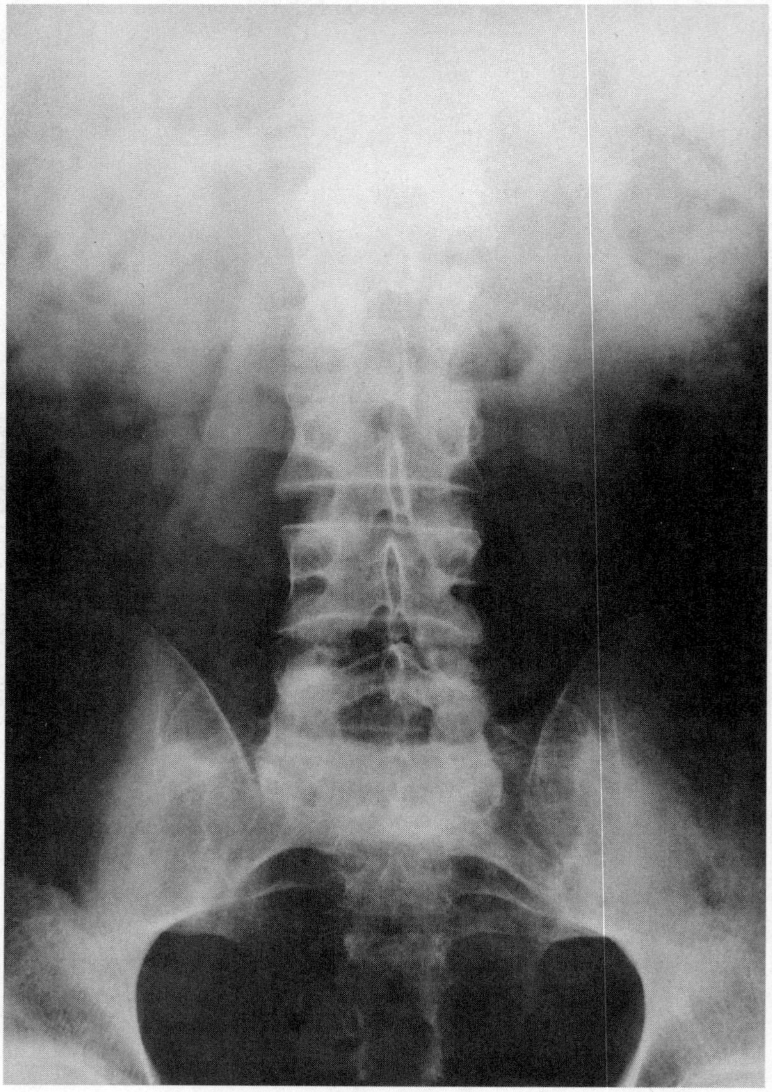

(A) a positive straight leg raising test
(B) limitation of chest expansion to 1 inch or less
(C) urethritis
(D) bilateral tightness of the hamstrings
(E) unilateral absence of the Achilles reflex

525. A 35-year-old woman who had undergone posterior spinal fusion from T7 to L4 with Harrington instrumentation for adolescent idiopathic scoliosis at age 13 complained of 18 months of back fatigue and right-sided low back pain. The pain was located in the mid to lower lumbar region, was worse with activity, and was relieved by rest. The neurologic examination was normal. Radiographs of the spine are shown below. The most likely source of her pain is

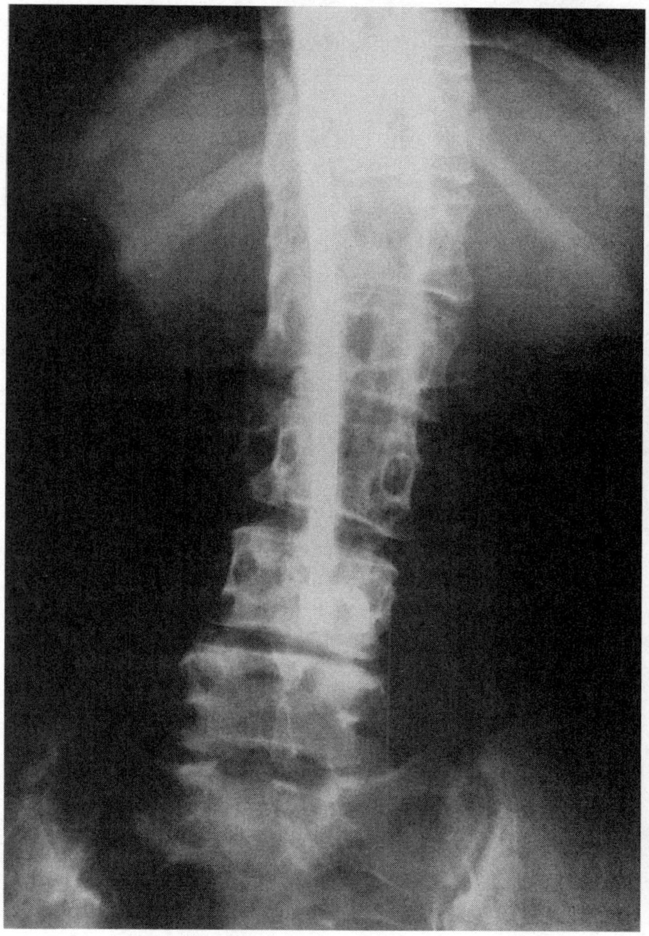

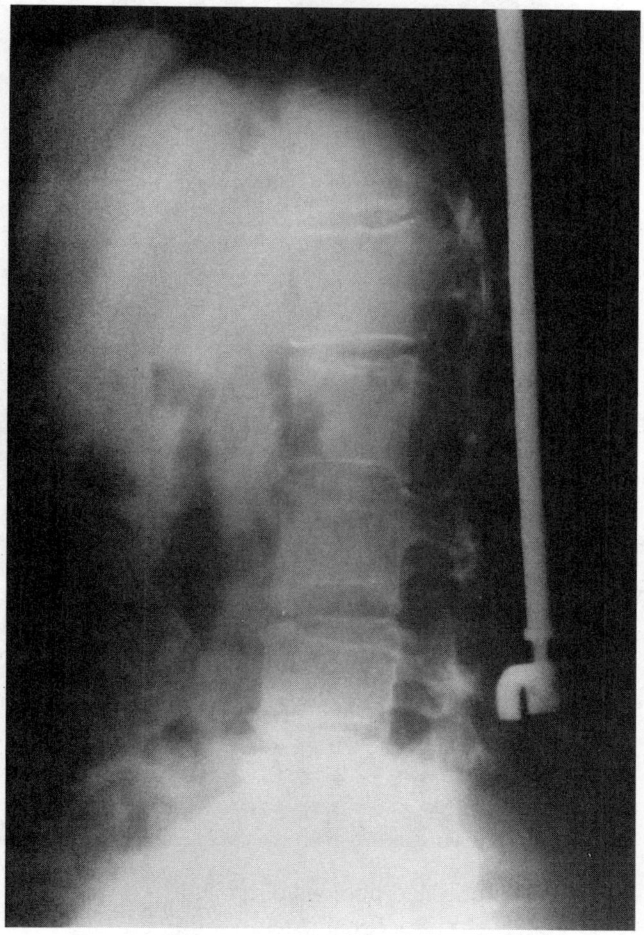

(A) degenerative disk disease
(B) degenerative arthritis of the facet joints
(C) pseudarthrosis of the fusion
(D) dislodgement of the instrumentation
(E) loss of the normal sagittal contour of the spine

526. A 57-year-old man has had 4 months of progressively worsening low back pain, which began 1 week after heavy lifting. The pain is dull, deep-seated, constant, and not relieved by rest, activity limitation, or NSAIDs. He also has had low-grade fevers and progressive fatigue. Sagittal MRI images are shown below. The most likely diagnosis is

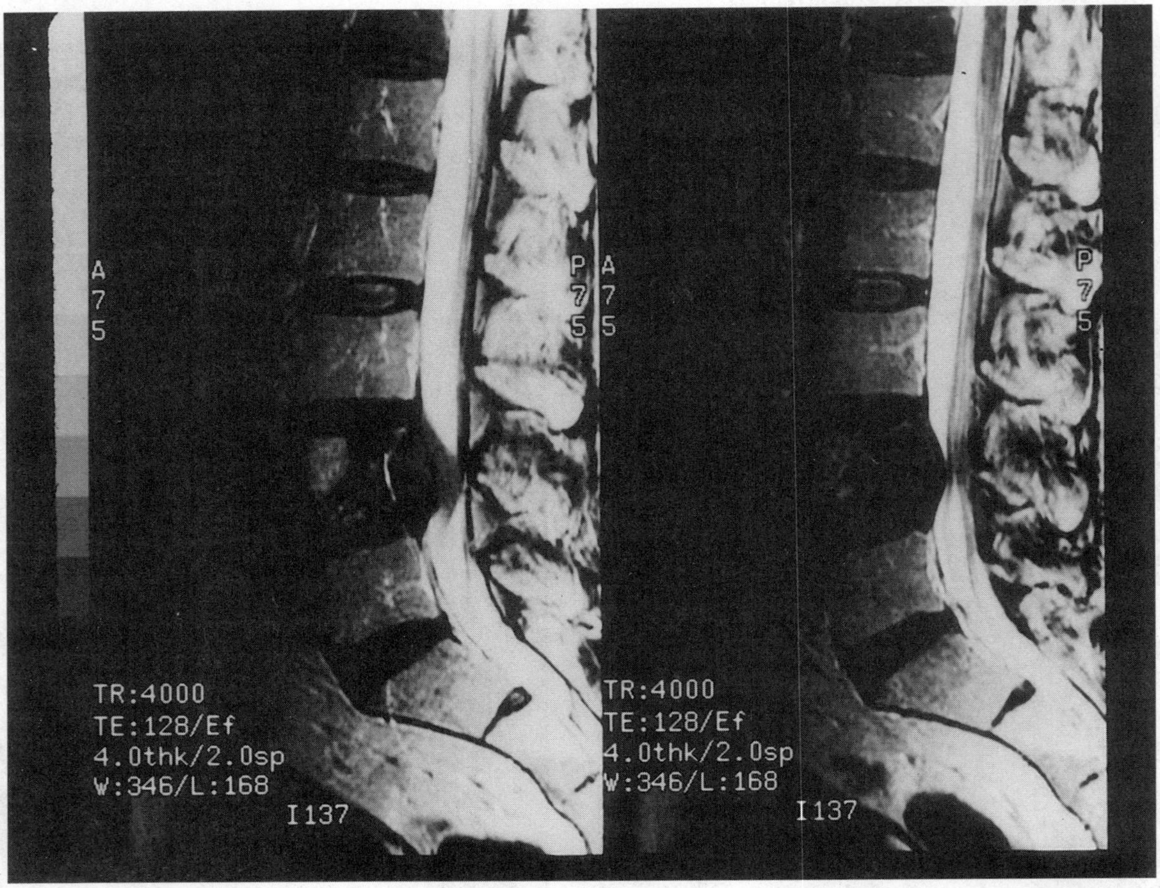

(A) herniated nucleus pulposus
(B) staphylococcal osteomyelitis
(C) osteogenic sarcoma
(D) chondrosarcoma
(E) osseous metastases

527. A 39-year-old man had 4 months of intermittent lumbosacral pain, which has now become constant and severe. Over the last 2 weeks, he has experienced paresthesias in both lower limbs. Examination revealed tenderness over the lumbar spine, paraspinous muscle spasm, a hip flexion contracture, a positive femoral stretch test, and a temperature of 38°C (100.4°F). Laboratory evaluation revealed an ESR of 60 mm/h and a WBC of 11,800. Figures A, B, and C on the following page are a lateral lumbosacral radiograph and T1- and T2-weighted sagittal MRI images, respectively. The most likely diagnosis is

(A) pyogenic osteomyelitis
(B) nonpyogenic osteomyelitis
(C) metastatic carcinoma
(D) Guillain-Barré syndrome
(E) an L2–3 herniated nucleus pulposus

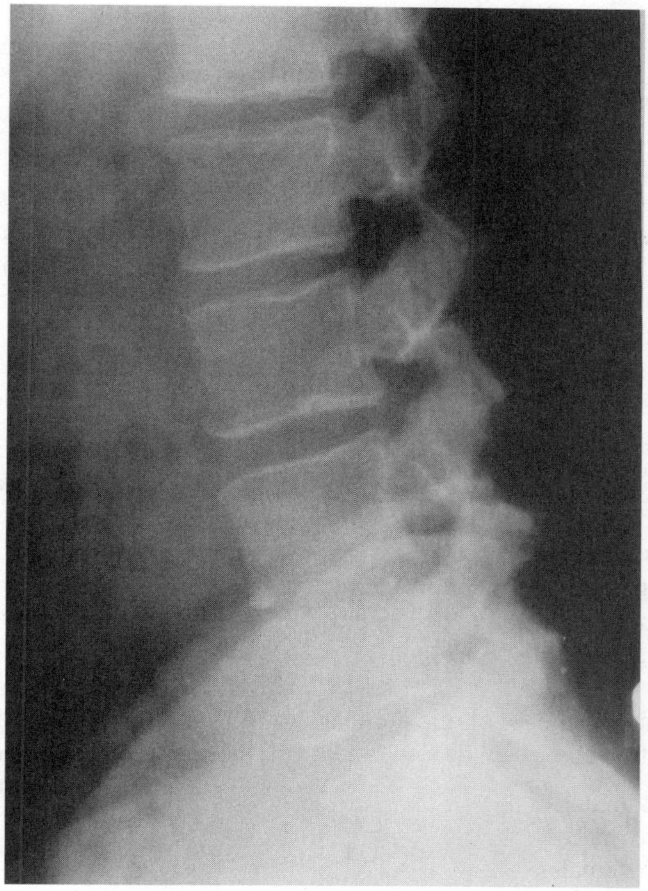

A

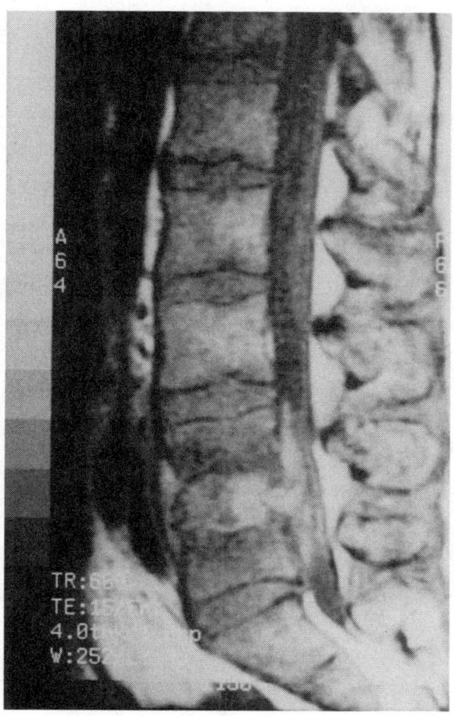

B

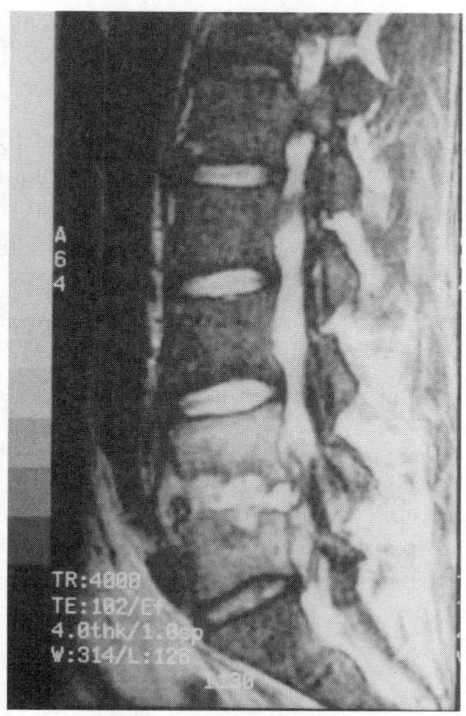

C

528. The imbibition pressure of the intervertebral disk is provided by the

(A) arrangement of collagen fibrils in the annulus
(B) negatively charged groups of proteoglycan side chains
(C) collagenase enzymes within the disk
(D) resistance of the vertebral end plates to compressive forces
(E) presence of collagen fibrils within the disk

529. The feature of degenerative disk disease most responsible for nerve root compression is

(A) increased lateral bulging of the annulus
(B) decreased disk height
(C) inward bulging of the inner annulus
(D) reduced internal pressure in the nucleus
(E) increased spinal mobility

530. Degenerative spondylolisthesis of the lumbar spine occurs most often at

(A) L3–4, in black males
(B) L3–4, in white males
(C) L3–4, in black females
(D) L4–5, in black females
(E) L5–S1, in white males

531. The pattern of neurologic findings most consistent with an acute herniation of the C4–5 disk is

(A) decreased sensation over the lateral forearm, weakness of wrist extension, absence of the brachioradialis reflex
(B) decreased sensation in the small finger, weakness of the interossei, absence of the triceps reflex
(C) decreased sensation in the middle finger, weakness of the triceps, absence of the triceps reflex
(D) decreased sensation over the lateral arm, weakness of the deltoid, absence of the triceps reflex
(E) decreased sensation over the lateral arm, weakness of the deltoid, no reflex asymmetry

532. Based on MRI studies, the maximum reduction in spinal cord volume encountered in asymptomatic patients with cervical spondylosis is approximately

(A) 3 percent
(B) 10 percent
(C) 15 percent
(D) 25 percent
(E) 30 percent

533. The primary advantage of MRI over contrast CT in the evaluation of cervical spondylosis is

(A) better localization of disease level
(B) less operator dependency
(C) more accurate identification of the cause of neural compression
(D) noninvasiveness
(E) better determination of lateral encroachment

534. In a patient with radiographic evidence of degenerative disk disease in the lumbar spine, pain referred to the medial aspect of the leg most likely results from

(A) compression of the L3 nerve root
(B) compression of the L4 nerve root
(C) compression of the L5 nerve root
(D) compression of the S1 nerve root
(E) abnormal stimulation of the annulus or facet joint capsule

Adult Diseases and Disorders: Spine and Pelvis

Answers

478. The answer is C. *(Frymoyer, Gordon, p 160.)* The primary effect of decreased disk height is increased loading of the facet joints, which increases the rate of degenerative change in the lumbar spine. Although these changes contribute to back pain, they usually do not in themselves cause nerve root compression. Motion in affected spinal segments may be reduced, but the clinical impact of this reduction is minimal.

479. The answer is A. *(Frymoyer, Gordon, p 142.)* Since irreversible nerve damage is unlikely before 3 months, and since nonoperative means are often successful in treating this condition, one is justified in continuing nonoperative therapy. Should the patient develop motor weakness or signs of cauda equina compression (bilateral leg pain and bowel or bladder dysfunction), prompt surgical decompression should be considered.

480. The answer is E. *(Frymoyer, Gordon, p 261.)* Only in a relatively small percentage of cases is the precise cause of low back pain known. Each of the choices listed in A through D may cause, either alone or in combination, low back pain. In most patients, however, the specific role played by each of these and other factors is unknown.

481. The answer is D. *(Frymoyer, Gordon, p 261.)* Spinal surgery (especially facetectomy), acute or chronic injury, degenerative disk disease, and muscular insufficiency are established causes of spinal instability. While bilateral spondylolysis often increases spinal instability, unilateral spondylolysis does not. In unilateral spondylolysis, the posterior vertebral ring is broken in only one place, so there is no potential for displacement of the spinal elements.

482. The answer is C. *(Frymoyer, Gordon, p 268.)* Scholten and associates showed that when forces of up to 1000 newtons were applied to the sacrum, the forces internal to the sacroiliac joints were always less than 530 newtons. Perhaps for this reason, degenerative changes in the sacroiliac joints are less prevalent and less marked than those in the lower lumbar spine. The perception that lower back pain resulted from pathology in the sacroiliac joints led, in the early part of the twentieth century, to many sacroiliac fusions. However, disappearance of the pain with appropriate treatment of the degenerative disk disease disproved the theory of primary sacroiliac disease as a major cause of low back pain.

483. The answer is B. *(Frymoyer, pp 1804–1805.)* The radiographs demonstrate the classic "hour glass" indentation of the thecal sac at L4–5 seen in lumbar spinal stenosis. They also reveal an L4–5 degenerative spondylolisthesis, which is frequently associated with the development of spinal stenosis and neurogenic claudication. Patients with spinal stenosis causing neurogenic claudication frequently do not have physical findings at rest; however, neurologic deficits can be elicited by provocative tests, such as the "walk test" (ambulation until symptoms arise).

484. The answer is A. *(Boden, pp 26–28).* The major biochemical events associated with degenerative disk disease are a loss of proteoglycans from both the disk and annulus, combined with calcification of the vertebral end plates. Water is lost from the nucleus as a result of the decrease in nuclear proteoglycans, which further reduces imbibition pressure. Loss of the ability of the disk to withstand loading increases stress on the facet joints, which increases degenerative changes in these articulations. Calcification of the vertebral end plates reduces nutrition to the disk, which potentiates other degenerative changes.

485. The answer is C. *(Boden, p 39).* As the disk ages, the annulus fibrosus becomes brittle and develops cracks and tears extending to the periphery. With disk herniation, nuclear material extrudes through such a tear. Between the ages of 30 and 50, the annulus becomes significantly weaker because of these cracks, and sufficient turgor remains in the nucleus to generate a protrusion. In the elderly, dessication and shrinkage of the nucleus reduces the likelihood of acute herniation.

486. The answer is B. *(Boden, p 30.)* Most lumbar disk herniations occur as a result of flexion injuries, which force the nuclear material posteriorly. While disk herniation can occur anteriorly, posteriorly, or laterally, the weakest portion of the annulus is posterolaterally, where reinforcement by the posterior longitudinal ligament is weakest.

487. The answer is E. *(Boden, p 30.)* Although disk herniations in the lumbar spine are most commonly posterolateral, herniations in the cervical spine are most often intraforaminal. Both posterolateral and midline protrusions also occur in the cervical area. Intraforaminal and posterolateral protrusions in the cervical spine are more likely to produce radicular symptoms, while midline protrusions often cause myelopathy because of the proximity of the spinal cord to the herniation.

488. The answer is A. *(Boden, p 35.)* Stenosis of the cervical spine may cause radiculopathy, myelopathy, or both. Although only 5 percent of patients with cervical spondylosis develop myelopathy, it is important to recognize these patients early because of their poorer prognosis and the need for prompt surgical decompression. Myelopathic changes are subtle, usually gradual in onset, and often associated with the formation of posterior osteophytes.

489. The answer is B. *(Boden, p 35.)* Acute myelopathy is most often the result of a central soft disk herniation, manifest as a complete or nearly complete block on a myelogram. The diameter of the cervical canal is an important predictor of spinal stenosis. Myelopathy is rarely seen, however, in patients with cervical canal diameters greater than 17 mm.

490. The answer is A. *(Boden, p 35.)* Cervical instability, defined as AP subluxation of more than 3.5 mm or sagittal angulation greater than 20° on flexion-extension radiographs, most commonly results from disk degeneration, with its attendant changes in the facet joints and loss of ligamentous support. In the cervical spine, it may occur at a single level but often involves multiple levels. Increased ligamentous laxity is the most common cause of cervical instability in children.

491. The answer is A. *(Boden, p 35.)* Spondylolisthesis at L4–5 occurs most commonly as a result of degeneration of the disk and facet joints. Unlike isthmic spondylolisthesis, which usually occurs at L5–S1 in young patients, degenerative spondylolisthesis does not involve a pars intraarticularis defect. Degenerative spondylolisthesis occurs six times more commonly at L4–5 than at L3–4.

492. The answer is C. *(Boden, p 36.)* Unlike isthmic spondylolisthesis, there is no pars defect in degenerative spondylolisthesis, which limits slippage in degenerative spondylolisthesis to 30 percent. Many patients with degenerative spondylolisthesis are asymptomatic, especially when vertebral instability is not demonstrable radiographically.

493. The answer is E. *(Boden, p 46.)* Compression of the C8 nerve root by a disk herniation at C7–T1 produces sensory changes in the ring and little fingers. Compression of C7 involves the index and middle fingers, and C6 the thumb and index finger. C5 compression involves the deltoid area, and C4 compression the back of the neck and anterior chest.

494. The answer is C. *(Rothman, p 555.)* The biceps possesses dual innervation but is commonly affected in a C6 radiculopathy. The radial wrist extensors share a C6 innervation. The extensor digitorum communis and triceps are primarily innervated by C7, while the deltoid is innervated by C5.

495. The answer is B. *(Boden, p 49.)* Traction on the cervical spine often increases and compression decreases radicular symptoms. Compression is performed by compressing the head with the neck slightly flexed laterally toward the affected side. The axial traction test is performed by applying 20 to 30 pounds of traction with the patient in the supine position. These tests are more specific than sensitive for the diagnosis of nerve root compression.

496. The answer is C. *(Boden p 55.)* In a radiographic study of asymptomatic patients between 30 and 70 years of age, Friedenberg and Miller found that 35 percent had spondylosis. This finding emphasizes the poor correlation between clinical and radiographic findings. The most common radiographic findings in cervical spondylosis are osteophyte formation and narrowing of the disk space.

497. The answer is B. *(Boden, pp 56–57.)* The major advantage of contrast CT over myelography in the evaluation of cervical radiculopathy is more accurate localization of the pathology. Because myelographic contrast medium extends only a short way along the nerve root sleeve, lateral lesions, such as foraminal herniations, cannot be readily visualized with routine myelography. Myelographic blockade is usually associated with myelopathy rather than radiculopathy. It is possible to measure spinal cord diameter more accurately with CT contrast studies; however, that information is more important for patients with myelopathic than with radicular findings. Since CT contrast studies are also invasive and are commonly preceded by routine myelographic films, contrast studies are not safer and simpler.

498. The answer is A. *(Boden, pp 57–58.)* MRI scanning is less sensitive than contrast CT for determination of soft tissues versus bone as the cause of neurologic encroachment. The tests are approximately equal in their ability to localize the level of disk disease. MRI has greater sensitivity and specificity for inflammatory processes and provides more accurate depiction of marrow changes associated with neoplasia than does contrast CT.

499. The answer is E. *(Boden, p 60.)* In patients with symptomatic cervical spondylolysis, electromyography is most valuable in helping localize the level of neural compression. It may also be helpful in delineating peripheral compressive neuropathies, although nerve conduction studies are also needed for accurate diagnosis in these cases. EMG changes in segments affected by anterior horn cell degeneration may be indistinguishable from those of upper motor neuron disease, and EMG is unable to detect cervical radiculopathies that affect only the sensory nerve root. Falsely negative EMG examinations are more likely during the first month following the onset of symptoms.

500. The answer is A. *(Boden, p 66.)* Immobilization is the cornerstone of treatment for acute cervical radiculopathy and is usually accomplished with a soft collar worn continuously at the outset. NSAIDs are used as a supplement rather than a substitute for immobilization. As symptoms improve, exercises to strengthen the paravertebral musculature should be instituted. If no improvement occurs in 3 to 4 weeks, trigger-point injection should be considered, followed, if symptoms persist, by cervical traction. With such a program, most patients with cervical radiculopathy will be able to return to normal activities within 2 months.

501. The answer is A. *(Boden, p 67.)* Cervical spondylosis is, in many cases, a normal feature of aging. Many asymptomatic patients show degenerative disk disease on plain radiographs, myelograms, and MRIs of the cervical spine. The finding most likely to be present in symptomatic patients is narrowing of the C5–6 or C6–7 disk space.

502. The answer is B. *(Boden, p 46.)* Pain from radiculopathy at C5–6 or lower is commonly referred to the interscapular area. Lesions involving the seventh nerve root also commonly cause hypesthesia in the long finger and weakness of wrist flexion, especially the flexor carpi radialis. C5–6 lesions, involving the sixth cervical root, involve loss of sensation in the lateral forearm, thumb, and index fingers, whereas C8 radiculopathy classically produces hypesthesia in the ring and little fingers and weakness of the intrinsic muscles of the hand.

503. The answer is D. *(Boden, p 88.)* The frequency of neurologic complications following surgery on the cervical spine is 1 to 2 percent and is slightly lower with anterior than posterior approaches. The anterior approach has a higher rate of complications related to bone grafts employed for fusion. Injuries to the spinal cord, nerve roots, and sympathetic chain do occur, but injury to the recurrent laryngeal nerve is the most common neurologic complication.

504. The answer is E. *(Boden, pp 84–85.)* The combination of spastic paralysis and the CT/myelogram study in the figure indicates cervical myelopathy, which requires prompt decompression to prevent progression of the neurologic deficit. Either anterior or posterior approaches may be used; however, most surgeons now avoid attempts to reconstruct the spinal canal.

505. The answer is E. *(Boden, p 97.)* The CT/myelogram reveals a central thoracic disk herniation with effacement of the anterior CSF and spinal cord compression. Unlike herniations in cervical and lumbar disks, symptomatic thoracic herniations are treated solely by surgical intervention. When the diagnosis is suspected and confirmed, surgical decompression is indicated as soon as possible to prevent irreversible spinal cord injury. Standard midline laminectomy is not indicated for this disorder, as the ventral disk is not accessible without manipulation of the spinal cord, which is associated with a high risk of neurologic deterioration. Disk excision has been safely performed using either an anterior thoracotomy or a posterior costotransversectomy. Each approach has advantages and disadvantages, and the approach selected should be based on the location of the herniation and experience of the surgeon.

506. The answer is A. *(Boden, p 103.)* Nachemson's studies showed the lowest intradiskal pressure occurred with the patient supine, followed by the lateral decubitus position. Sitting produced higher intradiskal pressures than standing, and pressures were increased in both positions by flexion of the trunk. The highest pressures encountered were with the patient sitting with the trunk flexed.

507. The answer is E. *(Boden, pp 104–105.)* Pain from degenerative disk disease referred to the sacroiliac joint and upper buttocks most commonly results from abnormal stimulation of local mesodermal elements: joint capsule, annulus, muscles, and ligaments. This sclerotogenous pain has the same embryonic origin as that of the mesodermal tissues stimulated. Radicular pain, on the other hand, is typically referred more distally to areas that correspond to the distribution of specific nerve roots.

508. The answer is D. *(Boden, p 107.)* Occupations requiring repetitive lifting in stooped or twisted positions have been shown in epidemiologic studies to correlate with a higher incidence of disk disease. Other associated risk factors include exposure to vibrations from vehicles or industrial machinery and cigarette smoking. The role of increased body height, obesity, and inequality of leg length in the development of disk disease is controversial. Pregnancy is associated with low back pain, but does not appear to cause an increased incidence of disk herniation.

509. The answer is C. *(Boden, p 112.)* The relationship of posture to symptoms is the most important aspect of the history in distinguishing neurogenic from vascular claudication. Extension of the lumbar spine is more likely to provoke neurogenic claudication, which is closely related to spinal stenosis. Rapid ambulation is likely to provoke or increase the neurologic deficit in neurogenic claudication, as is walking downhill, which is associated with increased extension of the spine. In the bicycle test of van Gelderan, claudication of neurogenic origin is not reproduced, since the trunk is flexed, which reduces lordosis and consequently increases the sagittal and foraminal dimensions of the spinal canal.

510. The answer is D. *(Rothman, pp 837–850.)* Until recently, myelography has been the "gold standard" for the confirmation of the diagnosis of acute herniation of a lumbar intervertebral disk. However, most authors now agree that MRI is the study of choice to confirm this diagnosis. MRI has the advantages of being noninvasive, not requiring ionizing radiation, offering multiplanar imaging, and evaluating the cause of the nerve root compression. All the tests listed have a significant number of positive findings in asymptomatic persons, which points out the importance of using these tests in a confirmatory way and closely correlating symptoms and signs with radiographic findings.

511. The answer is C. *(Boden, pp 118–119.)* The myelogram in the figure shows a cutoff of the L5 nerve root sleeve at the L4–5 interspace, suggesting compression of the L5 nerve root. The sensory distribution of L5 is the lateral calf and dorsum of the foot. L3 supplies the anterior knee, L4 the medial aspect of the leg, and S1 the posterior calf and lateral foot.

512. The answer is E. *(Boden, p 148.)* Early in the course of lumbar nerve root compression, EMGs show only muscle irritation; signs of denervation with fibrillation are not observed until after 3 weeks. The EMG is also abnormal in diabetic neuropathy and previous peripheral nerve disorders, so it is not a useful tool in differentiating these conditions from primary disk disease. EMG should be reserved for complex cases in which secondary nerve root involvement is suspected preoperatively, since it may be useful in detecting the existence of such a lesion.

513. The answer is A. *(Boden, p 160.)* Lumbar spondylolysis, with or without spondylolisthesis, is the structural abnormality most likely to be associated with significant low back pain. Approximately 5 percent of the population has this defect. Each of the other conditions has been implicated in the causation of low back pain, but none are as common as spondylolysis.

514. The answer is B. *(Boden, p 160.)* The nature of this patient's pain suggests a nonmechanical etiology, and its failure to respond to appropriate care is cause for concern. A bone scan is an excellent screening device, especially for tumors or infections. CT scanning has limitations as a broad screening test. The efficacy of gadolinium-enhanced MRI scans is still unknown. The nature of the symptoms does not suggest the facet joint as a cause.

515. The answer is D. *(Boden, pp 162–163.)* The next appropriate step in this patient with subjective sciatica but no objective findings (including a negative MRI) is continued nonoperative care, which may include formalized physical therapy and exercises or epidural steroid injections or both. Surgical intervention is not indicated in patients without objective findings or confirmatory diagnostic studies. Failure to respond to 3 months of nonoperative care in the face of no objective findings may indicate the need for psychosocial evaluation.

516. The answer is E. *(Boden, p 163.)* This patient has clinical and radiographic findings that support her complaints of radicular pain. If such patients are unimproved after 3 months of nonoperative treatment, they should be considered surgical candidates. When specific objective criteria for lumbar diskectomy are met, 95 percent of patients can expect satisfactory results.

517. The answer is E. *(Boden, pp 155–159.)* In the absence of symptoms or signs of cauda equina syndrome or a severe neurologic deficit, the initial treatment for all patients with radiculopathy should be nonoperative. At this stage, the specific diagnosis, whether an acute disk herniation or a simple strain, is not germane, since the initial treatment for both is the same. Routine AP and lateral radiographs are usually normal, and multiple studies have documented that they are not cost-effective and should be reserved for patients who fail initial therapy or have specific indications such as significant trauma, fever, weight loss, or a history of cancer. Oblique radiographs rarely reveal additional diagnostic information and should be reserved for patients with a suggestive history. MRI or CT myelography is indicated only for the patient with acute cauda equina compression or a significant neurologic deficit, or as a confirmatory diagnostic test in a patient with objective findings who has failed conservative care.

518. The answer is A. *(Frymoyer, Gordon, pp 746–747.)* All the listed abnormalities may be seen in rheumatoid arthritis as a direct result of rheumatoid destruction of the supporting joints, ligaments, and bone. However, atlantoaxial subluxation is the most common abnormality, being present in 19 to 71 percent of patients surveyed radiographically and in 11 to 46 percent of patients undergoing autopsy. An atlas-dens interval (ADI) of greater than 3.5 mm on flexion and extension lateral radiographs suggests failure of the entire atlantoaxial ligamentous complex. Atlantoaxial subluxation can result in compression of the spinal cord between the dens and the posterior arch of the atlas. Posterior atlantoaxial subluxation is a rare variant, accounting for approximately 7 percent of all C1–2 subluxations.

519. The answer is B. *(Frymoyer, pp 1776–1778.)* The MRI reveals a left L4–5 foraminal disk herniation. Foraminal disk herniations account for 3 to 10 percent of all disk herniations. Most foraminal herniations occur at the L4–5 or L3–4 levels in older patients (average age 50). They result in compression of the exiting nerve root, unlike classic posterolateral herniations that affect the traversing root. Thus, in this patient, findings on examination are those of compression of the left L4 nerve root.

520. The answer is C. *(Boden, pp 155–156.)* This patient has signs and symptoms of cauda equina syndrome. This typically results from pressure on the caudal sac, which contains the nerve roots to the lower limbs, bowel, and bladder. Cauda equina syndrome can result in paraplegia and bowel and bladder incontinence. The confirmatory MRI scan reveals a large, central L4–5 disk herniation. Cauda equina syndrome is the only indication for emergency disk surgery in the lumbar spine. Following immediate, definitive, diagnostic testing, patients require emergent surgical decompression. The goal of surgical intervention is to prevent progression of the neurologic deficit, since return of neurologic function is unpredictable.

521. The answer is C. *(Rothman, pp 1872–1875.)* The CT myelographic image depicts peripheral clumping of the intrathecal nerve roots surrounding a central space filled with cerebrospinal fluid consistent with adhesive arachnoiditis (AA). Historically, adhesive arachnoiditis was frequently seen following pantopague myelography, but many other agents may also cause AA. With the advent of metrizamide myelography, lumbar AA is now most commonly caused by previous lumbar disk surgery. The clinical picture of lumbar AA is that of low back pain with unilateral or bilateral sciatica. The sciatica is usually constant and often burning, tingling, or dysesthetic in quality. Both nonoperative and operative treatments have been proposed for AA; however, none have proved universally effective.

522. The answer is B. *(Frymoyer, pp 496, 1861.)* Recurrent herniated nucleus pulposus (HNP) is the most common cause of failure following surgical treatment of HNP. Recurrent herniation may occur at the same level on either the ipsilateral or contralateral side. Patients usually report complete resolution of symptoms following the initial surgical procedure, only to have subsequent recurrence of severe symptoms. Contrast-enhanced MRI scanning can help confirm the diagnosis of recurrent HNP. The hallmark of residual or recurrent HNP is a well-marginated, isointense or slightly hypointense region contiguous with the disk space that fails to enhance following gadolinium injection. Frequently, the recurrent fragment is surrounded by a rim of enhancing scar as seen in the current MRI.

523. The answer is D. *(Sherk, pp 678–680.)* The patient has early symptoms and signs of cervical myelopathy, and the CT myelogram demonstrates narrowing of the cervical canal with deformation of the spinal cord by a posterior ossified mass. This clinical and radiologic picture is characteristic of ossification of the posterior longitudinal ligament (OPLL), which is much more prevalent in Asiatic countries than in the United States. Radiographic studies have reported OPLL in 2 to 3 percent of the Japanese population as compared with 0.2 percent of Americans. The etiology of OPLL remains unclear, although there is some evidence to support a heritable cause.

524. The answer is B. *(Frymoyer, pp 699–705.)* The radiograph reveals bilateral symmetric sacroiliitis with near ankylosis, which, in association with decreased lumbar mobility and limited chest expansion, confirms the diagnosis of ankylosing spondylitis. Normal chest expansion in an adult man, measured at the nipple line, should be 5 cm. Involvement of the axial skeleton in ankylosing spondylitis can be quite severe. It causes inflammation of both joints and entheses (bony attachments of ligaments, tendons, and joint capsules), which results in ankylosis of the sacroiliac, apophyseal, and costovertebral joints. Urethritis is associated with Reiter's syndrome, which tends to be sudden in onset and have asymmetric sacroiliac involvement. Hamstring tightness is frequently associated with isthmic spondylolisthesis, while positive straight leg raising tests and absent reflexes are signs of radiculopathy.

525. The answer is E. *(Frymoyer, pp 1428–1435.)* Arthrodesis of the lower lumbar spine with distraction instrumentation frequently resulted in loss of the normal lumbar lordosis and the creation of an iatrogenic lumbar kyphosis. The "flat back" syndrome does not usually cause difficulties in the adolescent, but can become a significant problem when the patient reaches the third, fourth, and fifth decade of life. The typical symptoms are given in the question and tend to progressively worsen. To compensate for the loss of lordosis, patients frequently walk with hips and knees flexed and can develop fixed contractures, which can be striking and disabling. The optimum treatment is prevention by avoiding fusion of the lower lumbar spine or by preserving the normal sagittal contour when fusion to the lower lumbar region is necessary.

526. The answer is E. *(Frymoyer, pp 861–888.)* Metastatic lesions are by far the most common skeletal tumors and the spine is the most common site for skeletal metastasis. The MRI reveals a lesion at L4 with marrow changes as well as an extraosseous component. Additionally, there appear to be marrow signal intensity changes at T12, suggesting involvement of this vertebra. Multilevel involvement makes the other choices much less likely. Pain is the most universal symptom of metastatic disease; it is insidious in onset and relentlessly progressive. Patients may associate the onset with minor trauma; however, the temporal relationship is usually loose and vague. The pain of bony metastases is usually constant and fails to respond to rest or activity modification. These symptoms, in combination with constitutional symptoms such as fatigue, fever, and sweats, should result in a high index of suspicion for metastatic disease. While osteosarcoma and chondrosarcoma can involve the vertebral elements, metastatic disease is much more common at this site.

527. The answer is A. *(Rothman, pp 1319–1372.)* The radiograph reveals destruction of the disk space between L4 and L5 with involvement of the end plates; the T1-weighted MRI scan reveals a confluent decreased signal intensity of the vertebral bodies and adjacent disk, making the margin between the two indistinct; the T2-weighted scan reveals enhanced signal intensity of the vertebral bodies and disk. These findings, combined with the clinical history, are most consistent with a pyogenic spinal infection. Vertebral osteomyelitis represents 2 to 7 percent of all osteomyelitis. The infection is believed to begin with hematogenous seeding of the vertebral body near the end plate, with subsequent destruction of the disk. In contrast, nonpyogenic osteomyelitis usually destroys the vertebral bodies and spares the disk spaces. Laboratory evaluation can be equivocal, since the WBC is frequently normal and only the nonspecific ESR is consistently elevated. Despite characteristic radiographic findings, a definitive diagnosis can only be made by biopsy and tissue evaluation and culture.

528. The answer is B. *(Boden, p 26.)* The presence of negatively charged proteoglycan side chains within the nucleus pulposus help it develop the high imbibition pressure necessary to withstand loading. With aging, there is a loss of these negatively charged side chains and an increase in collagen content. The precipitating event for these changes is unknown.

529. The answer is A. *(Frymoyer, Gordon, p 160.)* Increased lateral bulging of the annulus is the most direct cause of nerve root compression in patients with degenerative disk disease. Decreased disk height causes increased loading of the facet joints, while inward bulging of the annulus leads to physical disruption of the disk. Reduced intradiskal pressure changes the load transmitted to the end plate, which may lead to osteophyte formation. Increased spinal mobility produces greater loading of adjacent structures.

530. The answer is E. *(Boden, p 35.)* Degenerative spondylolisthesis of the lumbar spine usually results from disk degeneration, erosion of cartilage in the intervertebral joints, and consequent laxity of the supporting structures of the spine. It is most common in older, black females, and occurs six times more frequently at L4–5 than at L3–4. Isthmic spondylolisthesis is more common in young patients and usually occurs at L5–S1.

531. The answer is E. *(Rothman, pp 554–555.)* Acute disk herniations in the cervical spine most commonly result in radicular findings. A C4–5 disk herniation would affect the C5 nerve root, most likely resulting in sensory changes in the lateral arm ("epaulet" pattern) and weakness of the deltoid and possibly the biceps. The biceps reflex is inconsistently affected by C5 root compression. Decreased sensation over the lateral forearm, weakness of wrist extension, and absence of the brachioradialis reflex represent a C6 radiculopathy. The C8 root supplies sensation to the small finger and innervation to the interossei. C7 radicular findings include middle finger numbness, triceps weakness, and asymmetry of the triceps reflex.

532. The answer is C. *(Boden, p 57.)* MRI studies have shown that spinal cord compression occurs in fewer than 5 percent of asymptomatic patients with cervical spondylosis and is due to disk protrusion. The reduction in cord volume averaged 7 percent and never surpassed 16 percent in these patients. Thus, it appears the cervical spinal cord can tolerate moderate volume loss before the occurrence of symptoms.

533. The answer is D. *(Boden, pp 57–58.)* While the techniques are approximately equal in their ability to localize the level of disk disease, contrast tomography is preferred for identifying the cause of neural compression and for delineating lateral encroachment. Since many options exist during the performance of MRI examinations, this technique is more operator-dependent than is contrast CT.

534. The answer is B. *(Boden, pp 104–105.)* Pain referred to the medial leg between the knee and the malleolus classically results from compression of the L4 nerve root. The L3 root involves the anterior knee; L5 the lateral calf, dorsum of the foot, and first toe; and S1 the posterior calf, lateral border of the foot, and fifth toe.

Adult Diseases and Disorders: Lower Limb

Frank C. Wilson, M.D.

DIRECTIONS: Each question below contains five suggested responses. Select the **one best** response to each question.

535. The rerupture rate following closed treatment (casting in equinus) of complete ruptures of the Achilles tendon is

(A) 1 to 5 percent
(B) 6 to 10 percent
(C) 11 to 15 percent
(D) 16 to 20 percent
(E) 21 to 25 percent

536. The preferred treatment of a 3-month-old rupture of the Achilles tendon in a 48-year-old laborer with a 2-cm palpable defect in the tendon is

(A) closed, with casting in equinus for 12 weeks
(B) operative, using a graft from the aponeurosis of the triceps surae
(C) operative, using a flexor digitorum longus tendon graft
(D) operative, using a posterior tibial tendon graft
(E) operative, using a dacron bridge

537. The primary indication for surgery in patients with hallux valgus is

(A) acute bursitis
(B) split-size shoe requirements
(C) metatarsus primus varus, with an angle between the first and second metatarsals of over 10°
(D) persistent symptoms with nonoperative management
(E) arthritic changes in the first metatarsophalangeal joint

538. The most important determinant of a successful outcome following surgery for hallux valgus is

(A) thorough preoperative assessment
(B) the technical skill of the surgeon
(C) the management during the first 2 postoperative weeks
(D) the long-term management
(E) avoidance of wound complications

539. Surgery for hallux valgus is *contraindicated* in the presence of

(A) a first metatarsal that is shorter than the second
(B) arthritis of the first metatarsophalangeal joint
(C) associated hallux rigidus
(D) an angle between the first and second metartarsals of over 10°
(E) gross ligamentous laxity

540. The most likely cause of pain following a Keller arthroplasty for correction of hallux valgus is

(A) failure to resect enough bone from the metatarsal head
(B) excessive resection of bone from the proximal phalanx
(C) lateral transfer metatarsalgia
(D) formation of a neuroma
(E) development of a hallux varus deformity

541. Which of the following patients best meets the indications for a Chevron distal metatarsal osteotomy for correction of a symptomatic bunion?

(A) Age 38, 1–2 intermetatarsal angle of 20°, hallux valgus of 35°, lateral subluxation of the sesamoids
(B) Age 62, 1–2 intermetatarsal angle of 15°, hallux valgus of 45°, normal sesamoid-metatarsal joints
(C) Age 66, 1–2 intermetatarsal angle of 9°, hallux valgus of 30°, normal sesamoid-metatarsal joints
(D) Age 57, 1–2 intermetatarsal angle of 18°, hallux valgus of 50°, lateral subluxation of the sesamoids
(E) Age 46, 1–2 intermetatarsal angle of 12°, hallux valgus of 27°, normal sesamoid-metatarsal joints

542. Which of the following conditions is most likely to predispose to plantar fasciitis?

(A) Equinovarus deformity
(B) Contracture of the Achilles tendon
(C) A plantar spur on the calcaneus
(D) An old fracture of the calcaneus
(E) Plantar fibromatosis

543. In plantar fasciitis, the location of the area of maximum tenderness is

(A) beneath the medial tuberosity of the os calcis
(B) on the medial surface of the os calcis just proximal to the origin of the plantar fascia
(C) on the inferior aspect of the os calcis proximal to the origin of the plantar fascia
(D) beneath the midportion of the longitudinal arch
(E) beneath the metatarsal heads

544. Pseudarthrosis of the talonavicular joint following triple arthrodesis

(A) is infrequent when the operation is performed for posttraumatic arthritis
(B) occurs in approximately 20 percent of cases
(C) may be minimized by the use of internal fixation
(D) is rare in the absence of postoperative infection
(E) is not affected by the period of non-weight-bearing postoperatively

545. The most significant etiologic factor in the development of forefoot deformity in patients with rheumatoid arthritis is

(A) shoes with narrow toeboxes
(B) spasm or contracture of the intrinsic muscles
(C) rupture of the long flexor and/or extensor tendons
(D) synovitis
(E) loss of articular cartilage

546. In order of decreasing frequency, the areas of initial complaint for which patients with rheumatoid arthritis consult physicians are

(A) knee, foot, hand
(B) hand, knee, hip
(C) knee, hand, hip
(D) hip, knee, hand
(E) hand, foot, knee

547. A 48-year-old male grocer had a painful hallux valgus deformity that had not responded to nonoperative measures. A standing AP radiograph of the foot is shown in the figure. The procedure that will likely result in the most patient satisfaction is

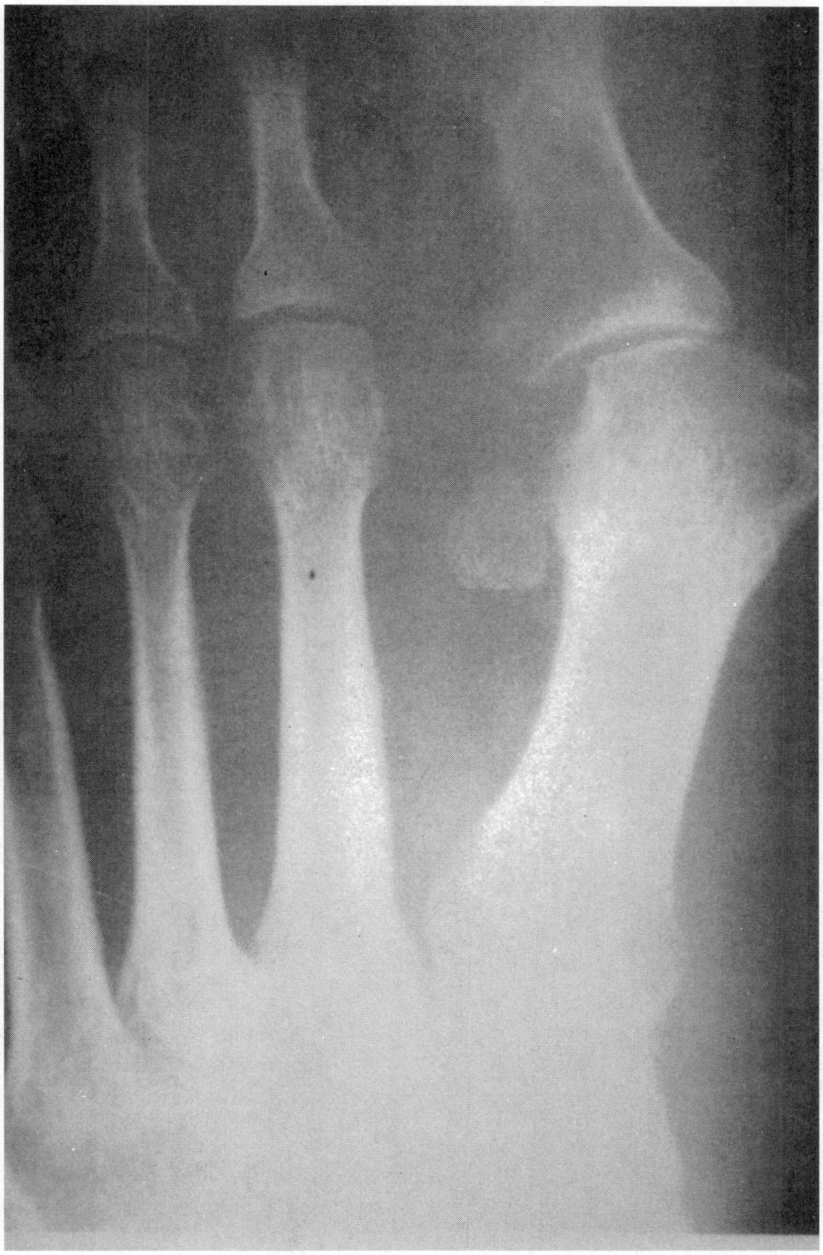

(A) Keller arthroplasty
(B) Mitchell osteotomy of the first metatarsal neck
(C) arthrodesis of the first metatarsophalangeal joint
(D) double-stemmed silastic implant arthroplasty of the first metatarsophalangeal joint
(E) fusion of the first metatarsocuneiform joint

548. A 35-year-old housewife had had rheumatoid arthritis for 2 years. Her only deformities were mild right hallux valgus and clawing of the right second toe. Both areas were intermittently symptomatic. An AP radiograph of the right foot is shown below. The most appropriate treatment is

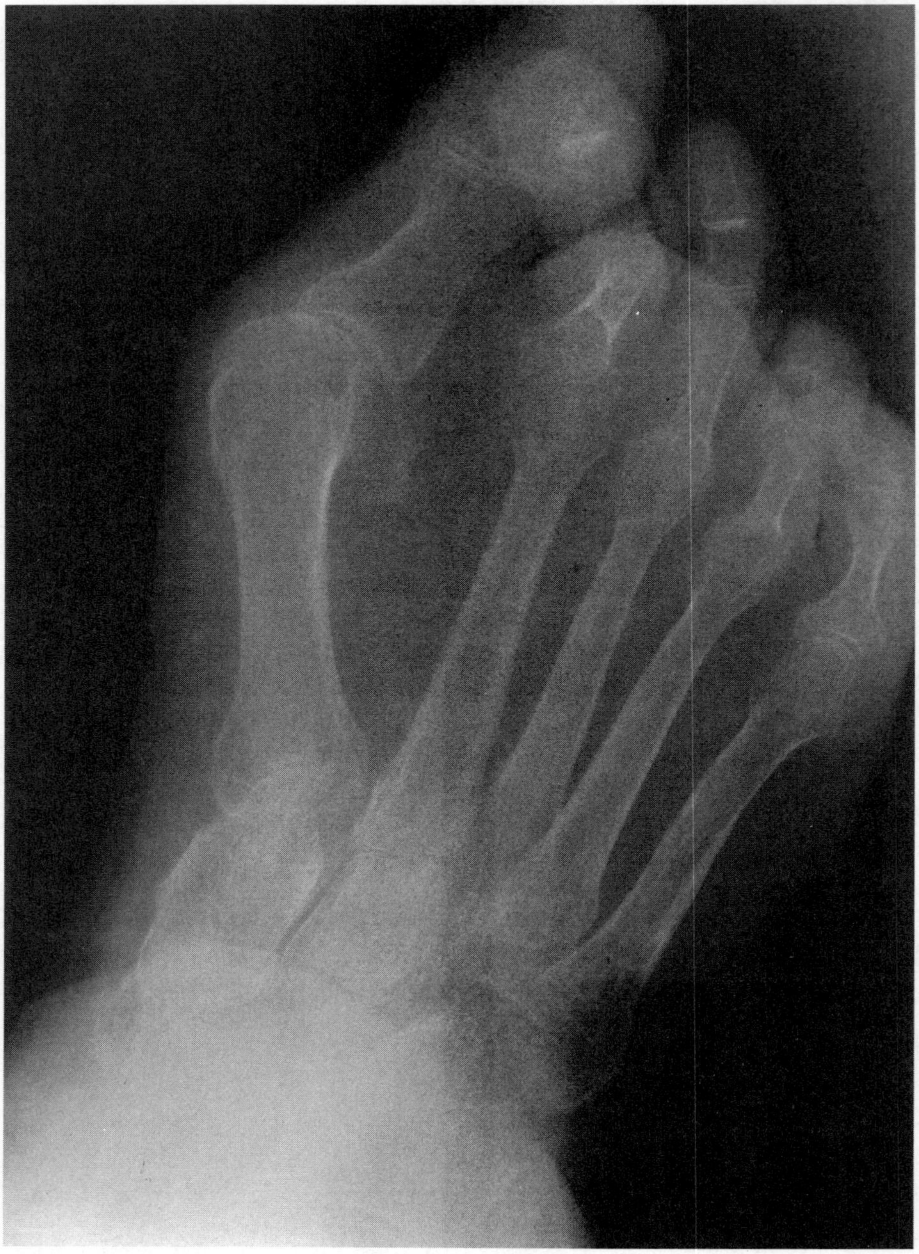

(A) resection of the medial eminence of the first toe and fusion of the PIP joint of the second toe
(B) fusion of the first metatarsophalangeal joint, dorsal capsulotomy of the second MTP joint, and pinning of the second toe
(C) Keller arthroplasty of the first toe and fusion of the PIP joint of the second toe
(D) fusion of the PIP joint of the second toe
(E) shoe modifications

549. In patients with rheumatoid arthritis, the most important mechanical factor in the development of painful callosities beneath the lateral metatarsal heads is

(A) inappropriate footwear
(B) hyperextension deformities of the metatarsophalangeal joints
(C) flexion contractures of the proximal interphalangeal joints
(D) thinning of the plantar fat pad
(E) distal displacement of the plantar fat pad

550. The factor most responsible for the development of hindfoot valgus in patients with rheumatoid arthritis is

(A) rupture of the posterior tibial tendon
(B) contracture of the peroneal muscles
(C) weight-bearing
(D) loss of articular cartilage in the subtalar joint
(E) a lateral compression fracture of the os calcis

551. The most common initial manifestation of rheumatoid disease in the forefoot is

(A) dorsal tenosynovitis
(B) lateral deviation of the toes
(C) fusiform swelling of the toes
(D) tender callosities over the PIP joints
(E) metatarsalgia

552. Long-standing rheumatoid deformity of the forefoot is most likely to show

(A) symmetric changes: hallux valgus, clawing and lateral deviation of the lateral four toes, and callosities over the dorsum of the PIP joints
(B) asymmetric changes: hallux valgus, clawing and lateral deviation of the lateral four toes, and a callus beneath the first metatarsal head
(C) symmetric changes: hallux varus, clawing and spreading of the middle three toes, and callosities at the tips of the lateral four toes
(D) symmetric changes: hallux valgus, clawing and lateral deviation of the middle three toes, and callosities beneath the metatarsal heads, over the dorsum of the PIP joints, and at the tips of the lateral four toes
(E) asymmetric changes: clawing and spreading of the lateral four toes, and a callus beneath the fifth metatarsal head

553. A 39-year-old patient with rheumatoid arthritis had a painful, nonfixed valgus deformity of the foot following rupture of the posterior tibial tendon. The optimal surgical management is

(A) debridement of the tendon ends and shoe modifications
(B) debridement of the tendon ends and primary repair
(C) tendon transference
(D) triple arthrodesis
(E) tenosynovectomy and free tendon grafting

554. In a patient with rheumatoid arthritis, the most important information to be obtained prior to performing a major surgical procedure is the

(A) activity of the patient's disease
(B) history with respect to steroid administration
(C) age of the patient
(D) stability of the cervical spine
(E) occupation of the patient

555. Which of the following provides the best description of the biochemical changes in osteoarthritic articular cartilage?

(A) Decreased water content, predominance of type I collagen, increased proteoglycan concentration
(B) Increased water content, predominance of type II collagen, decreased proteoglycan concentration
(C) Normal water content, predominance of type II collagen, increased proteoglycan concentration
(D) Decreased water content, approximately equal concentrations of type I and type II collagen, decreased proteoglycan concentration
(E) Increased water content, predominance of type II collagen, increased proteoglycan concentration

556. The condition most frequently associated with the development of osteoarthritis is

(A) obesity
(B) osteoporosis
(C) microfractures in the subchondral bone
(D) acute trauma
(E) advanced age

557. In the evaluation of a patient with osteoarthritis, MRI is of greatest value to

(A) distinguish genetic or metabolic disorders from primary osteoarthritis
(B) distinguish avascular necrosis from osteoarthritis
(C) establish the cause of radicular symptoms in spinal osteoarthritis
(D) distinguish between primary and secondary osteoarthritis
(E) assess more fully the extent of osteoarthritic changes in the joint

558. In patients with isolated osteophytosis of the hip, the percentage who will develop joint space narrowing and other changes of osteoarthritis within 10 years is

(A) less than 1 percent
(B) 1 to 20 percent
(C) 21 to 40 percent
(D) 41 to 60 percent
(E) over 60 percent

559. All the following factors have been implicated as causes of pain in osteoarthritis EXCEPT

(A) intraosseous venous congestion
(B) synovitis
(C) ligamentous stress
(D) irritation of endosteal nerve endings
(E) muscle strain

560. Which of the following statements best characterizes the effect of intraarticular corticosteroids for the treatment of osteoarthritis?

(A) Pain is relieved temporarily; they are "chondroprotective" if limited to six injections; exercise following injection improves the response
(B) Pain relief is unpredictable; they speed cartilage degeneration; rest after injection improves the response
(C) Pain is relieved temporarily; they do not damage cartilage significantly if used sparingly; rest after injection improves the response
(D) Pain is relieved permanently; their effect on cartilage is unpredictable; exercise after injection improves the response
(E) Pain decreases initially, then recurs in a more severe form; their effect on cartilage is related to preexisting joint damage; neither rest nor exercise after injection affects the response

561. Arthroscopy is most valuable in the treatment of the osteoarthritic knee when

(A) an internal derangement is present, with mechanical joint symptoms
(B) symptoms are related primarily to instability
(C) it is accompanied by chondral abrasion arthroplasty
(D) it is repeated regularly at 6-month intervals
(E) osteoarthritic changes are moderate and no mechanical symptoms are present

562. Osteopenia induced by the administration of glucocorticoids is best managed by

(A) adequate vitamin D and calcium intake, weight-bearing exercise, and correction of gonadal hormonal deficiencies
(B) adrenalectomy
(C) reduction of glucocorticoid dosage
(D) administration of diphosphonates or calcitonin
(E) hydrochlorothiazide

563. Optimal management of severe disuse osteopenia with hypercalcemia is

(A) mechanical compressive treatment; maintenance of water and electrolyte balance
(B) calcium and phosphate supplements
(C) calcitonin or diphosphonates; maintenance of water and electrolyte balance
(D) phosphate supplements; mechanical compressive treatment
(E) immobilization

564. The diagnosis of osteomalacia can be established with the greatest certainty by analysis of

(A) the serum 25-hydroxyvitamin D level
(B) the serum 1,25-dihydroxyvitamin D level
(C) the serum and urinary phosphate levels
(D) the patient's response to 400 to 1000 IU of vitamin D per day
(E) a bone biopsy after tetracycline labeling

565. Primary hyperparathyroidism is most commonly discovered as a result of

(A) routine biochemical screening
(B) nephrolithiasis
(C) generalized bone pain
(D) subperiosteal resorption of bone in the phalanges
(E) pathologic fracture

566. Which of the following best characterizes renal osteodystrophy?

(A) History of antacid intake, osteitis fibrosa cystica, osteoporosis, osteomalacia, and renal glomerular failure
(B) History of antacid intake, osteitis fibrosa cystica, osteomalacia, osteoporosis, osteosclerosis, and renal tubular failure
(C) History of malnutrition or previous gastrointestinal surgery, osteitis fibrosa cystica, and osteomalacia
(D) History of preexisting renal disease, osteomalacia, and secondary hyperparathyroidism
(E) Primary hyperparathyroid disease, hypercalcemia, hypophosphatemia, and osteoporosis

567. A 46-year-old woman of European descent had had 6 years of intermittent leg pain and slowly increasing deformity of her tibia. An anteroposterior radiograph is shown below. The most likely diagnosis is

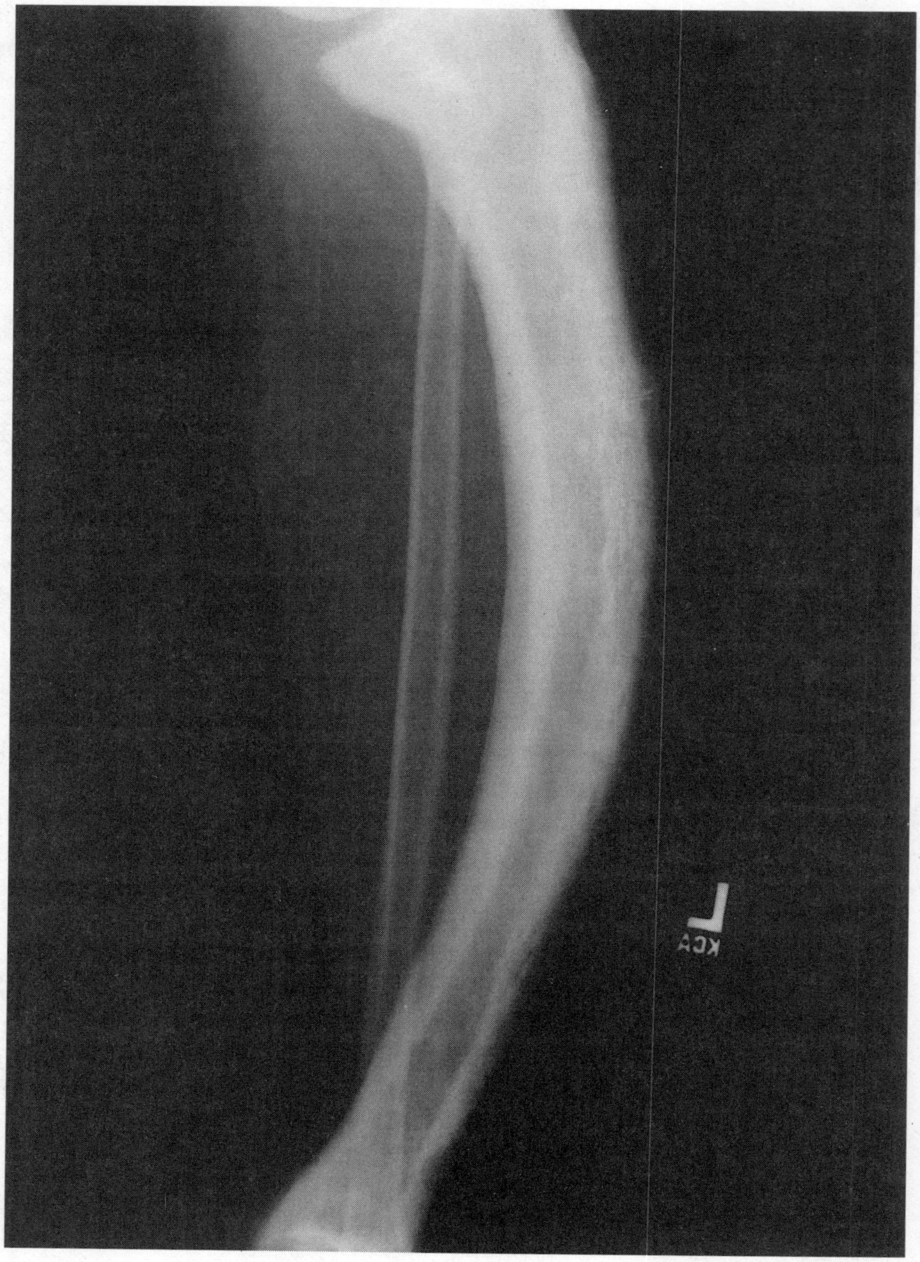

(A) secondary hyperparathyroidism
(B) renal osteodystrophy
(C) vitamin D–resistant rickets
(D) Paget's disease
(E) hypophosphatasia

568. Which of the following nontraumatic conditions is LEAST likely to play a major role in the development of avascular necrosis (AVN) of bone?

(A) Excessive intake of alcohol
(B) Sickle cell disease
(C) Decompression sickness
(D) Osteopenia
(E) Chronic liver disease

569. The usual sequence of pathologic events in the development of symptomatic avascular necrosis (AVN) of the hip is

(A) multiple vascular insults, bone death, repair, microfractures, collapse of the articular surface, degeneration of articular cartilage, osteoarthritis
(B) a single vascular insult, bone death, repair, no structural sequelae
(C) multiple vascular insults, bone death, microfractures, collapse of articular surface, osteoarthritis
(D) a single vascular insult, bone death, repair, residual "bone infarct"
(E) multiple vascular insults, bone death, collapse, repair, residual subchondral sclerosis

570. The most reliable imaging technique for the early diagnosis of AVN of bone is

(A) routine radiography
(B) radionuclide bone scanning
(C) CT
(D) single-photon emission computed tomography (SPECT)
(E) MRI

571. A 46-year-old office worker with a history of alcohol abuse had hip pain of 2 months' duration. A radiograph and MRI scan of the affected hip are shown below. The most appropriate treatment for this patient is

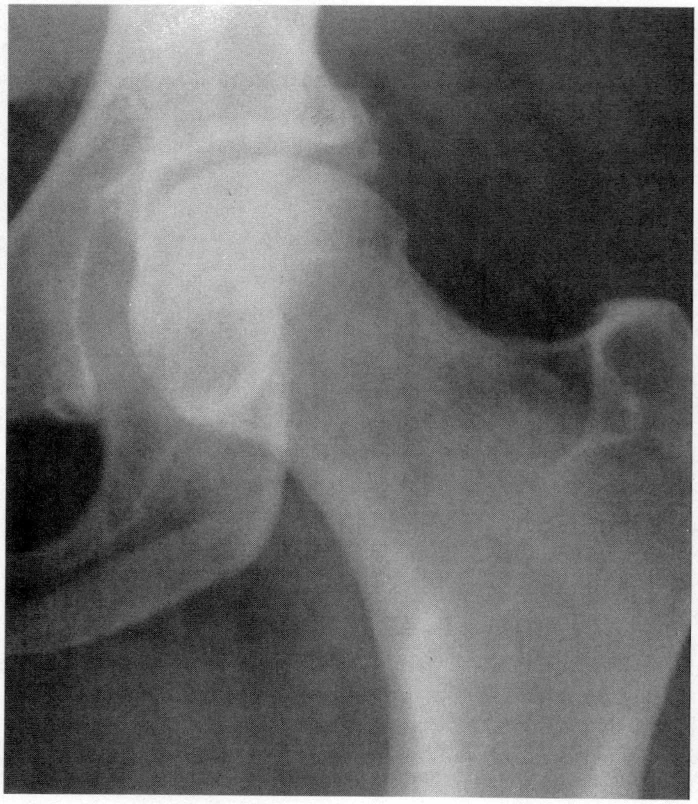

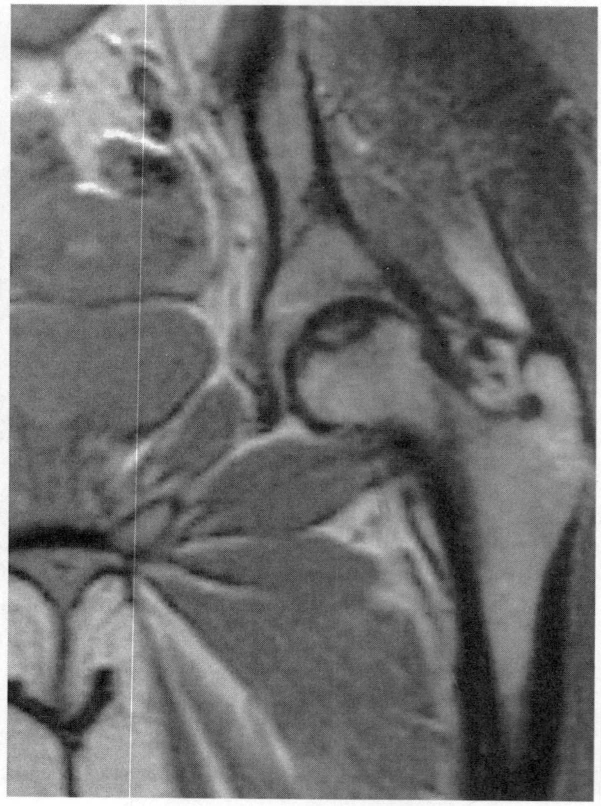

(A) non-weight-bearing with crutches
(B) core decompression of the femoral head
(C) core decompression and bone grafting of the femoral head
(D) transtrochanteric rotational osteotomy of the femur
(E) prosthetic replacement of the femoral head

572. A 37-year-old housewife had a 3-month history of pain in the sole of her left foot. Examination and electrodiagnostic studies confirmed the diagnosis of tarsal tunnel syndrome. The most appropriate management is

(A) a medial arch support
(B) a medial arch support and NSAIDs
(C) a medial arch support, NSAIDs, and instillation of a local anesthetic
(D) a medial arch support, NSAIDs, and instillation of a local anesthetic mixed with corticosteroids
(E) surgical decompression of the posterior tibial nerve

573. The type of toxicity most frequently encountered in postoperative patients receiving NSAIDs is

(A) gastrointestinal dysfunction
(B) renal dysfunction
(C) hepatic dysfunction
(D) dermatologic disorders
(E) hematologic disorders

574. Failure of total knee arthroplasties incorporating the latest prosthetic designs is most often attributable to

(A) malposition
(B) loosening
(C) infection
(D) subluxation
(E) errors in technique

575. Which of the following statements most accurately describes the results of synovectomy of the knee joint for early rheumatoid arthritis?

(A) No subjective (pain and swelling), objective (motion and stability), or radiographic (bone erosions) differences from controls at either 2 or 5 years
(B) Subjective improvement only at both 2 and 5 years
(C) Objective improvement only at both 2 and 5 years
(D) Radiographic improvement only at both 2 and 5 years
(E) Subjective, objective, and radiographic improvement at 2 years; results similar to controls at 5 years

576. A *contraindication* to surgical synovectomy in rheumatoid arthritis is the presence of

(A) active disease
(B) intraarticular loculations
(C) stage III destruction of the joint
(D) rheumatoid nodules
(E) a poorly motivated patient

577. A *contraindication* to replacement arthroplasty of the hip in patients with rheumatoid arthritis is

(A) atlantoaxial subluxation
(B) severe bilateral hand deformities
(C) temporomandibular arthritis with limited mandibular motion
(D) asymptomatic bacteriuria
(E) valgus deformity of the ipsilateral knee

578. Modern cementing techniques have improved the results of cemented total hip arthroplasty by decreasing

(A) loosening of the acetabular component
(B) loosening of the femoral component
(C) breakage of the femoral component
(D) polyethylene wear
(E) "cement disease"

579. Deep wound infection following primary total hip arthroplasty occurs in approximately

(A) 1 percent of cases, of which 15 percent develop after 24 months
(B) 2 percent of cases, of which 25 percent develop after 24 months
(C) 3 percent of cases, of which 35 percent develop after 24 months
(D) 4 percent of cases, of which 45 percent develop after 24 months
(E) 5 percent of cases, of which over 50 percent develop after 24 months

580. Optimal treatment for a short, slightly obese 32-year-old male surveyor with disabling posttraumatic arthritis of the hip, as shown in the figure, is

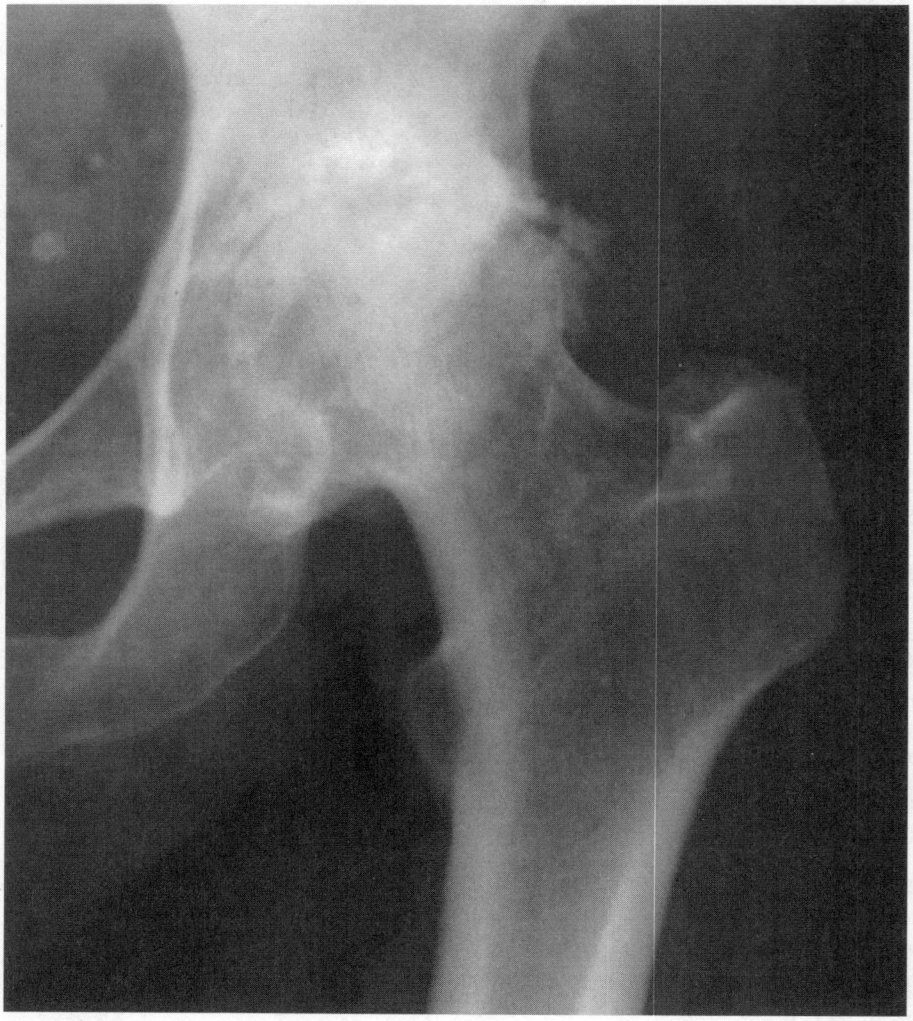

(A) intertrochanteric rotational osteotomy
(B) intertrochanteric angulation osteotomy
(C) cemented total hip arthroplasty
(D) cementless total hip arthroplasty
(E) arthrodesis of the hip

581. During the performance of a total knee arthroplasty, trial reduction revealed the knee to be excessively tight in flexion and loose in extension. These findings are best corrected by

(A) resecting more of the distal femur
(B) resecting more of the proximal tibia
(C) using a smaller femoral component
(D) using a smaller femoral component and a thicker polyethylene insert
(E) using a smaller femoral component and a thinner polyethylene insert

582. During the performance of a total knee arthroplasty, trial reduction revealed the knee to be excessively loose in flexion and tight in extension. These findings are best corrected by

(A) releasing the posterior capsule or resecting more of the distal femur or both
(B) using a smaller femoral component
(C) using a larger femoral component
(D) resecting more of the proximal tibia
(E) using a thinner polyethylene insert

583. During the performance of a total knee arthroplasty, trial reduction revealed excessive tightness in both flexion and extension. These findings are best corrected by

(A) using a smaller femoral component
(B) resecting more bone from the proximal tibia
(C) resecting more bone from the proximal tibia and releasing the posterior capsule
(D) resecting more bone from the posterior femur and using a thinner polyethylene component
(E) resecting more bone from the distal femur

584. A high tibial osteotomy performed for degenerative joint disease of the knee is most likely to succeed in

(A) young patients with rheumatoid arthritis and varus deformities under 10°
(B) old patients with osteoarthritis and varus deformities over 10°
(C) young patients with osteoarthritis and valgus deformities under 10°
(D) old patients with rheumatoid arthritis and varus deformities under 10° whose disease is confined to the medial compartment
(E) young patients with osteoarthritis and varus deformities under 10°

585. High tibial osteotomy is NOT usually recommended for disabling arthritis of the knee for patients with

(A) osteoarthritis
(B) posttraumatic arthritis
(C) a varus deformity over 10°, even if the knee is stable
(D) a valgus deformity over 15°, even if the knee is stable
(E) a fixed flexion contracture over 5°

586. The clinical deformities most commonly encountered in knees affected by long-standing rheumatoid arthritis are

(A) varus, internal rotation, and medial subluxation of the tibia
(B) varus, external rotation, and rotatory subluxation of the tibia
(C) valgus, external rotation, and lateral subluxation of the tibia
(D) valgus, external rotation, and medial subluxation of the tibia
(E) valgus and recurvatum of the tibia

587. The most frequent cause of marked (over 60°) fixed flexion deformities of the knees in patients with rheumatoid arthritis is

(A) rheumatoid involvement of the quadriceps mechanism
(B) an ipsilateral hip flexion contracture
(C) an ipsilateral hamstring contracture
(D) changes in joint architecture
(E) nonambulatory status

588. An otherwise healthy 61-year-old executive had had 7 years of increasing pain and stiffness in an osteoarthritic knee. He complained of medial joint line pain with every step and pain at rest, both of which were unrelieved by NSAIDs. Examination revealed a stable knee with a range of motion from 5 to 120°. Weight-bearing radiographs are shown below. The preferred management is

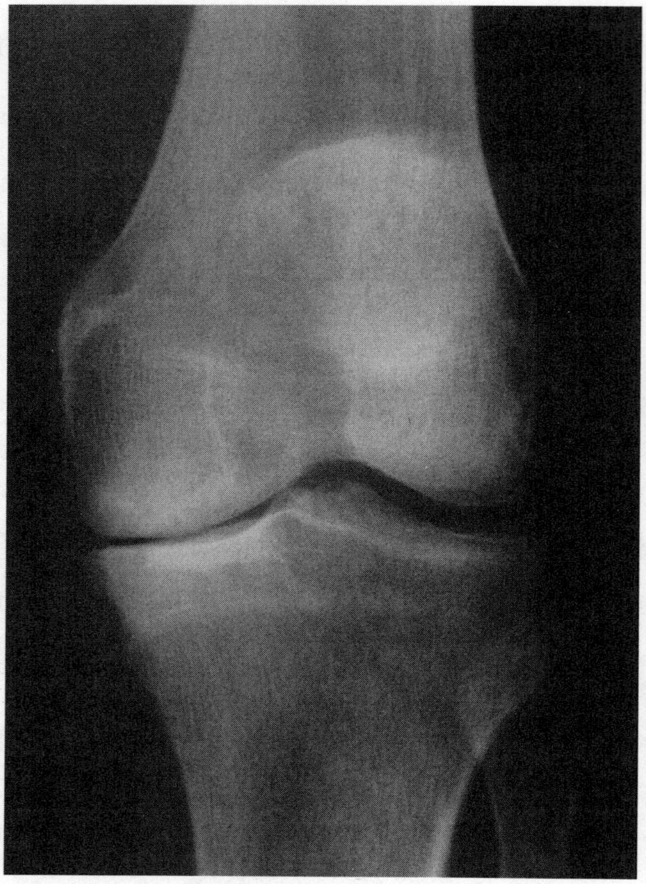

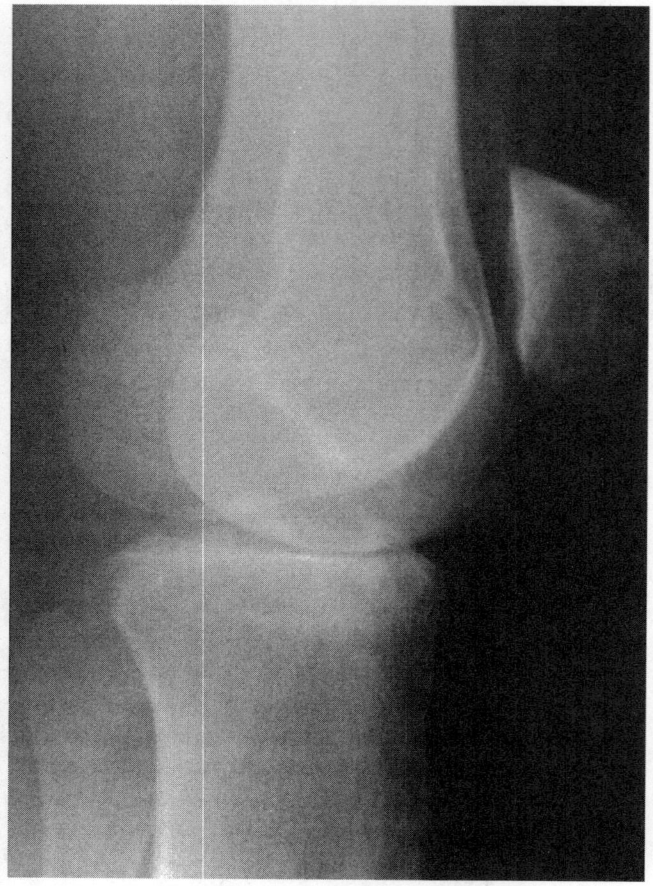

(A) arthroscopic debridement
(B) unicondylar arthroplasty of the medial compartment
(C) total knee arthroplasty without patellar resurfacing
(D) total knee arthroplasty with patellar resurfacing
(E) arthrodesis of the knee

589. During the exposure for a total knee arthroplasty in a patient with osteoarthritis and minimal deformity, the lateral collateral ligament was inadvertently divided. The most appropriate management of this complication is

(A) primary repair of the ligament, wound closure, and casting, followed by reoperation for knee arthroplasty in 6 weeks
(B) primary repair of the ligament after completion of the knee arthroplasty
(C) primary repair of the ligament after distal transfer of its origin
(D) primary repair of the ligament, reinforced by a fascia lata graft
(E) use of a constrained condylar prosthesis

590. A *contraindication* to total knee replacement is the presence of

(A) grade IV quadriceps strength
(B) a past history of sepsis in the involved knee
(C) an angular deformity greater than 35°
(D) a flexion deformity greater than 60°
(E) a sound arthrodesis

591. During total knee arthroplasty, after correcting an angular deformity by appropriate soft-tissue releases, the prosthesis selected should

(A) be posteriorly stabilized
(B) provide firm mediolateral stability
(C) be fully constrained
(D) have a relatively flat polyethylene surface
(E) be slightly oversized

592. Following total knee replacement and postoperative anticoagulation with warfarin, the incidence of deep venous thrombosis, as determined by venography, is approximately

(A) 15 percent
(B) 30 percent
(C) 45 percent
(D) 60 percent
(E) 75 percent

593. Following total knee arthroplasty, patients with venograms positive for deep venous thrombosis should be anticoagulated with therapeutic doses of

(A) heparin for 3 weeks
(B) heparin for 3 months
(C) heparin for 6 months
(D) warfarin (Coumadin) for 3 weeks
(E) warfarin (Coumadin) for 3 months

594. Loosening of the tibial component following total knee arthroplasty has been associated primarily with

(A) poor surgical technique
(B) poor prosthetic design
(C) marked preoperative varus deformity
(D) marked preoperative valgus deformity
(E) preoperative recurvatum deformity

595. The major disadvantage of arthroscopic synovectomy of the knee is the

(A) technical difficulty
(B) prolongation of operative time
(C) difficulty in achieving hemostasis
(D) damage to articular cartilage
(E) inability to remove an adequate amount of synovium

Adult Diseases and Disorders: Lower Limb

Answers

535. The answer is D. *(Pfeffer, p 208.)* The literature shows a rerupture rate averaging 18 percent following prolonged immobilization in equinus for the treatment of ruptures of the Achilles tendon. The rate of rerupture following operative treatment is about 1 percent. Complications of *open* treatment are primarily those of surgery: sural nerve injury, wound necrosis, skin slough, and infection.

536. The answer is B. *(Pfeffer, pp 213–214.)* Patients with old ruptures of the Achilles tendon and defects in the tendon greater than 1 cm should be treated surgically. A defect of 1 to 3 cm can be effectively bridged by turning down a flap from the aponeurosis of the triceps surae in the manner of Lindholm. Use of the flexor digitorum longus tendon is more complicated and usually reserved for repair of an old tendon *avulsion* from the os calcis. Use of the posterior tibial tendon is not recommended because of the foot imbalance created by its loss. Synthetic materials have biocompatibility problems that threaten the normal healing process.

537. The answer is D. *(Pfeffer, p 220.)* Surgery for hallux valgus should be done for symptoms rather than for appearance or radiographic findings. The primary justification for surgical intervention is continued pain after an adequate trial of nonoperative management. The need for split-size shoes is infrequent, although, when present, it supports the case for operative management.

538. The answer is A. *(Pfeffer, p 221.)* Although all the factors listed influence the outcome following surgery for hallux valgus, selection of the wrong patient or the wrong operation is the most frequent error. The decision whether or not to operate must be made on the basis of a comprehensive evaluation that includes assessment of the patient's personality and expectations and careful evaluation of preoperative radiographs.

539. The answer is E. *(Pfeffer, p 226.)* The first metatarsal is normally shorter than the second, so this is not a contraindication to surgery for hallux valgus. MTP arthritis, a first and second intermetatarsal angle of over 10°, and hallux rigidus are *indications* for hallux valgus surgery. Patients with gross ligamentous laxity (e.g., Ehlers-Danlos syndrome) have a high failure rate following surgery for hallux valgus; with the possible exception of fusion operations, surgery should be avoided in these patients.

540. The answer is C. *(Pfeffer, p 224.)* Neither failure to resect enough of the metatarsal head nor excessive resection of bone from the proximal phalanx are commonly associated with significant pain following a Keller arthroplasty. Neuroma formation is rare, as is postoperative hallux varus deformity. The shortening of the first toe that results from a Keller arthroplasty is often associated with lateral transfer metatarsalgia, especially in high-demand patients. This procedure is indicated primarily for low-demand patients or as a salvage procedure after failed bunion surgery in the older patient.

541. The answer is E. *(Pfeffer, p 229.)* Patients most suited for a Chevron osteotomy are under the age of 50, have an angle between the first and second metatarsals of less than 15°, a hallux valgus deformity of less than 40°, and normal sesamoid-metatarsal joints. This operation is less effective in older patients (osteoporosis makes fixation difficult), and those with greater deformity, which cannot be adequately corrected by this procedure. Patients with more severe deformity are usually best managed by an osteotomy at the base of the first metatarsal.

542. The answer is B. *(Pfeffer, p 249.)* Tightness of the Achilles tendon is related to the development of plantar fasciitis. Normally, ankle dorsiflexion increases after heel strike in the stance phase of gait. If dorsiflexion is limited by tightness in the Achilles tendon, stress is transferred to the plantar fascia. Acquired planovalgus deformities have also been shown to be associated with increased incidence of plantar fasciitis. Plantar calcaneal spurring is an incidental finding.

543. The answer is A. *(Pfeffer, p 250.)* The most characteristic finding in plantar fasciitis is tenderness at the origin of the plantar fascia from the medial tubercle of the os calcis. Pain on the *medial* surface of the os calcis superior to the tubercle suggests entrapment of the first branch of the lateral plantar nerve. If the tenderness is proximal to the medial tubercle, it may represent a stress fracture of the os calcis. Tenderness in the midportion of the longitudinal arch is more likely to reflect arthritic changes in the midtarsal joints, and tenderness beneath the metatarsal heads is not associated with plantar fasciitis.

544. The answer is C. *(Wilson, J Bone Joint Surg 47-A:340–348, 1965.)* The talonavicular joint is the joint most prone to pseudarthrosis following triple arthrodesis, with an incidence of 10 percent. Internal fixation reduces the frequency of pseudarthrosis, as does delaying weight-bearing for at least 6 weeks postoperatively. Except for patients with neuropathic joints or spasticity, where the pseudarthrosis rate is higher, no connection between the preoperative diagnosis and the rate of fusion has been shown; nor has a higher rate of pseudarthrosis been documented following postoperative wound infection.

545. The answer is D. *(Kelley, pp 818–820.)* All the factors listed may contribute to the development of forefoot deformity in patients with rheumatoid arthritis; however, the most critical factor is synovitis. Synovitis causes swelling, which produces capsular and ligamentous stretching, with the loss of static joint supports. The joints are then susceptible to the development of deformity from external forces. With disease progression, loss of articular cartilage contributes to joint instability.

546. The answer is A. *(Kelley, p 819.)* Rheumatoid arthritis affects approximately 2 or 3 per 1000 people in the general population. Although most well known for its crippling hand deformities, the disease can affect any diarthrodial joint. The knee is the area for which physicians are most frequently consulted, followed by the foot and hand.

547. The answer is C. *(Pfeffer, p 221.)* Resection arthroplasty (Keller procedure) is not indicated in a high-demand, relatively young patient. The Mitchell osteotomy is technically demanding, shortens the first metatarsal, and risks avascular necrosis. For these reasons, it is employed infrequently. Silastic implants have a high rate of failure in weight-bearing joints, and fusion of the first metatarsocuneiform joint does not adequately address the arthritis and deformity at the first MTP joint. Arthrodesis in 15° of valgus and 25° of dorsiflexion may be expected to provide a stable, pain-free first ray and a buttress against further deformity of the lesser toes. In addition, the likelihood of lateral transfer metatarsalgia is small.

548. The answer is E. *(Kelley, p 818.)* The important principle in the treatment of rheumatoid arthritis of the forefoot is to delay surgery whenever possible until the disease has run its course, providing comprehensive surgical management on a rational basis. In a young woman with disease for only 2 years, further deformities will almost assuredly evolve as the disease progresses. Shoe modifications, such as a larger toebox, an arch support, or a metatarsal bar, should provide adequate relief of symptoms until the final extent of her forefoot deformity is clearer.

549. The answer is B. *(Kelley, p 620.)* As a result of stretching of the capsular and volar plate at the MTP joints, there is progressive dorsal subluxation of these joints. This increases tension in the long flexors, leading to secondary PIP joint flexion contractures. With dorsal displacement of the MTP joint, the proximal phalanx becomes more vertically aligned with respect to the metatarsal and acts as a piston, in response to shoe pressure, to depress the metatarsal head. Whether the subsequent loss of fat pad beneath the metatarsal heads is related to thinning of the fat pad from increased pressure or to distal displacement resulting from MTP hyperextension is not clear. Both factors probably contribute.

550. The answer is C. *(Kelley, p 820.)* An increase in the normal valgus posture is the most common deformity of the hindfoot in patients with rheumatoid arthritis. Weakening of the static supports of the subtalar joint by synovitis allows weight-bearing to cause displacement of the os calcis into excessive valgus. In fact, rheumatoid patients who are bedridden are more likely to develop varus deformities of the heel. Rupture of the posterior tibial tendon, which has been reported in 5 percent of rheumatoid patients, contributes to the development of valgus deformity, as does loss of articular cartilage in the subtalar joint. Contracture of the peroneal muscles is more often a result of increased valgus than a cause of it.

551. The answer is E. *(Kelley, p 821.)* The most common presenting manifestation of rheumatoid disease of the forefoot is metatarsalgia. The MTP joints are the earliest and most frequently affected joints in the forefoot in rheumatoid patients. Synovitis involving these joints causes pain (metatarsalgia) with weight-bearing. Patients may also complain that their shoes have become too tight, and MTP swelling may cause separation of the toes. The other findings listed occur later in the course of the disease.

552. The answer is D. *(Kelley, p 822.)* End-stage rheumatoid disease of the forefoot, described by Michotte as *pied rond rheumatismal*, is classically manifest by marked hallux valgus, clawing and lateral deviation of the middle three toes, and callosities under the metatarsal heads, over the PIP joints, and at the tips of the toes. Deviation of the first toe is produced by shoe pressure after the joint supports are weakened by capsular distention. Pressure from the great toe forces the middle toes laterally over the fifth toe. Intrinsic spasm causes clawing, which leads to callosities from shoe pressure.

553. The answer is E. *(Kelley, p 829.)* Debridement alone is indicated primarily for partial ruptures of the posterior tibial tendon, which are seldom diagnosed. Primary repair is seldom possible because of the degenerated tendon ends. There are no tendons readily available for transference to replace the posterior tibial tendon. Triple arthrodesis is indicated for a fixed deformity with destruction of the subtalar joints. Tenosynovectomy with free tendon grafting after the tendon ends are resected to normal tendon is the procedure of choice in this young patient.

554. The answer is D. *(Kelley, p 827.)* Lateral radiographs of the cervical spine in flexion and extension are critical prior to intubation of patients with rheumatoid arthritis. Approximately 40 percent of patients have atlantoaxial subluxation, which may, if unrecognized prior to surgery, result in serious neurologic injury. If atlantoaxial instability is present, nasotracheal intubation or stabilization of the cervical spine may be necessary prior to surgery on the limbs. All the other conditions should be evaluated, but they are rarely a contraindication to surgery.

555. The answer is B. *(Kelley, p 452.)* The water content of osteoarthritic cartilage is increased, especially early in the course of the disease. Although some studies have shown the presence of type I collagen in osteoarthritic cartilage, the predominant collagen type remains that of normal cartilage, or type II. The most pronounced biochemical change in osteoarthritic cartilage is a sharp decrease in the concentration of mature proteoglycans.

556. The answer is E. *(Kelley, pp 459–464.)* The strongest risk factor for the development of osteoarthritis is age. While obese patients have more symptomatic osteoarthritis, especially of the knee, the role of obesity in the *production* of osteoarthritis is unclear. Repetitive trauma may cause microfractures in the subchondral bone, which, with healing, stiffen the bone and increase the stress on the articular cartilage, but this cause-and-effect relationship has not been proved. Osteoporosis with weakening of the underlying bone may actually protect against the development of osteoarthritis.

557. The answer is C. *(Kelley, pp 475–479.)* Radionucleotide bone scanning is more helpful than MRI in distinguishing genetic or metabolic disorders from primary osteoarthritis. MRI may demonstrate bone infarction before changes are seen on routine radiographs, but the development of symptoms is most often associated with characteristic findings on routine radiographs. The need to exclude causes of secondary osteoarthritis, such as pigmented villonodular synovitis or synovial chondromatosis, is rare, and other techniques, such as CT scanning or arthroscopy, are more specific and may be therapeutic as well as diagnostic. MRI is, however, very sensitive and specific in determining the site of nerve root or cord compression in patients with spinal osteoarthritis.

558. The answer is A. *(Kelley, p 481.)* The presence, on radiographs, of osteophytes surrounding the hip is not diagnostic for osteoarthritis. Rather, it is related to age. Of patients who have osteophytes as the only abnormality on a radiograph of the hip, fewer than 1 percent develop other roentgenographic changes of osteoarthritis within 10 years.

559. The answer is D. *(Kelley, p 484.)* Irritation of endosteal nerve endings has not been identified as a cause of pain in osteoarthritis. Venous congestion is the basis for *forage* in the treatment of osteoarthritis of the hip. Ligamentous stress and muscle strain may result from bone deformity and osteophytosis. Synovitis is a common finding in patients with osteoarthritis, accounting for warmth, effusion, and erythema in addition to pain.

560. The answer is C. *(Kelley, p 488.)* Following intraarticular injection of corticosteroids, pain is relieved temporarily, and in some cases pain appears to be permanently reduced. Clinical experience supports the safety of intraarticular steroid use; however, rapid progression of joint degeneration has been observed after frequent, repeated injections. For this reason, it is recommended that intraarticular corticosteroids not be used at intervals of less than 4 to 6 months. Studies also support the value of rest following injection in potentiating the response. For this reason, it is advisable to caution patients to minimize joint loading for a period following injection.

561. The answer is A. *(Kelley, p 489.)* Although controlled studies are lacking, osteoarthritic patients with symptoms suggestive of internal derangement seem to benefit most from arthroscopic debridement. Those whose symptoms are related primarily to instability seem to benefit least, along with those who have moderate changes without internal derangement. The benefit of arthroscopic debridement tends to lessen with subsequent procedures. No long-term studies have supported the efficacy of shaving fibrillated articular cartilage; it may, in fact, cause increased cartilage fibrillation.

562. The answer is A. *(Kelley, p 555.)* Each of the choices listed may be helpful in the management of glucocorticoid-induced osteopenia. Adrenalectomy results in both increased bone formation and decreased resorption; however, bone mass does not return to normal. Reduction of glucocorticoid medication to the lowest possible level is also important; however, dosages low enough to allow return to normal bone mass will usually not effectively treat the underlying disorder. Diphosphonates and calcitonin are theoretically useful; however, their efficacy in steroid-induced osteopenia has not been well documented. Hydrochlorothiazide reduces the urinary loss of calcium, but does not in itself constitute adequate treatment for this disorder.

563. The answer is C. *(Kelley, p 557.)* Immobilization induces a rapid decrease in bone formation without affecting bone resorption. This leads to hypercalcemia and increased urinary excretion of calcium, which may produce as much as a 20 percent decrease in bone mass within 4 months. Mechanical compressive therapy does not improve calcium balance, and calcium and phosphate supplements are of no benefit. Hypercalcemia may be controlled with calcitonin or diphosphonates. Adequate water intake and electrolyte balance are important adjuncts to other measures.

564. The answer is E. *(Kelley, p 559.)* In its fully developed form, osteomalacia is easily diagnosed. Early in the course of the disease, however, the diagnosis can be best established by means of a bone biopsy after tetracycline labeling. The number and thickness of osteoid seams per unit area of bone may be assessed by this technique, and tetracycline labeling will confirm decreased mineralization of osteoid seams, which defines osteomalacia. Most, but not all, forms of osteomalacia are characterized by reduced serum levels of phosphate. Other forms have normal serum levels of vitamin D. Vitamin D–dependent osteomalacia does not respond to physiologic doses (400 to 1000 units per day) of vitamin D.

565. The answer is A. *(Kelley, p 562.)* Almost one-half of patients with hyperparathyroidism are asymptomatic, the diagnosis having been made from biochemical abnormalities on routine screening examinations. Nephrolithiasis occurs in 20 percent of patients, usually as a later manifestation of the disease. Bone disease is clinically evident in 5 to 10 percent of patients, and subperiosteal resorption is the most common radiologic finding, most frequently in the middle phalanges and clavicles. Even so, subperiosteal resorption is a rare finding in *primary* hyperparathyroidism. Cystic lesions in bone ("brown tumors"), through which pathologic fractures occasionally occur, are very rare, especially as the presenting finding.

566. The answer is B. *(Kelley, pp 565–566.)* In its fully developed form, renal osteodystrophy is characterized by osteitis fibrosa cystica, osteoporosis, osteosclerosis, osteomalacia, and chronic renal tubular failure. Ingestion of aluminum-containing antacids, combined with deposition of aluminum in bone as a result of renal failure, is diminishing as a result of the use of calcium carbonate instead of aluminum as the primary phosphate-binding agent for reducing serum phosphate levels in patients with renal failure. Osteomalacia is common and results both from decreased deposition of vitamin D and increased deposition of aluminum in bone. With progression of renal disease, osteitis fibrosa cystica becomes evident. Elevated serum levels of parathyroid hormone, combined with hypocalcemia, produce osteoporosis. Osteosclerosis is seen in uremic patients, most characteristically in the vertebrae, where alternating bands of osteoporosis produce the "rugger-jersey spine."

567. The answer is D. *(Kelley, pp 566–567.)* The classic radiographic findings in Paget's disease are bowing of the limbs, enlargement of the skull, and kyphosis. The figure shows the characteristic "saber shin" pattern of tibial bowing with evidence of numerous stress fractures on the convex side of the deformity, which can be the source of intermittent, severe pain. Pain is more common in Paget's disease of bone than in any of the other conditions listed. A biopsy of the tibia would reveal bone formation and destruction, with prominent cement ("reversal") lines, which produce the classic mosaic pattern of Paget's disease.

568. The answer is D. *(Kelley, pp 576–577.)* Although osteopenia could in theory predispose to microfractures and subsequent avascularity, few elderly patients with osteopenia develop AVN. The mechanisms by which excessive intake of alcohol and chronic liver disease cause AVN have not been clearly established, but they are thought to be related to alternations of the circulating lipids with formation of microemboli. Abnormal cell forms in sickle cell disease are thought to cause sludging in the circulation, and the nitrogen bubbles of decompression sickness form intraluminal emboli.

569. The answer is A. *(Kelley, pp 578–579.)* Although AVN may result from a single, massive vascular disruption, it is more commonly the result of a series of lesser insults incurred over a period of weeks or months. Bone death stimulates the process of repair, which may be complete if the lesion is small, leaving only a residual bone infarct or "bone island." Such lesions are usually asymptomatic and seen as incidental findings on x-ray. Larger lesions are more likely to be symptomatic and exceed the capacity of the repair process to revascularize the infarct. With continued stress on dead bone, microfractures occur, and, with subsequent collapse, the overlying cartilage is subjected to abnormal stress and more rapid wear. Eventually, the acetabular side of the joint is involved, and osteoarthritis ensues.

570. The answer is E. *(Kelley, pp 581–583.)* While routine radiographs are the simplest, best, and least expensive means for diagnosing *established* AVN, MRI is the best single method for the *early* diagnosis of AVN. Increased radioisotope uptake is a nonspecific finding. Although bone scanning is a relatively quick and inexpensive method for scanning the entire skeleton, it must be remembered that increased uptake of the isotope reflects simply increased vascularity or new bone formation and is not specific for AVN or other conditions.

571. The answer is C. *(Kelley, pp 584–587.)* The figure shows precollapse (Ficat stage II) AVN of the femoral head. Decompression and cancellous bone grafting of the femoral head results in 70 percent of patients having functional hips at a mean follow-up of 3 years, compared with 31 percent of patients treated nonoperatively. Decompression of the femoral head relieves what many believe is an important component in the propagation of the disease. Cortical strut grafting provides a mechanical buttress against collapse of the articular surface, whereas cancellous grafting serves as a scaffold to enhance repair. Osteotomy and femoral head replacement should be considered after collapse of the femoral head. Total hip replacement is more ideally suited for the older patient with destruction on both sides of the joint.

572. The answer is B. *(Kelley, p 629.)* Supporting the foot with medial arch supports is the cornerstone of the nonoperative management of tarsal tunnel syndrome. The tenosynovitis associated with this condition will be relieved by NSAIDs. Instillation of local anesthetics rarely produces permanent benefit, and local corticosteroids are dangerous if injected into adjacent tendons. Although surgical decompression may be necessary in up to 60 percent of patients, it should be recommended only after failure of nonoperative treatment.

573. The answer is B. *(Kelley, pp 669–670.)* Although a major concern with the postoperative administration of NSAIDs is inhibition of platelet aggregation, renal dysfunction is the most frequent postoperative type of toxicity encountered. In postoperative patients who are volume-depleted, inhibition of prostaglandin synthesis by an NSAID can lead to a decline in renal perfusion and glomerular filtration rate, with a rise in serum creatinine levels. Fluid retention and hyperkalemia may also occur.

574. The answer is E. *(Kelley, p 813.)* While early failures were primarily related to loosening of poorly designed components, failure of late models results, in approximately equal numbers, from malposition, loosening, infection, and subluxation. Since each of these is caused primarily by errors in technique, this is the best choice.

575. The answer is E. *(Kelley, pp 689–690.)* A study of synovectomy by the Arthritis Foundation showed improved clinical and radiographic results 2 years following synovectomy. At 5 years, however, there was no statistically significant difference between patients undergoing synovectomy and control patients. Interestingly, the patients themselves were overwhelmingly satisfied with their results, both early and late. It has been hard to assess accurately the value of synovectomy in rheumatoid arthritis because of the natural fluctuations in disease activity; however, if performed before significant articular erosions have occurred, the procedure has value for at least 2 or 3 years.

576. The answer is E. *(Kelley, p 691.)* In patients with rheumatoid arthritis, results following synovectomy are dependent upon sufficient patient motivation for prolonged compliance with a physical therapy program. Synovectomy is appropriate for patients with stage I, II, or III joint disease but should not be carried out in patients with stage IV articular destruction. Rheumatoid nodules per se are not a contraindication to synovectomy; however, they should be avoided in any operative approach. It is not necessary to await a normal sedimentation rate to carry out synovectomy, although the procedure should not be done in the face of floridly active disease and a "toxic" patient.

577. The answer is D. *(Kelley, p 783.)* The presence of infection anywhere in the body should be considered a contraindication to joint replacement surgery. The other conditions listed require modification of operative or postoperative protocols. The anesthesiologist must be made aware of C1–2 changes or of temporomandibular arthritis, so that nasotracheal intubation or regional anesthesia may be used. Forearm crutches may be necessary when hand function is severely compromised. An ipsilateral valgus knee deformity should be appreciated by the surgeon; failure to do so may result in malpositioning of the femoral component.

578. The answer is B. *(Kelley, pp 786–788.)* Modern cementing techniques, including plugging of the intramedullary canal, irrigation with pulsatile lavage, and pressurization of the cement have significantly improved the results of cemented total hip arthroplasty. The primary reason for this improvement has been a reduction in the rate of femoral loosening. In one study, the femoral loosening rate at 5 years was 24 percent with older cement techniques, compared with 4 percent with modern techniques.

579. The answer is A. *(Kelley, pp 789–790.)* The incidence of deep infection following hip arthroplasty was found by the NIH Consensus Panel to be approximately 1 percent, of which 15 percent developed after 24 months, presumably as a result of hematogenous spread. The high incidence of late hematogenous seeding underscores the need for prompt antibiotic treatment of infection elsewhere in the body and for prophylaxis when dental extractions or urinary tract manipulations are to be performed.

580. The answer is E. *(Kelley, p 791.)* Young patients who place heavy demands on their weight-bearing joints and who have advanced degenerative changes and little motion should be strongly considered for arthrodesis, especially when the opposite hip is disease-free. As can be seen from the radiograph, no part of the joint is spared, so osteotomy could not be expected to position uninvolved parts of the joint into a weight-bearing position. It is unlikely that total hip arthroplasty would enable this patient to work at his present occupation for more than 10 years without further surgery. Finally, short patients are less disabled by arthrodesis of the hip than are tall patients.

581. The answer is D. *(Kelley, p 794.)* In this situation, the anteroposterior dimension of the femoral component is too large. Using a femoral component one size smaller will increase the flexion space by 3 to 5 mm while not altering the extension space. Soft-tissue balance of the knee should be obtained by use of a thicker polyethylene insert.

582. The answer is A. *(Kelley, p 794.)* This combination of findings often occurs in patients with uncorrected flexion contractures of the knee. In such cases, the posterior capsule should be released from the distal femur; however, care should be taken not to disrupt the origins of the gastrocnemius muscles, which will produce postoperative spasm and difficulty obtaining extension. If release of the posterior capsule does not balance the knee in flexion and extension, more bone should be resected from the distal femur.

583. The answer is B. *(Kelley, p 794.)* As a general rule, if trial reduction reveals excessive tightness in both flexion and extension, corrective measures should be undertaken on the tibial side. In most other circumstances, changes should be made on the femoral side. If the tightness is minimal, correction may be obtained simply by increasing the posterior slope of the tibia. In the vast majority of cases, however, resection of a small amount of additional bone from the proximal tibia is the preferred solution.

584. The answer is E. *(Kelley, p 796.)* High tibial osteotomy is a very good means of buying time in the younger patient with osteoarthritis, minimal varus deformity, a stable knee, and disease that is confined largely to the medial compartment. If slight overcorrection (9 to 10°) valgus is obtained and the knee is stable, good results may be expected in approximately 90 percent of patients. Even though rheumatoid arthritis may appear to be limited to only one compartment, such is never the case, and the results following high tibial osteotomy in these patients are not as good as in patients with osteoarthritis.

585. The answer is D. *(Kelley, p 796.)* Osteoarthritis and posttraumatic arthritis, especially in younger patients, are ideal indications for high tibial osteotomy, since they involve primarily only one compartment of the joint. The results following this procedure are less satisfactory in patients who have a varus deformity in excess of 10°, largely because of the greater difficulty in obtaining the correct postoperative alignment. In patients with a severe deformity, especially severe valgus, correction through the tibia leaves persistent joint obliquity, which may lead to recurrence of the deformity. Such patients are usually better managed by distal femoral osteotomy, which corrects the joint obliquity.

586. The answer is C. *(Kelley, p 797.)* Rheumatoid knees are characterized by valgus deformity associated with external rotation and lateral subluxation of the tibia. These deformities create changes in ligamentous length, particularly attenuation of the medial collateral ligament, that must be balanced at surgery. Varus angulation is relatively uncommon in rheumatoid patients, though it is the typical deformity in patients with osteoarthritis.

587. The answer is E. *(Kelley, p 797.)* Mild flexion deformities of the knee in patients with rheumatoid arthritis arise because the distended, inflamed joint is more comfortable in this position. The flexion deformity becomes fixed with the development of contracture of the posterior capsule. Patients who continue to walk, however, rarely develop flexion deformities in excess of 30°.

588. The answer is B. *(Kelley, pp 798–800.)* Among the choices listed, the preferred management is medial compartment replacement since neither the lateral nor the patellofemoral compartment appears to be significantly involved. Also, this procedure would offer the shortest rehabilitation for a busy executive who is only 4 years from retirement. It has also been observed that better motion is achieved with unicondylar than with total knee replacement; and, with preservation of the cruciate ligaments, patients retain the sensation of a normal knee.

589. The answer is E. *(Kelley, p 802.)* A constrained condylar prosthesis is the best choice for this complication, since stability of the knee is enhanced by the fit of a tibial post into the femoral component. Additional stability is provided by stems on both components. This prosthesis may also be used in knees with severe valgus or flexion deformities, correction of which may cause instability.

590. The answer is E. *(Kelley, p 804.)* As a general rule, a painless arthrodesis in acceptable position should not be converted to a knee arthroplasty. The results of such procedures are substandard, and failure of the arthroplasty makes reconversion to arthrodesis more difficult. Grade IV quadriceps strength is adequate to extend the knee against gravity and is the minimum strength required for acceptable results following total knee arthroplasty. While active sepsis is a contraindication to surgery, old sepsis is not.

591. The answer is A. *(Kelley, p 808.)* Correction of angular deformities by ligamentous releases almost invariably involves excision of the cruciate ligaments, for which a posterior stabilized prosthesis is recommended. More, rather than less curvature of the polyethylene surface of the tibial implant is required in cruciate-sacrificing designs. Fully constrained prostheses are seldom necessary. There is no reason for use of an oversized total knee prosthesis.

592. The answer is D. *(Kelley, p 809.)* In a recent study of anticoagulated patients who underwent total knee arthroplasty at the Hospital for Special Surgery, 64 percent had venographic evidence of deep venous thrombosis on the fifth postoperative day. In this study, there was poor correlation between the clinical and venographic diagnoses of deep venous thrombosis.

593. The answer is E. *(Kelley, p 809.)* Therapeutic heparinization is not recommended in the first week following total knee arthroplasty because of the high incidence of hemarthrosis. Anticoagulation with warfarin (coumadin) is recommended and should be continued for 2 to 3 months unless there is an associated pulmonary embolus, in which case warfarin is continued for 6 months.

594. The answer is B. *(Kelley, p 81.)* The incidence of loosening of the tibial component following total knee arthroplasty has been reduced by improvements in design, such as the addition of metal backing to the tibial component, which increases the stiffness of the polyethylene. Another beneficial change has been the advent of a one-piece tibial component with a central fixation peg. In a recent series of total knee arthroplasties with these tibial design features, only two cases of tibial component loosening were identified in 100 osteoarthritic knees that had been followed from 5 to 9 years. One of the two cases of loosening was due to poor surgical technique.

595. The answer is A. *(Kelley, p 688.)* Arthroscopic synovectomy is a technically demanding procedure, requiring patience and persistence by the surgeon. It does, however, offer lower morbidity and the opportunity for a more complete synovial resection than does open synovectomy.

Adult Trauma

Douglas R. Dirschl, M.D.

DIRECTIONS: Each question below contains five suggested responses. Select the **one best** response to each question.

596. In the field, basic management priorities for emergency medical technicians (EMTs) include all the following EXCEPT

(A) management of the airway
(B) safe extrication of the patient
(C) transport to an appropriate trauma center
(D) stabilization of fractures
(E) determination of the trauma score

597. The use of pneumatic antishock garments (PASGs) is absolutely *contraindicated* in which of the following situations?

(A) Pelvic fractures
(B) Fractures of the lower limb
(C) Diaphragmatic ruptures
(D) Spinal fractures
(E) Traumatic amputations of the lower limb

598. Physical findings consistent with tension pneumothorax include all the following EXCEPT

(A) paradoxical motion of the thoracic cage
(B) decreased breath sounds
(C) tympany on chest percussion
(D) distended neck veins
(E) hypotension

599. The amount of blood loss a healthy 70-kg man must sustain before a significant drop in systolic pressure occurs is approximately

(A) 500 mL
(B) 1000 mL
(C) 1500 mL
(D) 2000 mL
(E) 3000 mL

600. Initial management of a traumatized adult in shock consists of insertion of at least two large-bore peripheral intravenous catheters and administration of

(A) Ringer's lactate, 1 L over a 1 h period
(B) Ringer's lactate, 1 L bolus
(C) normal saline, 1 L bolus
(D) Ringer's lactate, 2 L bolus
(E) normal saline, 2 L bolus

601. The most commonly injured intraabdominal organ by blunt trauma is the

(A) liver
(B) kidney
(C) pancreas
(D) small intestine
(E) prostate

602. The maximum amount of sagittal plane deformity that is acceptable for a fracture in the middle third of the proximal phalanx is

(A) 5°
(B) 10°
(C) 20°
(D) 30°
(E) 40°

603. In applying a halo ring, location of the anterior pins too far anteriorly is most likely to result in injury to the

(A) temporal artery
(B) temporalis muscle
(C) supratrochlear nerve
(D) supraorbital nerve
(E) frontal sinus

604. In the use of a halo ring and vest in an adult patient, the lowest rates of pin loosening and infection follow initial tightening torques of

(A) 4 inch-pounds
(B) 8 inch-pounds
(C) 12 inch-pounds
(D) 16 inch-pounds
(E) 20 inch-pounds

605. All the following are characteristics of a complete rupture of the pectoralis major muscle EXCEPT that

(A) the deformity is obvious when the muscle contracts
(B) pain is the patient's greatest concern
(C) late repair is impractical
(D) early surgical repair is effective
(E) rupture usually occurs near the humeral insertion of the muscle

606. Compared with nonoperative treatment of grade 3 acromioclavicular separations, operative treatment results in

(A) greater strength
(B) improved motion
(C) greater long-term relief of pain
(D) a higher incidence of complications
(E) more rapid return to athletic activities

607. Which of the following is most commonly associated with displaced fractures of the scaphoid?

(A) Negative ulnar variance
(B) Positive ulnar variance
(C) Fractures of the radial styloid
(D) Fractures of the ulnar styloid
(E) Disruption of the scapholunate ligament

608. One month after a fall onto an outstretched hand, a 40-year-old man complained of weakness and stiffness of the wrist and pain in the radial snuff box. Radiographs showed a nondisplaced fracture through the waist of the scaphoid. The most appropriate management is

(A) application of a thumb spica cast
(B) electrical stimulation
(C) internal fixation
(D) internal fixation and bone grafting
(E) CT of the wrist

609. A 21-year-old woman injured her knee while skiing. The only detectable injury was a complete tear of the medial collateral ligament. The optimal treatment is

(A) a compressive wrap and early motion
(B) a hinged knee brace and early motion
(C) an above-knee cast
(D) operative repair of the medial collateral ligament
(E) operative repair of the medial collateral ligament and the posteromedial corner

610. An 18-year-old wrestler sustained a posterolateral dislocation of the elbow. Examination after reduction of the elbow revealed that the elbow could be easily redislocated. Radiographs obtained after reduction showed a concentric reduction with anatomic alignment. Further treatment should consist of

(A) immobilization at 90° for 1 week
(B) immobilization at 90° for 3 weeks
(C) immobilization at 90° for 6 weeks
(D) operative repair of the medial collateral ligament
(E) operative repair of the medial and lateral collateral ligaments

611. The most common problem associated with removal of a Zickel nail after healing of a subtrochanteric fracture of the femur is

(A) inability to remove the triflanged nail from the femoral neck and head
(B) inability to remove the nail from the femoral canal
(C) fracture of the distal femur
(D) refracture of the proximal femur
(E) breakage of the nail

612. The most significant risk factor for a poor result following prompt reduction of a traumatic posterior dislocation of the hip is

(A) advanced age of the patient
(B) open reduction of the hip joint
(C) instability after closed reduction
(D) full weight-bearing within 4 weeks of injury
(E) early motion of the hip

613. After closed reduction of a posterior dislocation of the hip in the operating room under general anesthesia, intraoperative radiographs show concentric reduction of the hip joint, and physical examination reveals excellent stability. The next step in the management of this patient should be

(A) bed rest in skin traction
(B) bracing of the hip in abduction
(C) early motion, with weight-bearing as tolerated
(D) application of a hip spica cast
(E) CT of the hip

614. For stabilization of comminuted subtrochanteric fractures, the highest torsional stiffness may be achieved with

(A) five Ender's nails
(B) a conventional locked intramedullary nail
(C) a Zickel nail
(D) a compression hip screw and side plate
(E) a blade plate

615. The single most important aspect of treatment in attaining good results following open tibial fractures is

(A) prophylactic antibiotics
(B) thorough irrigation
(C) adequate debridement
(D) rigid skeletal stabilization
(E) early soft-tissue coverage

616. Which of the following is the most appropriate initial antibiotic treatment of grade III open tibial fractures?

(A) First-generation cephalosporin
(B) Second-generation cephalosporin
(C) First- or second-generation cephalosporin with an aminoglycoside
(D) Penicillin G with an aminoglycoside
(E) Penicillin G and a first- or second-generation cephalosporin

617. Two days after being bitten by a cat, a 25-year-old man had painful flexor tenosynovitis of his left index finger. The organism most likely to be responsible for this inflammation is

(A) *Staphylococcus aureus*
(B) *Eikenella* species
(C) *Staphylococcus epidermidis*
(D) *Pasteurella multocida*
(E) *Streptococcus pyogenes*

618. A 19-year-old man sustained a 1-cm laceration over the right fifth metacarpophalangeal joint when he struck someone in the mouth. Treatment should consist of

(A) oral antibiotics and loose closure of the wound
(B) intravenous antibiotics, loose closure of the wound, and observation
(C) oral antibiotics, debridement, and open treatment of the wound
(D) intravenous antibiotics, debridement, and loose closure of the wound
(E) intravenous antibiotics, surgical exploration, and open treatment of the wound

619. The diagnosis of posttraumatic adult respiratory distress syndrome (ARDS) following multiple trauma is best made by

(A) a chest radiograph
(B) arterial blood gases
(C) coagulation studies
(D) a sputum smear
(E) a complete blood count

620. After open reduction and internal fixation of an intertrochanteric fracture, a 70-year-old patient had minimal serosanguinous drainage from the incision for 6 weeks. Cultures of the drainage grew *Staphylococcus epidermidis*. The next step in management should be

(A) a bone scan
(B) an MRI scan
(C) a complete blood count
(D) aspiration for culture and sensitivity
(E) surgical debridement and hardware removal

621. The procedure that provides the best initial evaluation of lower genitourinary tract injuries following displaced fractures of the anterior pelvis is

(A) a retrograde urethrogram
(B) an excretory urethrogram
(C) insertion of a Foley catheter
(D) a cystogram
(E) cystoscopy

622. Optimal internal fixation of a femoral neck fracture is achieved by

(A) three cancellous screws or pins
(B) five to seven cancellous screws or pins
(C) a sliding hip screw
(D) a sliding hip screw supplemented with pins
(E) Ender's nails

623. The most useful test for the diagnosis of a posterior pelvic ring injury is

(A) an AP radiograph of the pelvis
(B) pelvic inlet and outlet radiographs
(C) a CT scan of the pelvis
(D) a CT scan of the pelvis with three-dimensional reconstruction
(E) an MRI scan of the pelvis

624. The greatest delay in revascularization of the diaphysis of a long bone following internal fixation of a fracture is associated with which of the following fixation devices?

(A) A standard plate and screws
(B) A low-contact plate and screws
(C) An unreamed intramedullary nail
(D) A reamed intramedullary nail
(E) An external fixator

625. A 35-year-old man sustained a posterior dislocation of the hip with a shearing fracture of the femoral head. The most critical factor in minimizing the risk of osteonecrosis of the femoral head is the

(A) interval between injury and reduction of the dislocation
(B) surgical approach chosen for internal fixation of the fracture
(C) type of internal fixation used for the fracture
(D) presence of other musculoskeletal injuries
(E) type of femoral head fracture

626. The method of skeletal stabilization chosen for an open tibial fracture should be based primarily on the

(A) age of the patient
(B) fracture pattern
(C) soft-tissue injury
(D) amount of bone loss
(E) severity of other musculoskeletal injuries

627. Six hours following closed reduction and above-elbow casting of a Colles' fracture, a patient complained of numbness in the index and long fingers. Examination revealed decreased sensation to light touch in the index and long fingers. The most appropriate initial treatment is

(A) observation
(B) univalving the above-elbow cast
(C) removing the cast and extending the wrist
(D) measuring interstitial pressure in the carpal canal
(E) performing open release of the transverse carpal ligament

628. Five weeks after treatment of an extraarticular fracture of the distal radius in a below-elbow cast, a 70-year-old woman was suddenly unable to extend her thumb. The most likely diagnosis is

(A) compression of the posterior interosseous nerve
(B) rupture of the extensor pollicis longus
(C) displacement of the fracture
(D) compartment syndrome in the forearm
(E) osteoarthritis of the basilar joint of the thumb

629. A 35-year-old man fell from a roof onto his outstretched hand. Radiographs of the elbow revealed a markedly comminuted fracture of the radial head. Six months after radial head resection, the patient complained of ipsilateral wrist pain and weakness of grip. The most likely diagnosis is

(A) posttraumatic arthritis of the elbow
(B) entrapment of the posterior interosseous nerve
(C) nonunion of an unrecognized scaphoid fracture
(D) proximal migration of the radius
(E) compression of the median nerve at the elbow

630. In patients sustaining closed tarsometatarsal fracture-dislocations, the factor most closely associated with a poor functional outcome is the

(A) fracture pattern
(B) method of internal fixation
(C) extent of damage to the articular surfaces
(D) length of postoperative cast immobilization
(E) age of the patient

631. A 21-year-old college student with a symptomatic nonunion of the scaphoid but no degenerative arthritis should be treated by

(A) observation
(B) bracing of the wrist for heavy labor
(C) radial styloidectomy
(D) bone grafting and internal fixation
(E) radiocarpal arthrodesis

632. Indications for operative treatment of a hypertrophic nonunion of a fracture of the clavicle include all the following EXCEPT

(A) pain
(B) cosmetic deformity
(C) loss of shoulder function
(D) brachial plexus compression
(E) thoracic outlet compression

633. Following closed reduction of an anterior dislocation of the shoulder, radiographs revealed a fracture of the greater tuberosity that is displaced 2 cm superiorly. The most appropriate treatment is

(A) sling and swathe immobilization
(B) immobilization in an abduction orthosis
(C) percutaneous pin fixation of the greater tuberosity
(D) open reduction and internal fixation of the tuberosity
(E) late excision of the tuberosity fragment if symptomatic

634. A 45-year-old woman sustained a closed, minimally displaced midshaft fracture of the humerus. She had no associated injuries. The best management for this fracture is

(A) a hanging arm cast
(B) a Velpeau dressing
(C) a shoulder spica cast
(D) a functional brace
(E) an intramedullary nail

635. A 20-year-old man fell on his outstretched hand during an intramural football game. Examination revealed tenderness in the radial snuff box, but radiographs were normal. After 2 weeks in a thumb spica cast, he continued to have tenderness in the radial snuff box. Repeat radiographs were normal. The next step in evaluating this patient should be

(A) fluoroscopy of the wrist
(B) trispiral tomography of the wrist
(C) a three-phase bone scan
(D) a CT scan of the scaphoid
(E) arthroscopy of the wrist

636. The earliest finding in a developing compartmental syndrome of the leg is

(A) pain disproportionate to the injury
(B) numbness or tingling in the great toe
(C) pain with stretching of the extensor hallucis longus tendon
(D) decreased capillary refill
(E) increased intracompartmental pressure

637. Following a period of unconsciousness, a multiply traumatized patient was coherent and cooperative but complained of swelling and pain in the volar forearm. One hour later, the patient developed sluggish capillary refill in the fingers and pain in the volar forearm with passive finger extension. The measured intracompartmental pressure was 45 mmHg. The most appropriate management is

(A) strict elevation of the limb
(B) observation and repeat measurement of intracompartmental pressure in 1 h
(C) immediate fasciotomy of the superficial volar compartment of the forearm
(D) immediate fasciotomy of the deep volar compartment of the forearm
(E) immediate fasciotomy of all volar compartments of the forearm

638. Three hours after closed reduction and above-knee casting for a tibial shaft fracture, a 25-year-old patient complained of increasing pain in the leg. Capillary refill was sluggish and passive motion of the toes caused pain in the leg. The most appropriate initial management of this patient is

(A) elevating the limb and performing serial examinations
(B) univalving the cast
(C) bivalving the cast and dividing the cast padding
(D) removing the cast
(E) measuring intracompartmental pressure

639. A 28-year-old man sustained a pneumothorax, a closed fracture of the femur, and closed, displaced fractures of the ipsilateral humerus, radius, and ulna. The patient was resuscitated and taken to the operating room. After femoral fracture stabilization, the humeral and forearm fractures should be treated by

(A) skeletal traction
(B) closed reduction and plaster immobilization
(C) internal fixation of the forearm fractures and immobilization of the humeral fracture
(D) internal fixation of the humeral fracture and immobilization of the forearm fractures
(E) open reduction and internal fixation of the humeral and forearm fractures

640. A 32-year-old unbelted driver involved in a head-on motor vehicle accident had a blood pressure of 110/60 mmHg, a pulse of 110 beats per minute, and a P_{O_2} of 90 mmHg in the emergency department. The patient had multiple facial lacerations and bruising over his right clavicle. The chest radiograph was unremarkable. A radiograph should now be obtained of the

(A) skull
(B) face
(C) cervical spine
(D) abdomen
(E) pelvis

641. A patient involved in a motor vehicle accident had an initial Pa_{O_2} of 50 mmHg. The patient was intubated and placed on 50% FI_{O_2}. Repeat arterial blood gas showed a Pa_{O_2} of 70 mmHg. Auscultation of the chest revealed diminished breath sounds over the left chest. The most appropriate initial management of this patient is to

(A) obtain a chest radiograph
(B) increase inspired oxygen
(C) perform a needle thoracostomy
(D) insert a chest tube
(E) measure central venous pressure

642. A patient involved in a motor vehicle accident arrived at the trauma center with a blood pressure of 80/60 mmHg and a pulse of 150 beats per minute. Fluid resuscitation was begun with 2000 mL of Ringer's lactate over 15 min. The patient's blood pressure rose to 110/60 mmHg, but then dropped again to 80/60 mmHg. The next step in management should be

(A) administration of albumin
(B) administration of normal saline
(C) transfusion of blood
(D) insertion of a central venous catheter
(E) intubation

643. After initial fluid resuscitation, arterial blood gases for a traumatized patient revealed a pH of 7.26, a P_{CO_2} of 28, a P_{O_2} of 70, and a bicarbonate of 16. The most appropriate next step in management is to

(A) administer more intravenous fluid
(B) increase the inspired oxygen concentration
(C) administer dopamine
(D) administer bicarbonate
(E) intubate the patient

644. A 32-year-old man involved in a head-on motor vehicle accident had a blood pressure of 90/60 mmHg, a pulse of 110 beats per minute, a Pa_{O_2} of 80 mmHg, and bilateral clavicular fractures. The radiograph of his chest is shown below. The next step in management should be

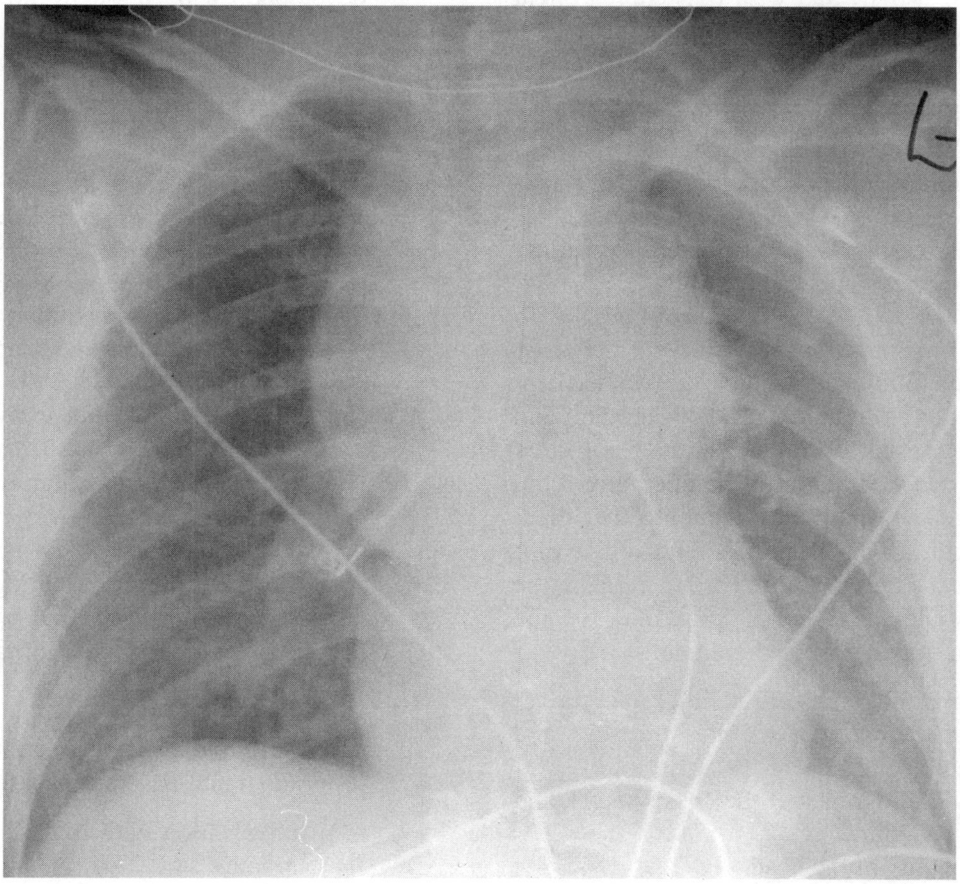

(A) endotracheal intubation
(B) chest tube thoracostomy
(C) needle thoracostomy
(D) arch aortogram
(E) CT scan of the chest

---

645. A 19-year-old man involved in a motorcycle accident sustained an injury to the right lower limb. Radiographs revealed a posterior dislocation of the knee. The most appropriate initial management is

(A) application of an above-knee cast
(B) application of an external fixator
(C) an arteriogram
(D) closed reduction
(E) open reduction

646. Endotracheal intubation of a patient with a probable cervical spine injury is best accomplished by

(A) orotracheal intubation
(B) nasotracheal intubation
(C) needle tracheostomy
(D) tracheostomy
(E) cricothyroidotomy

647. A 38-year-old man sustained a tibial fracture when his leg was run over by a truck. He subsequently developed acute compartmental syndrome and was treated with four-compartment fasciotomies. The most appropriate management of the tibial fracture is

(A) application of an above-knee cast
(B) application of skeletal traction
(C) an unreamed, locked, intramedullary nailing
(D) a reamed, locked, intramedullary nailing
(E) plate osteosynthesis

648. A 25-year-old man brought to the emergency department following a motor vehicle accident had a blood pressure of 60/40 mmHg and rapidly increasing abdominal girth. The patient was transported directly to the operating room for emergency laparotomy without other diagnostic studies. The surgeons removed a ruptured spleen and diagnosed a fracture of the tibia. The next diagnostic procedure in the evaluation of this patient should be

(A) plain radiographs of the tibial fracture
(B) plain radiographs of the thoracic and lumbar spines
(C) plain radiographs of the chest, pelvis, and cervical spine
(D) a CT scan of the head
(E) a CT scan of the pelvis

649. After intramedullary nailing of a fracture of the femoral shaft, the surgeon noticed an ipsilateral, nondisplaced fracture of the femoral neck. The risk of avascular necrosis associated with the missed femoral neck fracture is

(A) less than 5 percent
(B) 10 percent
(C) 25 percent
(D) 40 percent
(E) 60 percent

650. Ten weeks after reamed, interlocked, intramedullary nailing of a closed femoral shaft fracture in a 35-year-old man, a deep infection developed, with purulent drainage from the surgical incision that communicated with the proximal tip of the femoral nail. After debriding and culturing the wound, intravenous antibiotics were begun. The most appropriate treatment of the fracture would be to

(A) leave the nail in place until fracture union, then remove it
(B) remove the nail, ream the femoral canal, and repeat intramedullary nailing
(C) remove the nail and place the patient in traction
(D) remove the nail and apply an external fixator
(E) remove the nail and apply a cast brace

651. A 21-year-old college student who underwent locked, intramedullary nailing of a femoral fracture 6 months ago, and who was bearing full weight, complained of occasional aching at the fracture site. Radiographs showed excellent alignment of the femur, but no evidence of union at the site of the fracture. The most appropriate treatment for this patient is

(A) observation with repeat radiographs in 2 months
(B) pulsed electromagnetic field stimulation of the thigh
(C) open bone grafting with autogenous iliac crest
(D) exchange nailing with a reamed, unlocked, intramedullary nail
(E) exchange nailing with a reamed, locked, intramedullary nail

652. All the following observations about medial subtalar dislocations are correct EXCEPT that

(A) avascular necrosis of the talus is uncommon following this injury
(B) they heal less rapidly than do lateral subtalar dislocations
(C) closed reduction is usually stable
(D) late talonavicular arthrosis is uncommon
(E) the outcome of this injury is related to the mechanism

653. The risk of which of the following is most likely to be minimized when a fracture of the femur in a polytraumatized patient is stabilized in the first 24 h after injury?

(A) Infection
(B) Shortening
(C) Nonunion
(D) Pulmonary complications
(E) Heterotopic ossification

654. A 35-year-old woman sustained a closed, oblique fracture of the humerus at the junction of the middle and lower thirds and had a complete radial nerve palsy. The fracture was anatomically reduced and immobilized in a brace. The most appropriate management of the radial nerve palsy is

(A) immediate exploration and repair of the radial nerve; continued nonoperative fracture treatment
(B) immediate exploration and repair of the radial nerve; open reduction and internal fixation of the humerus
(C) exploration and repair of the radial nerve 3 weeks after injury if no improvement is seen
(D) exploration and repair of the radial nerve 6 weeks after injury if complete denervation is present
(E) tendon transfers 3 months after injury if no improvement is seen following electromyographic studies

655. While cleaning a barn, a farmer fell and sustained a grade IIIB open fracture of the tibial shaft. The most appropriate initial intravenous antibiotic therapy is

(A) penicillin
(B) a cephalosporin
(C) penicillin and a cephalosporin
(D) a cephalosporin and an aminoglycoside
(E) a cephalosporin, an aminoglycoside, and penicillin

656. While reaming the intramedullary canal during treatment of a fracture of the femoral shaft, the surgeon noticed a nondisplaced fracture of the ipsilateral femoral neck. The most appropriate management would be

(A) intramedullary nailing of the shaft fracture; nonoperative treatment of the neck fracture
(B) intramedullary nailing of the shaft fracture, followed by stabilization of the neck fracture
(C) stabilization of the neck fracture, followed by completion of intramedullary nailing of the shaft fracture
(D) stabilization of the neck fracture, followed by plate osteosynthesis of the shaft fracture
(E) plate osteosynthesis of the shaft fracture, followed by stabilization of the neck fracture

657. The most common thoracic injury following blunt trauma is

(A) myocardial contusion
(B) pulmonary contusion
(C) pneumothorax
(D) aortic arch rupture
(E) rib fracture

658. A 21-year-old man sustained a grade IIIB open tibial fracture in a motorcycle accident. After debridement and skeletal stabilization, the patient had a 5 × 5 cm soft-tissue defect that left the anteromedial surface of the proximal tibia exposed. The most appropriate treatment of the soft-tissue defect is a

(A) medial gastrocnemius muscle flap
(B) lateral gastrocnemius muscle flap
(C) soleus muscle flap
(D) free latissimus dorsi muscle flap
(E) skin graft after the granulation tissue matures

659. A 38-year-old woman who sustained a fracture of the mid humerus 6 months ago had a painful, hypertrophic nonunion with 23° of lateral angulation. The most appropriate treatment is

(A) application of an above-elbow cast
(B) application of an above-elbow cast and electrical stimulation
(C) application of a polypropylene splint with collar and cuff
(D) open reduction, bone grafting, and plate osteosynthesis
(E) open reduction, bone grafting, and intramedullary nailing

660. A polytraumatized patient, whose injuries included an L1 burst fracture, underwent an uncomplicated, closed nailing of a fracture of the tibial shaft. Six hours following the procedure the anterior compartment of the leg felt tense. The patient was comfortable and had no change in his neurologic status and no pain with passive plantar flexion of the great toe. The most appropriate management is to

(A) elevate the extremity and reexamine in 2 h
(B) order arteriography
(C) measure the anterior compartment pressure
(D) measure the pressure in all four compartments of the leg
(E) perform immediate fasciotomy of all four compartments

661. A 32-year-old woman sustained a closed Lisfranc (tarsometatarsal) fracture-dislocation. After closed reduction, a 5-mm offset remains at the first metatarsocuneiform joint. The most appropriate treatment is

(A) application of a below-knee, non-weight-bearing cast
(B) application of a below-knee walking cast
(C) application of a bulky dressing and early motion
(D) percutaneous pinning in situ
(E) open reduction and internal fixation

662. A 17-year-old inadvertently stepped into a hole, forcing his ankle into dorsiflexion and inversion. The ankle ligament most likely damaged is the

(A) anterior talofibular
(B) posterior talofibular
(C) posterior tibiofibular
(D) calcaneofibular
(E) deltoid

663. A posterior dislocation of the shoulder is most commonly associated with a fracture of the

(A) surgical neck of the humerus
(B) greater tuberosity
(C) lesser tuberosity
(D) neck of the scapula
(E) clavicle

664. A displaced fracture of the greater tuberosity of the humerus is most likely to block which of the following shoulder motions?

(A) Forward elevation
(B) Flexion
(C) Extension
(D) Internal rotation
(E) External rotation

665. A 20-year-old college student involved in a motor vehicle accident sustained a closed head injury, fractures of multiple ribs, and bilateral, closed fractures of the femoral shafts. The most appropriate management of the femoral fractures is

(A) immediate fixation of both femoral fractures with Ender's nails
(B) immediate fixation of both femoral fractures with unreamed, interlocked femoral nails
(C) immediate fixation of both femoral fractures with reamed, interlocked femoral nails
(D) delayed fixation of both femoral fractures with unreamed, interlocked femoral nails
(E) delayed fixation of both femoral fractures with reamed, interlocked femoral nails

666. A 25-year-old man sustained a grade IIIB open tibial fracture in an automobile accident. Management consisted of debridement, administration of intravenous antibiotics, and fracture stabilization. Five days later, the patient had a clean 6×6 cm wound over the anteromedial surface of the distal third of the tibia with exposed bone. The most appropriate treatment for the soft-tissue defect is a

(A) split thickness skin graft
(B) medial gastrocnemius muscle flap
(C) soleus muscle flap
(D) flexor hallucis longus muscle flap
(E) free muscle flap

667. A 15-year-old boy involved in a motorcycle accident sustained closed head trauma, blunt abdominal trauma, and a closed, transverse fracture of the femoral shaft. The most appropriate treatment of the femoral fracture would consist of

(A) immediate application of a spica cast
(B) skeletal traction for 3 weeks, followed by a spica cast
(C) skeletal traction for 6 weeks, followed by a cast brace
(D) open reduction and internal fixation with a plate and screws
(E) closed reduction and intramedullary nail fixation

668. A 30-year-old laborer had complete loss of the skin and extensor tendons over the dorsum of his hand from the wrist to the metacarpophalangeal joints after his hand was caught in a piece of factory machinery. Following debridement, the dorsal periosteum of all four metacarpals was exposed. The most appropriate soft-tissue coverage would be a

(A) split thickness skin graft
(B) full thickness skin graft
(C) local rotation skin flap
(D) local muscle flap
(E) pedicle groin flap

669. The best modality for evaluating the congruity of the posterior facet of the subtalar joint in a patient with a calcaneal fracture is

(A) an axial radiograph of the heel
(B) a Broden's radiograph
(C) a lateral radiograph of the foot
(D) a CT scan
(E) an MRI scan

670. Excessive tightening of transiliac bars used for posterior fixation of a pelvic fracture is most likely to result in

(A) loosening of the anterior pelvic plate and screws
(B) injury to a lumbosacral nerve root
(C) inequality of leg-lengths
(D) further damage to the gluteal musculature
(E) a greater likelihood of failure of posterior pelvic fixation

671. A 34-year-old man fell 30 feet from a roof. Immediate postinjury radiographs of the lumbar spine and an axial CT scan of the area of injury are shown below. The patient is neurologically intact. The most appropriate management of this injury is

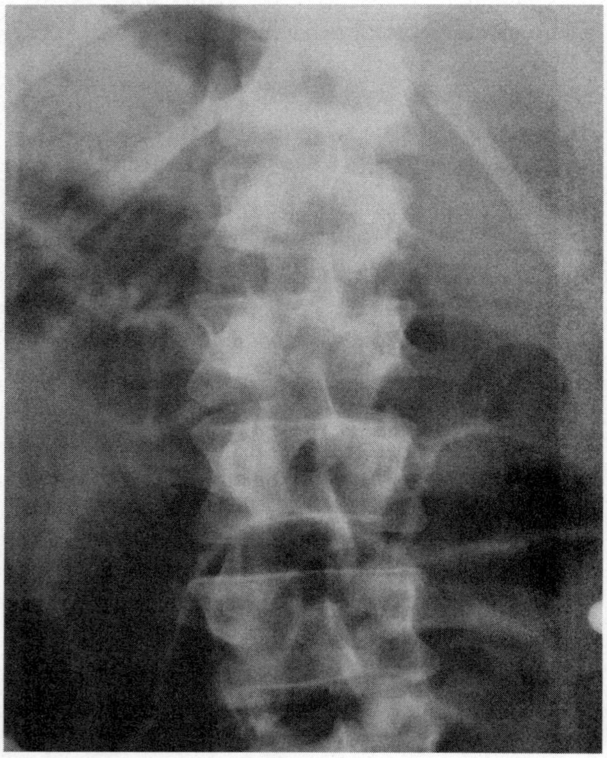

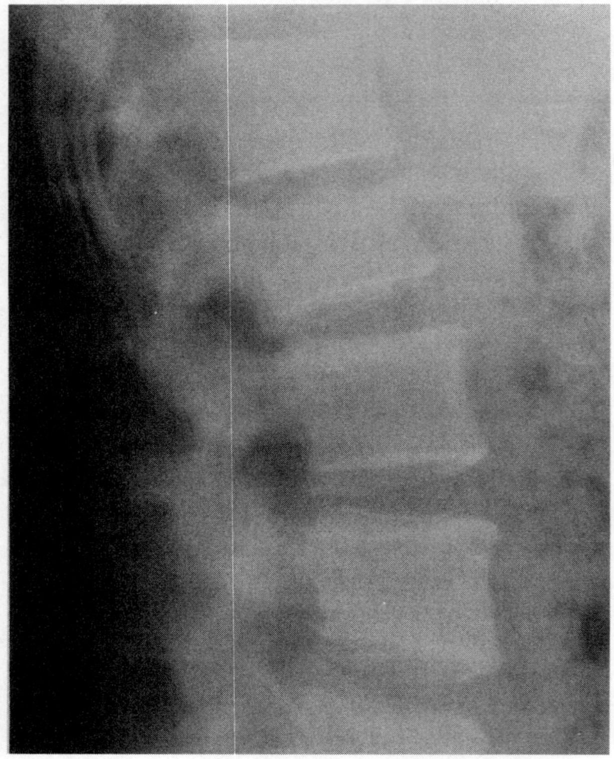

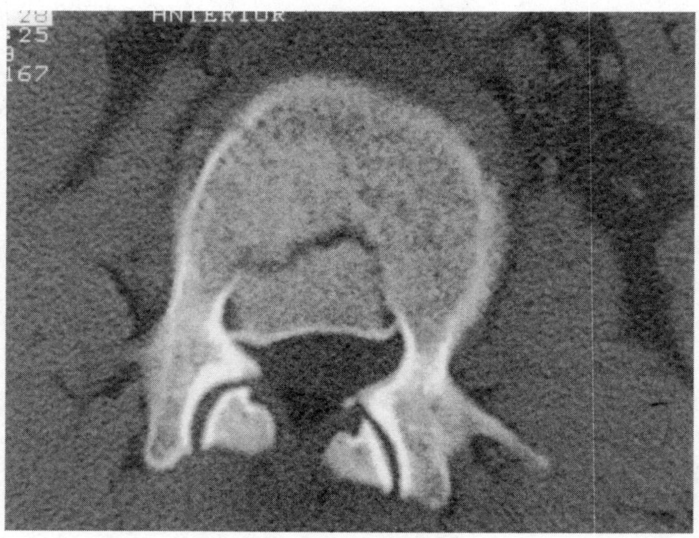

(A) bed rest for 6 weeks and application of a thoracolumbar orthosis
(B) decompressive laminectomy
(C) indirect reduction and posterior instrumentation
(D) anterior decompression and instrumentation
(E) anterior decompression and anterior and posterior instrumentation

672. A 42-year-old mason fell from a scaffolding and sustained the injury in the figure. Upon arrival in the emergency room, his blood pressure was 90/60 mmHg. After administration of a 2-L bolus of Ringer's lactate solution, his blood pressure remained 90/60, and his pulse was 140. The most appropriate immediate management is

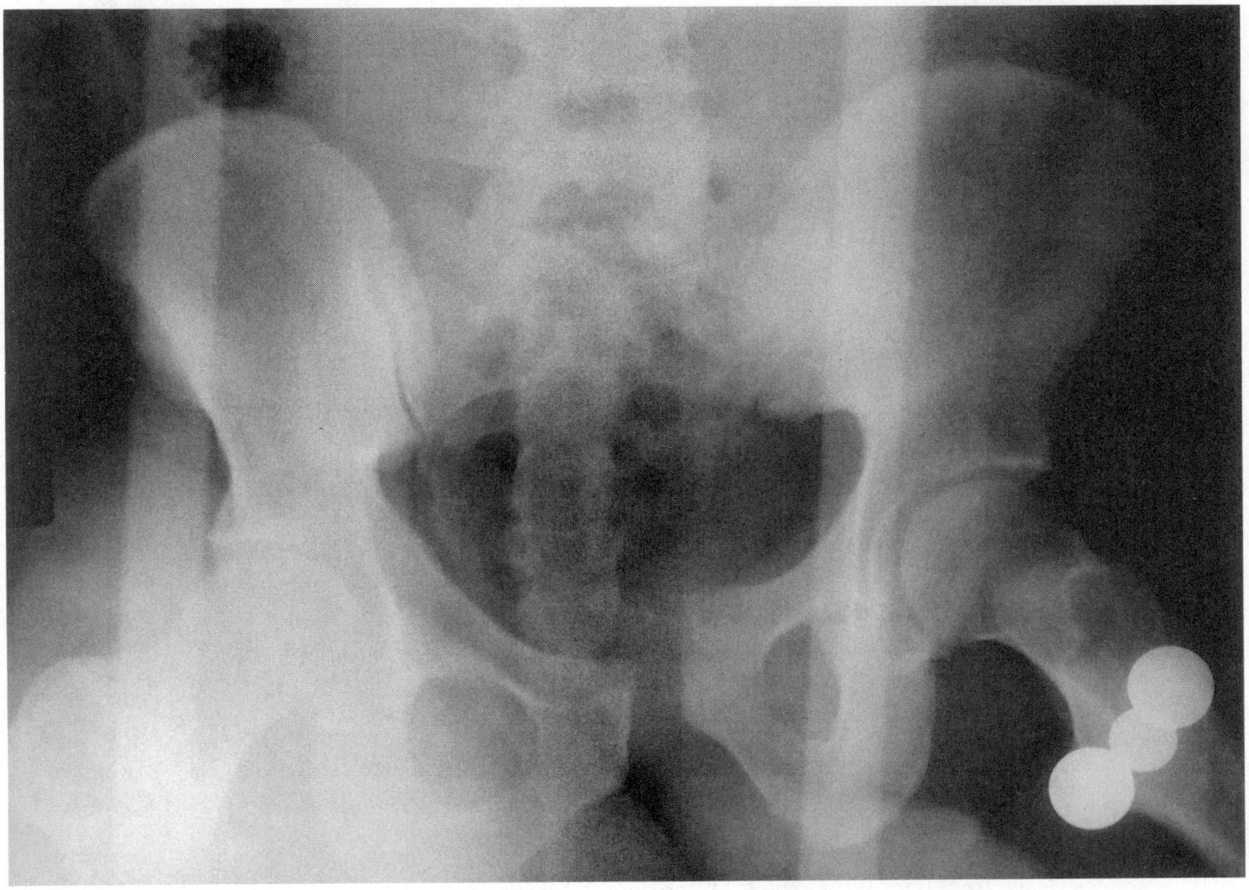

(A) application of MAST trousers
(B) exploratory laparotomy
(C) anterior external skeletal fixation of the pelvis
(D) internal fixation of the anterior and posterior pelvic fractures
(E) application of a pelvic sling

673. A 17-year-old boy sustained the pelvic injury in the figure in a motor vehicle accident. The most appropriate management of the posterior pelvic injury is

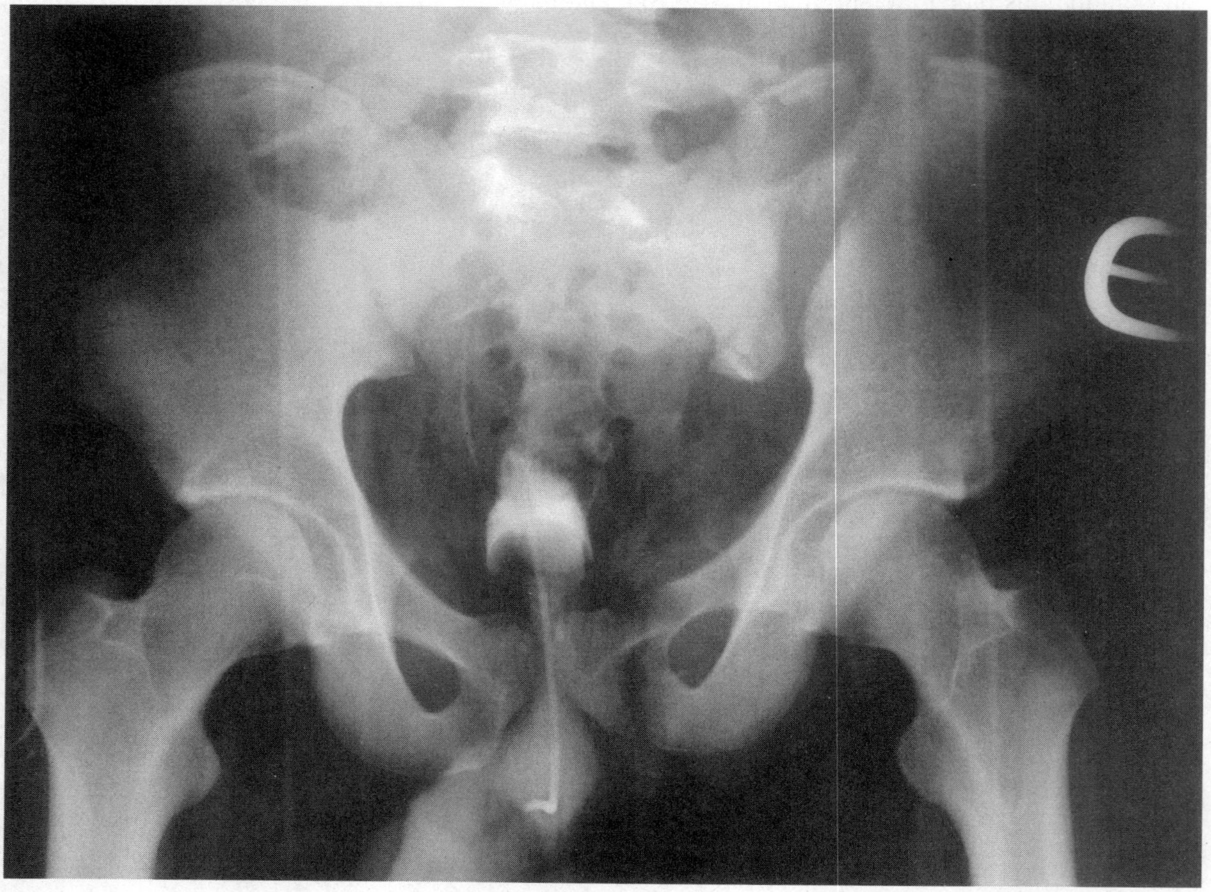

(A) nonoperative treatment with early mobilization
(B) nonoperative treatment with skeletal traction
(C) open reduction and fixation with transilial bars
(D) open reduction and internal fixation with transiliac sacral screws
(E) open reduction and internal fixation with a plate and screws

674. The mechanism by which the injury depicted in the radiographs below occurs is

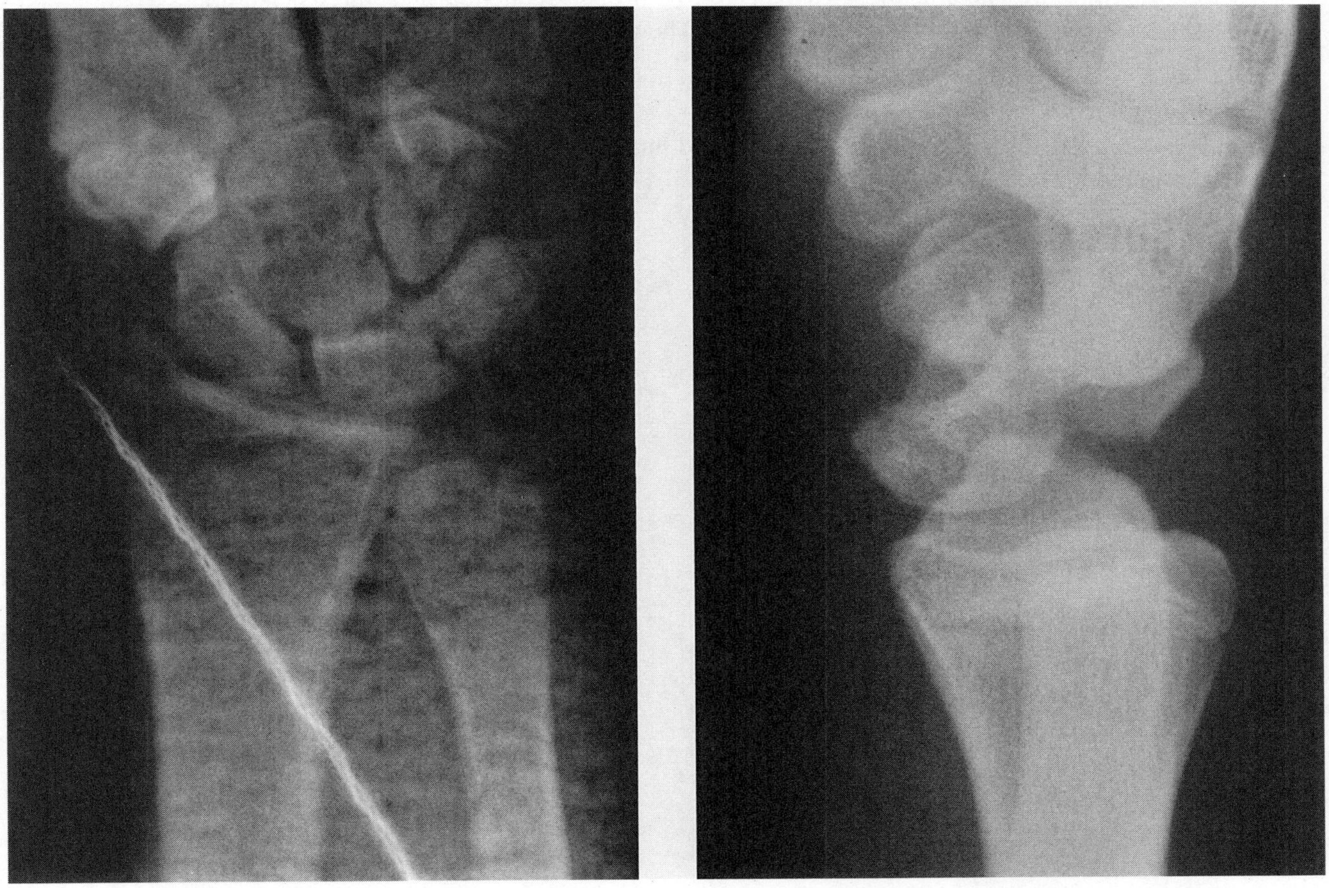

(A) wrist extension
(B) wrist flexion
(C) axial loading with the wrist extended
(D) axial loading with the wrist flexed
(E) forced rotation of the wrist

675. A 27-year-old man involved in a motorcycle accident sustained a severe, closed head injury and the injuries in figures *A* and *B*. The fractures were treated with open reduction and internal fixation. A radiograph 6 months following surgery is shown in figure *C*. The most likely cause of the radiographic result is

(A) excessive periosteal stripping at the time of operation
(B) prolonged postoperative immobilization
(C) excessive delay prior to open reduction and internal fixation
(D) failure to bone graft at the time of operation
(E) the presence of a severe, closed head injury

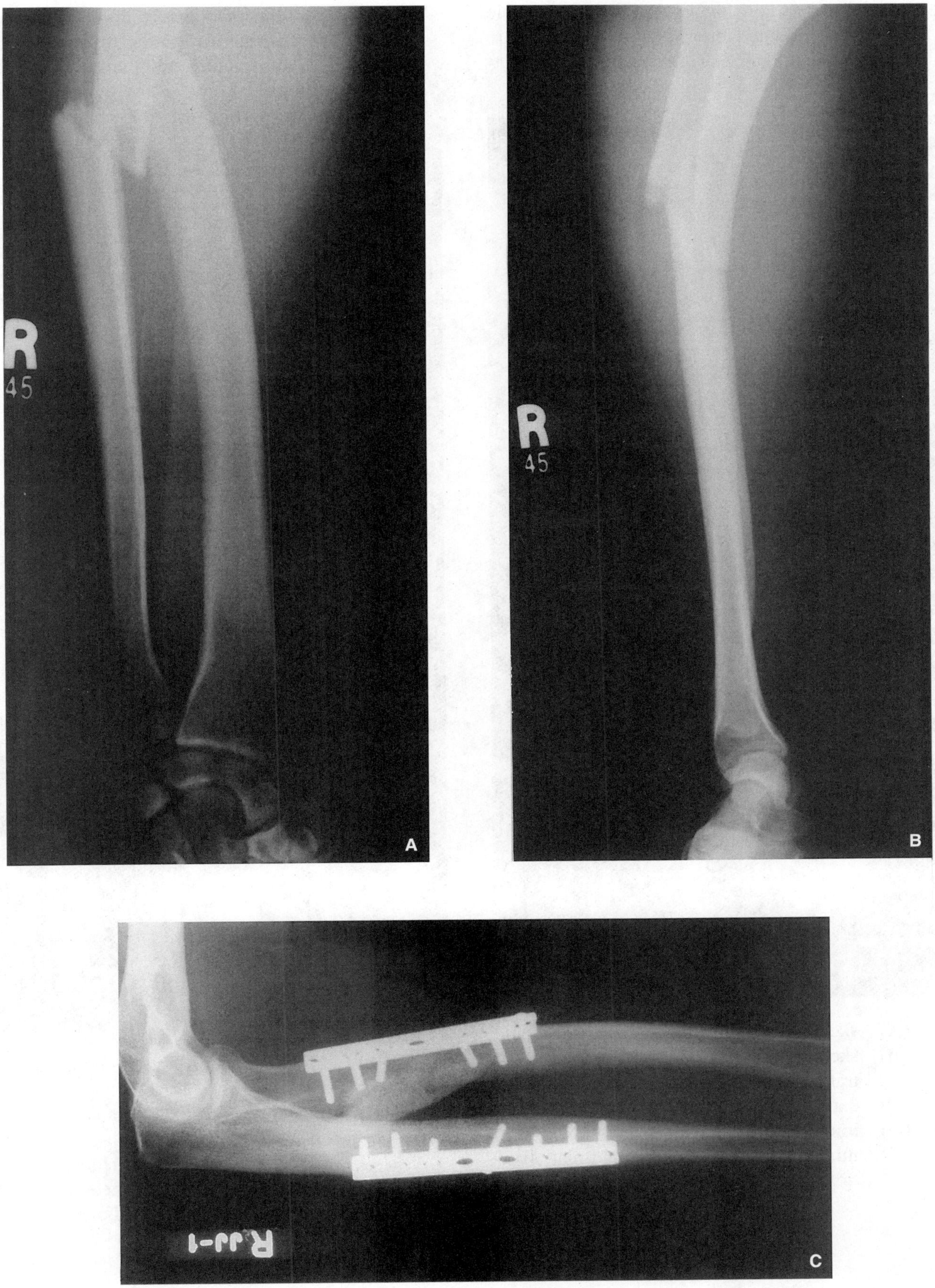
R
45
A
R
45
B
C

676. A 17-year-old girl involved in a motor vehicle accident sustained the grade II open fracture shown in the figure. The most appropriate treatment of this fracture is

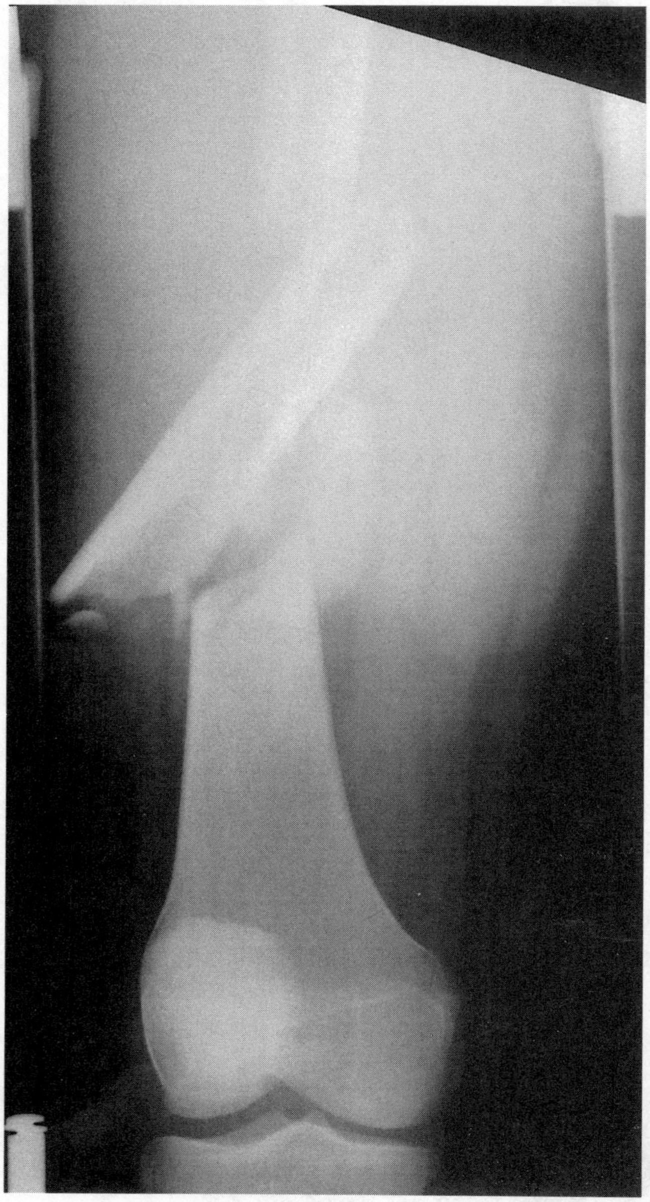

(A) skeletal traction followed by cast bracing
(B) skeletal traction followed by delayed intramedullary nailing
(C) external skeletal fixation
(D) immediate intramedullary nailing
(E) immediate open reduction and plate fixation

677. A 19-year-old man involved in a motorcycle accident sustained a splenic rupture, a closed femoral shaft fracture, and the ipsilateral grade II open injury shown in the figure. The most appropriate management of this injury is

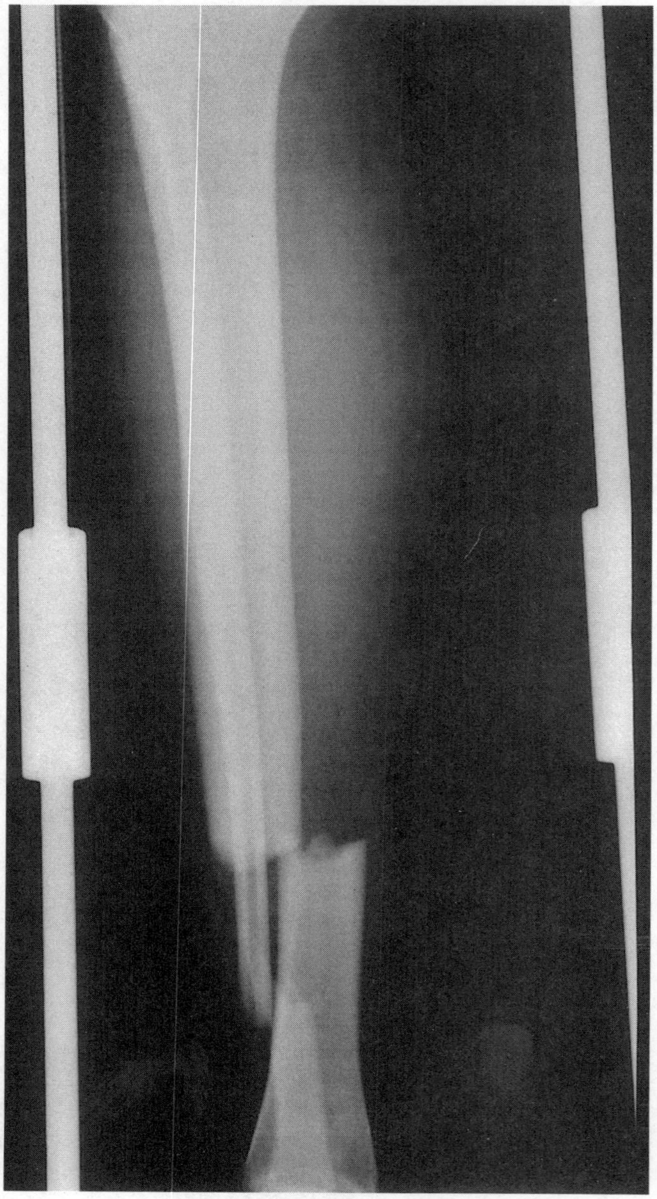

(A) closed reduction and immobilization in plaster
(B) immediate unreamed intramedullary nailing
(C) immediate reamed intramedullary nailing
(D) delayed, unreamed intramedullary nailing
(E) delayed, reamed intramedullary nailing

678. A healthy 50-year-old woman fell 10 feet and sustained the closed fracture depicted below. The most appropriate method of treatment for this fracture is

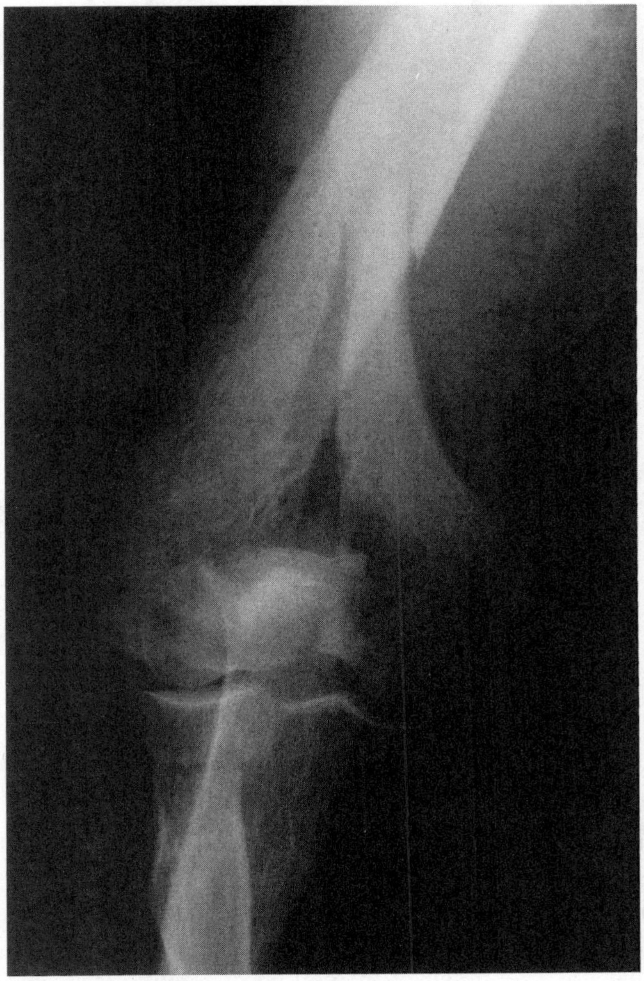

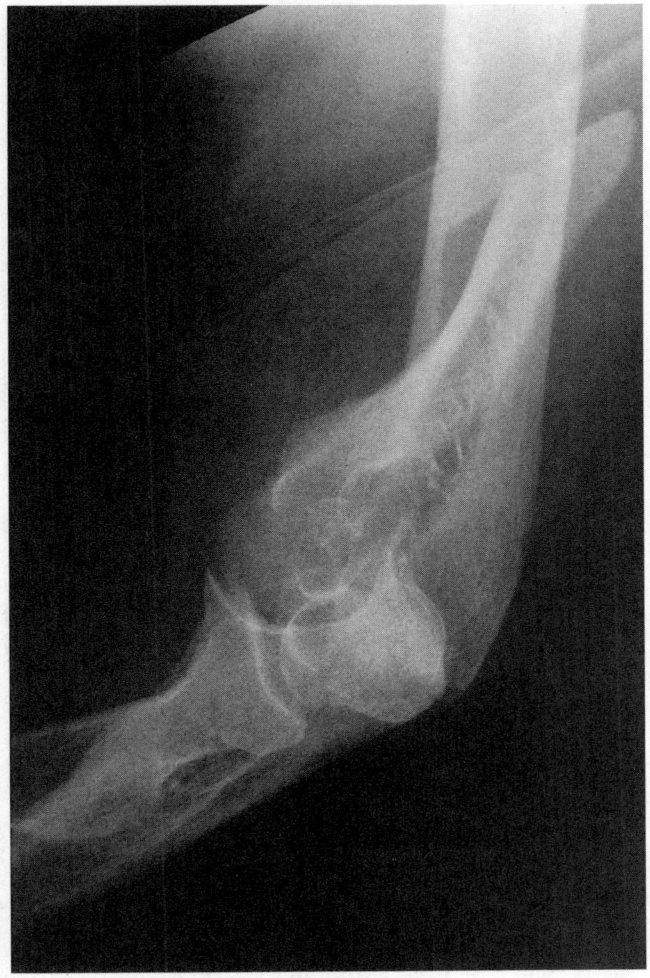

(A) cast immobilization for 8 weeks
(B) protective bracing with early mobilization
(C) closed reduction and percutaneous pin fixation
(D) open reduction and internal fixation of the lateral column
(E) open reduction and internal fixation of medial and lateral columns

679. A 54-year-old woman sustained the ankle injury depicted below. The most appropriate treatment for this injury is

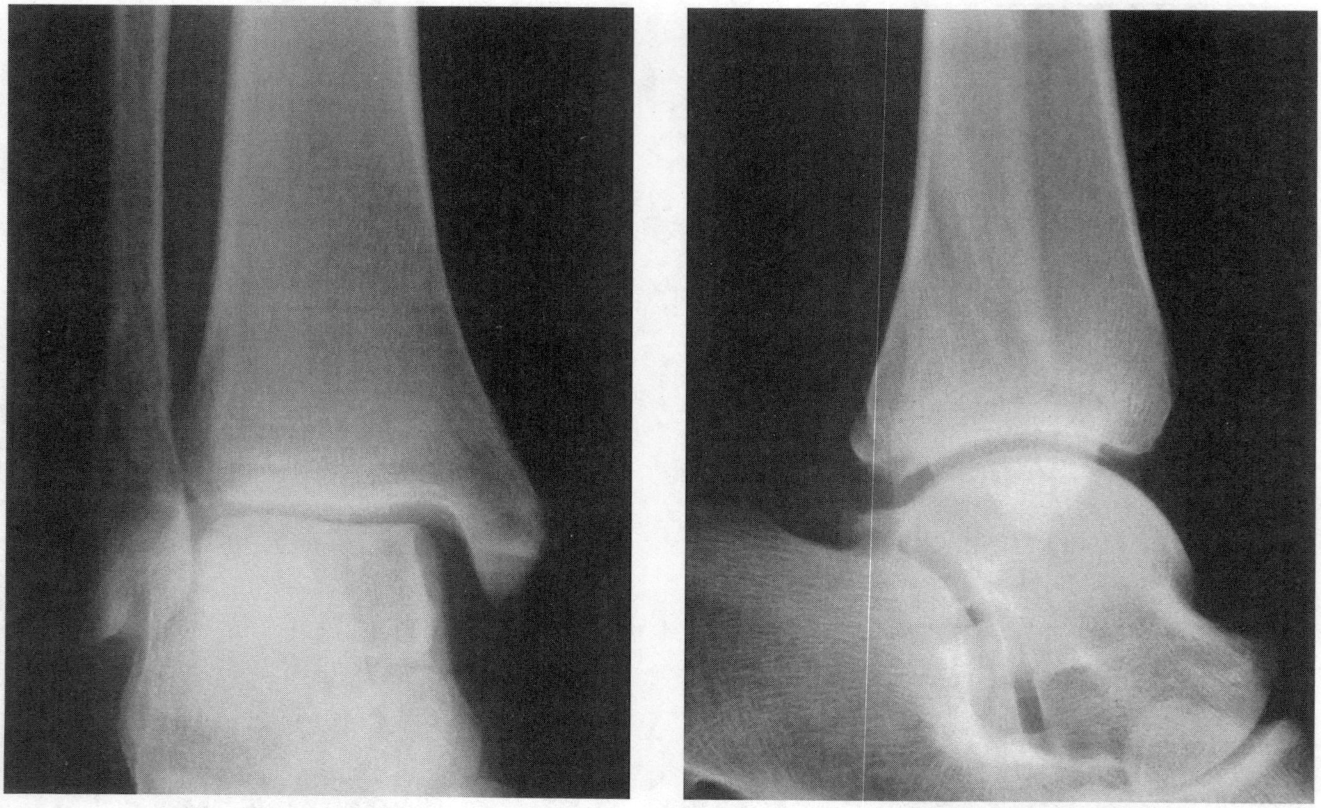

(A) closed reduction and application of a below-knee cast
(B) open reduction and internal fixation of the fibular fracture
(C) open reduction and internal fixation of the fibular fracture; insertion of a transsyndesmotic screw
(D) open reduction and internal fixation of the fibular fracture; repair of the deltoid ligament
(E) open reduction and internal fixation of the fibular fracture; repair of the deltoid ligament; insertion of a transsyndesmotic screw

680. Three weeks after a motor vehicle accident, a 21-year-old woman complained of continued lateral knee pain with ambulation. Radiographs are shown below. The most appropriate treatment is

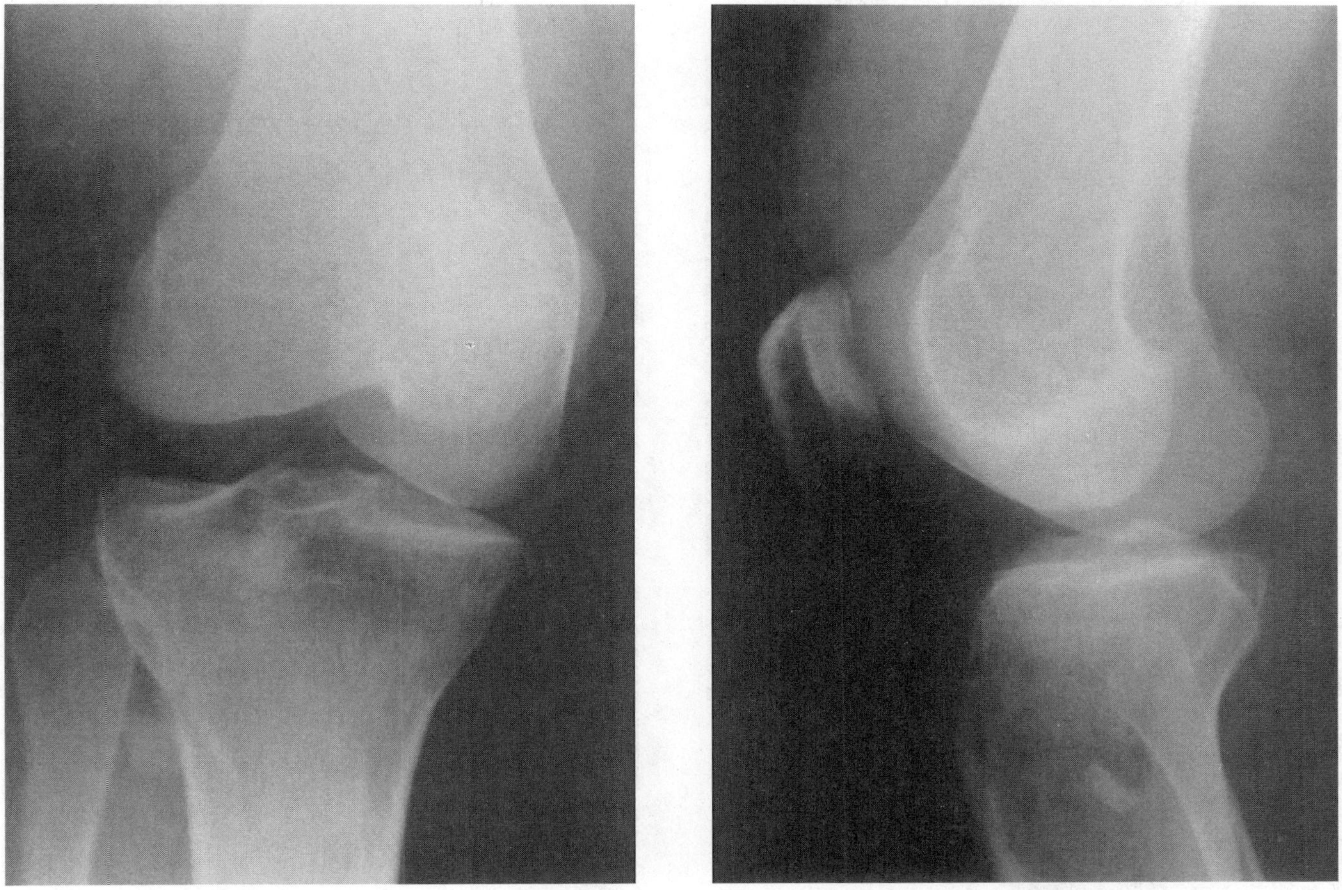

(A) application of an above-knee cast; no weight-bearing
(B) protective bracing; range of motion exercises; no weight-bearing
(C) protective bracing; range of motion exercises; partial weight-bearing
(D) open reduction and internal fixation; no weight-bearing
(E) open reduction and internal fixation; partial weight-bearing

681. A 44-year-old man sustained a severe, closed, distal tibial fracture in a fall. Preoperative (*left*) and immediate postoperative (*right*) radiographs are shown below. The most common complication associated with this method of treatment is

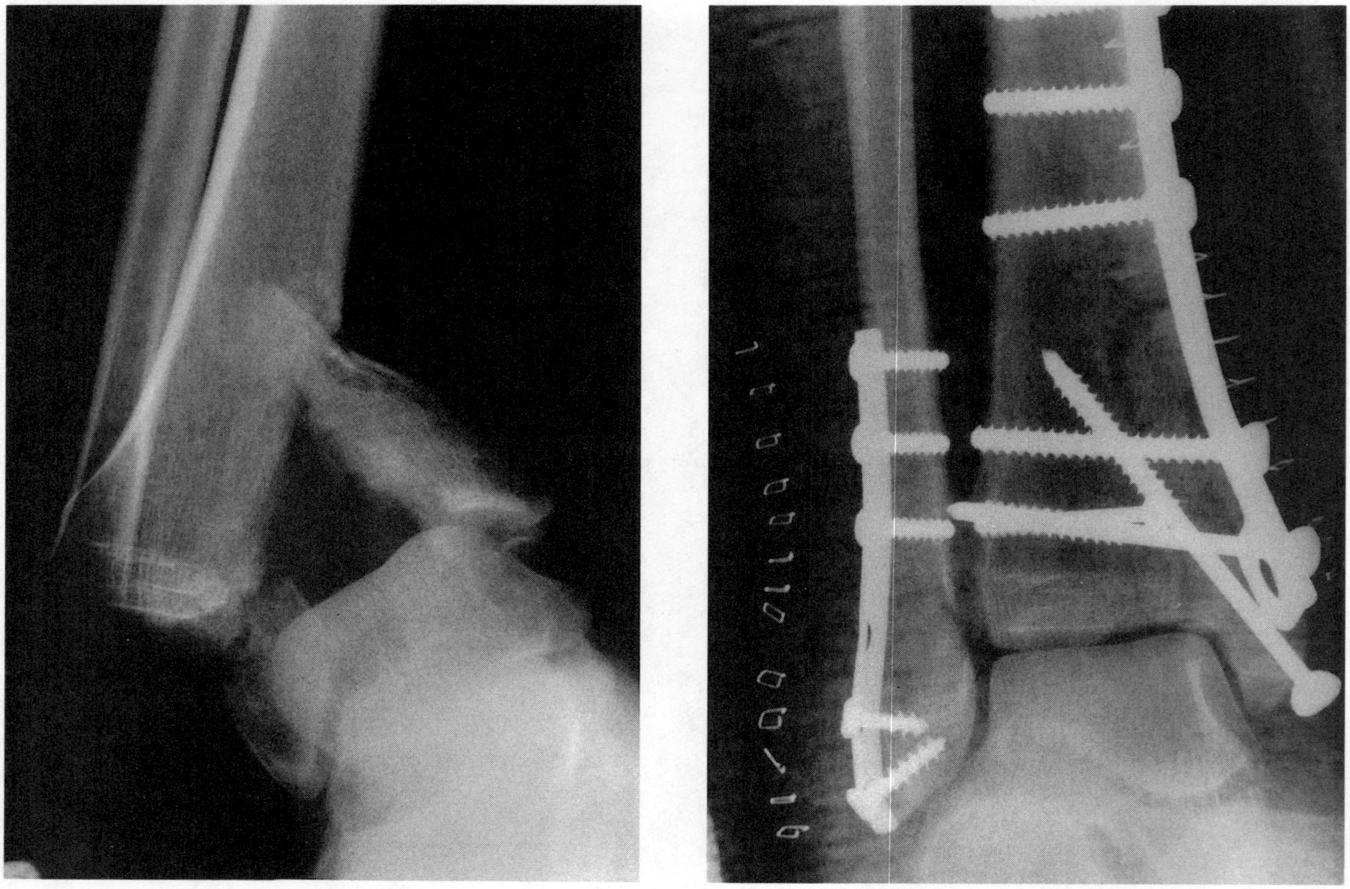

(A) failure of fixation
(B) nonunion
(C) neurologic injury
(D) sloughing of the skin edges
(E) osteomyelitis

682. One month after a fall onto his shoulder, a 35-year-old man had persistent shoulder pain and weakness. Passive external rotation was limited to 5°. Radiographs and a CT scan are shown. The most appropriate treatment is

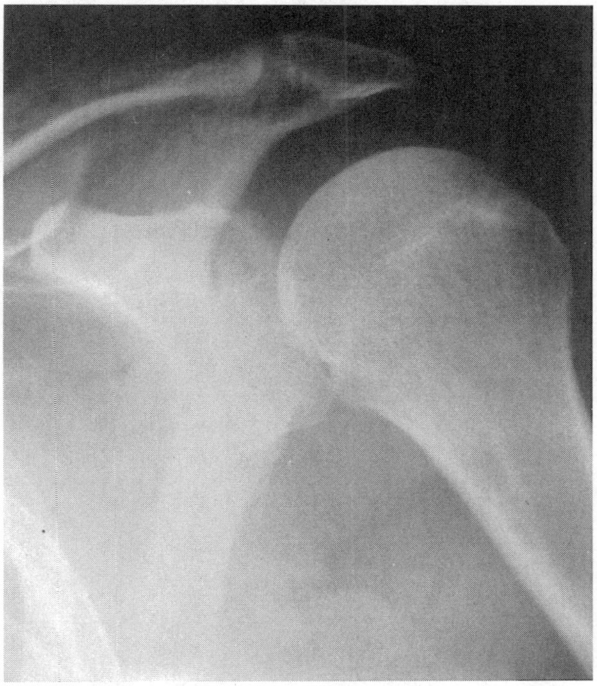

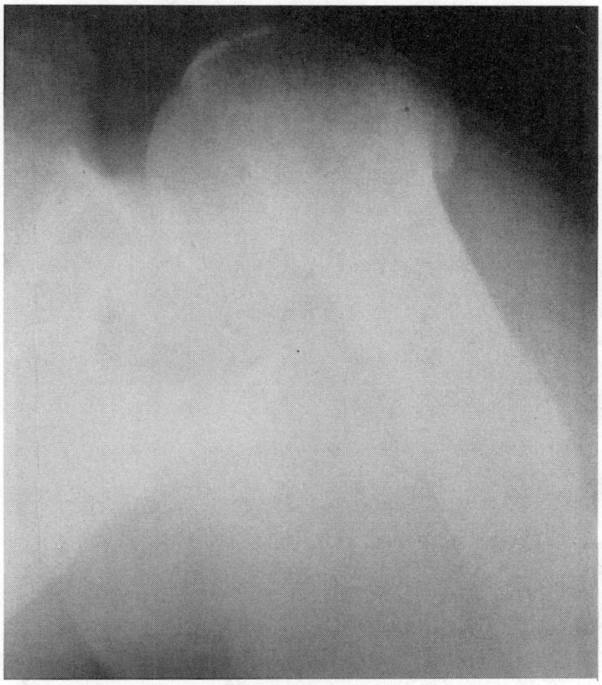

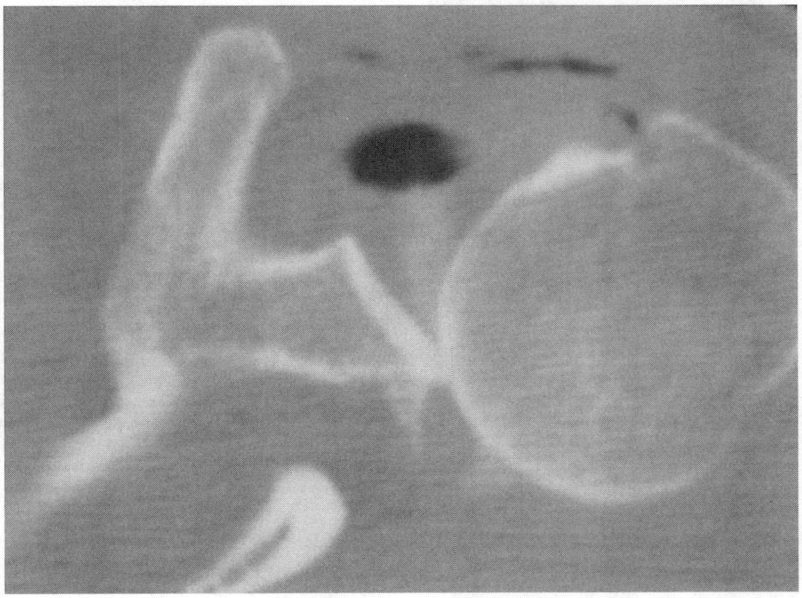

(A) institution of a vigorous physical therapy program
(B) closed reduction; immobilization in external rotation
(C) open reduction through an anterior approach; immobilization in internal rotation
(D) open reduction through an anterior approach; immobilization in external rotation
(E) open reduction through a posterior approach; immobilization in internal rotation

683. A 50-year-old man sustained the injury shown below. The most appropriate method of treatment for this fracture is

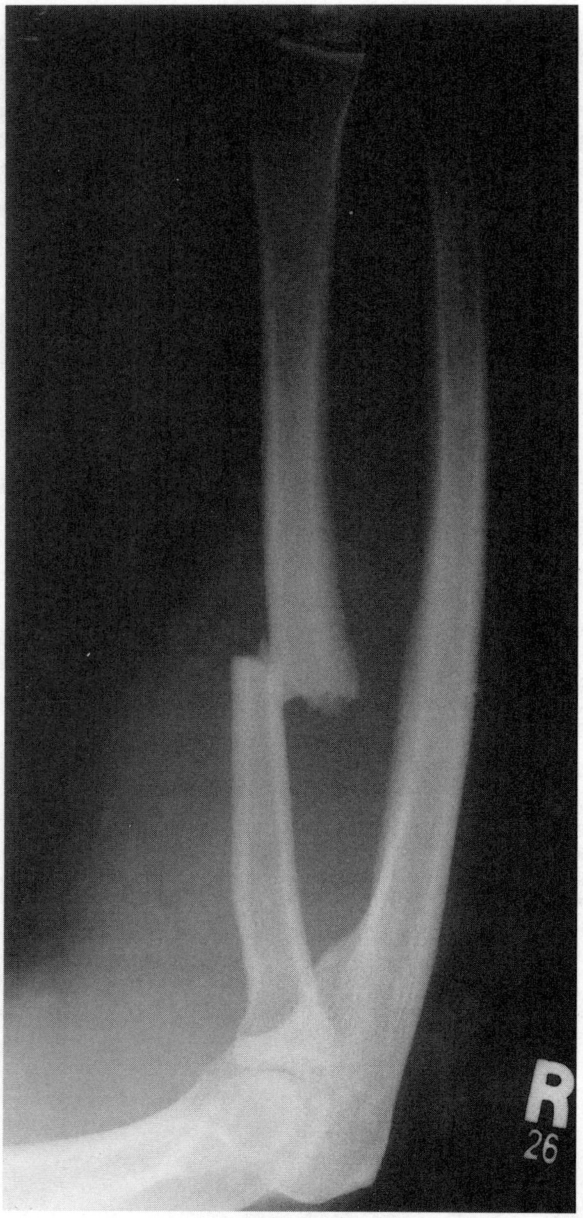

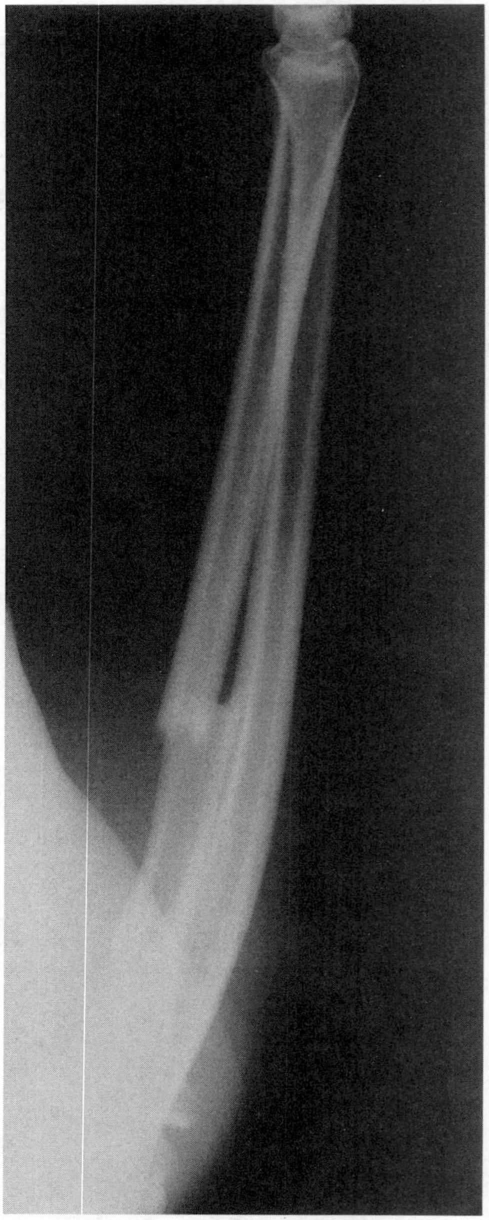

(A) closed reduction; immobilization in supination
(B) closed reduction; immobilization in neutral rotation
(C) open reduction and internal fixation; immobilization in supination
(D) open reduction and internal fixation; immobilization in neutral rotation
(E) open reduction and external skeletal fixation

684. A 55-year-old woman involved in a motor vehicle accident sustained a right calcaneal fracture, a left tibial shaft fracture, a right distal radial fracture, and the fracture of her left humerus shown below. The most appropriate treatment of this fracture is

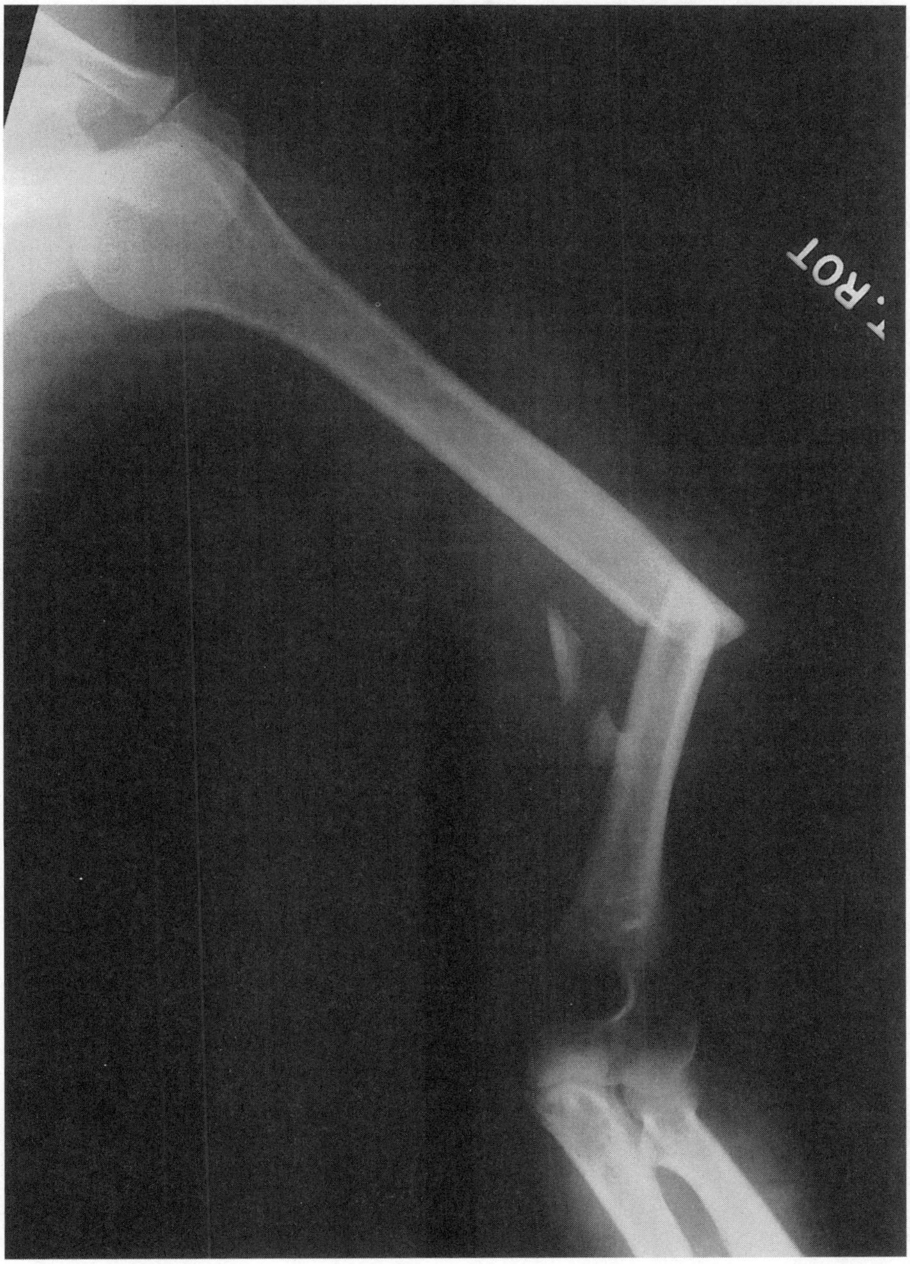

(A) a functional brace
(B) a shoulder spica cast
(C) a hanging-arm cast
(D) external skeletal fixation
(E) plate osteosynthesis

685. A 20-year-old laborer complained of 3 months of pain on the lateral border of his foot with ambulation. The symptoms gradually increased until he was unable to work because of pain. Radiographs are shown on the following page. The most appropriate treatment is

(A) immobilization in a non-weight-bearing cast
(B) immobilization in a walking cast
(C) iliac crest bone grafting
(D) intramedullary screw fixation and bone grafting
(E) intramedullary screw fixation alone

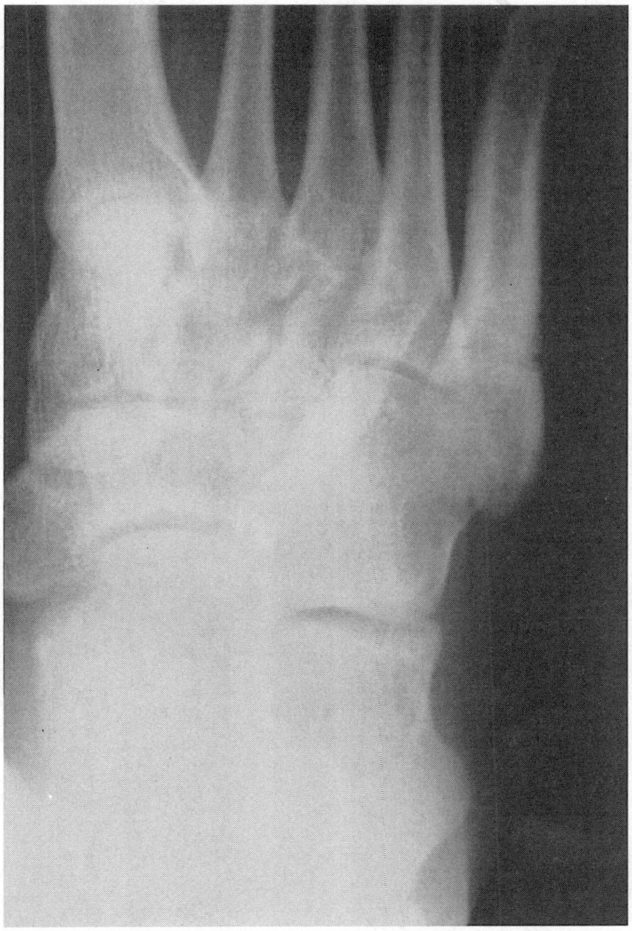

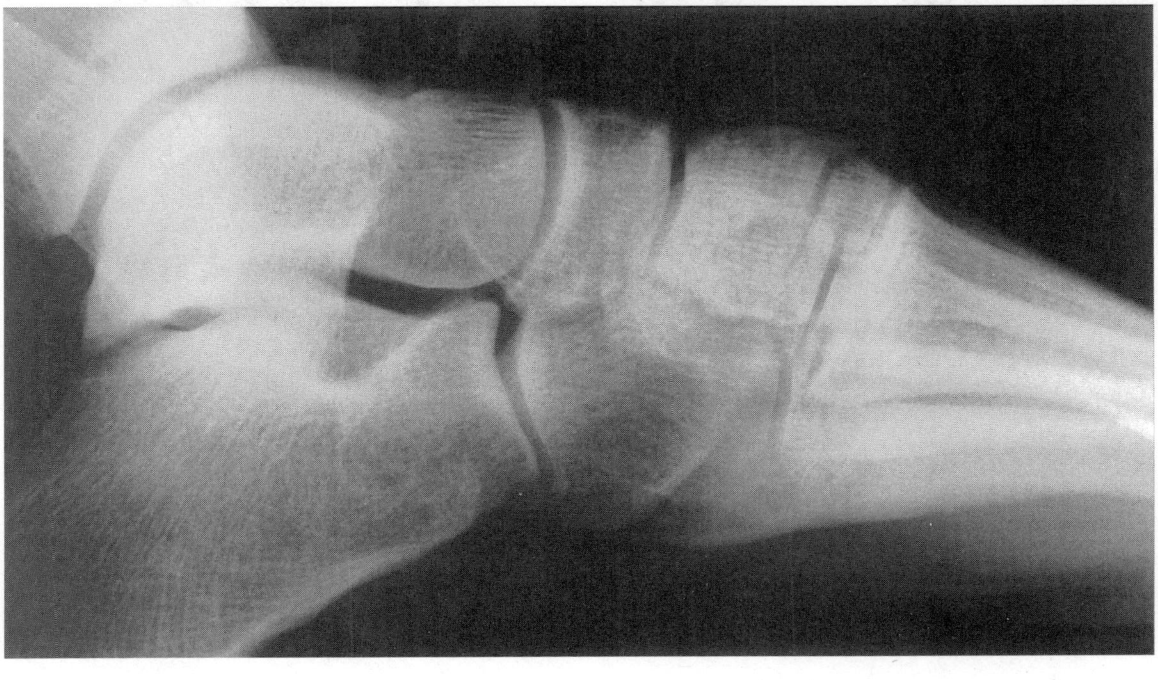

686. The radiographs below were taken 19 days after treatment of an extraarticular distal radial fracture by closed reduction, insertion of percutaneous pins, and casting. The most appropriate treatment at this time is to

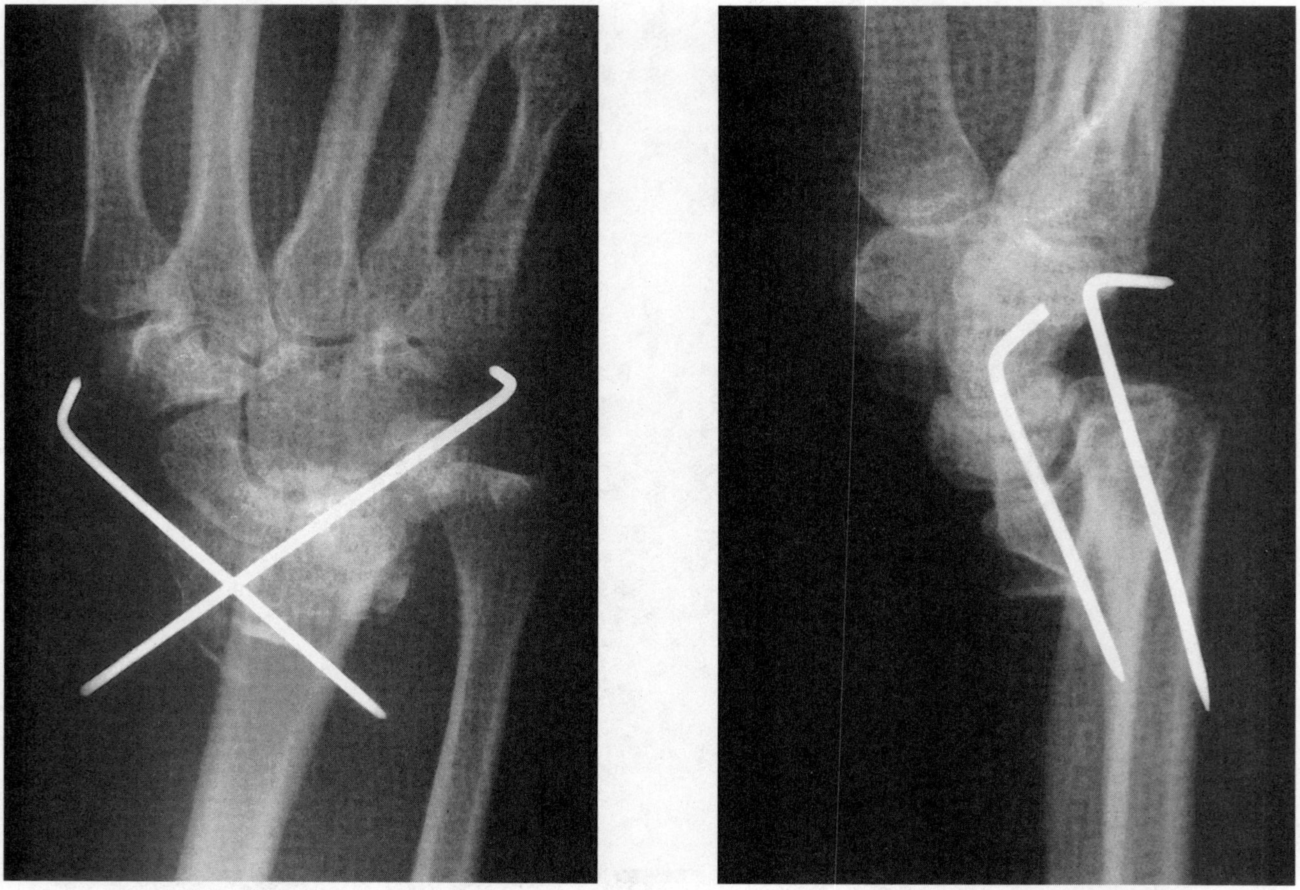

(A) observe the fracture until union occurs
(B) repeat closed reduction and cast immobilization
(C) repeat closed reduction and percutaneous pin fixation
(D) repeat closed reduction and external skeletal fixation
(E) perform open reduction and internal fixation

687. A 21-year-old woman sustained an external rotation injury to her ankle. She had marked swelling over the medial ankle and anterolateral portion of the distal tibia. Radiographs of the ankle are shown below. The next step in the management of this patient is

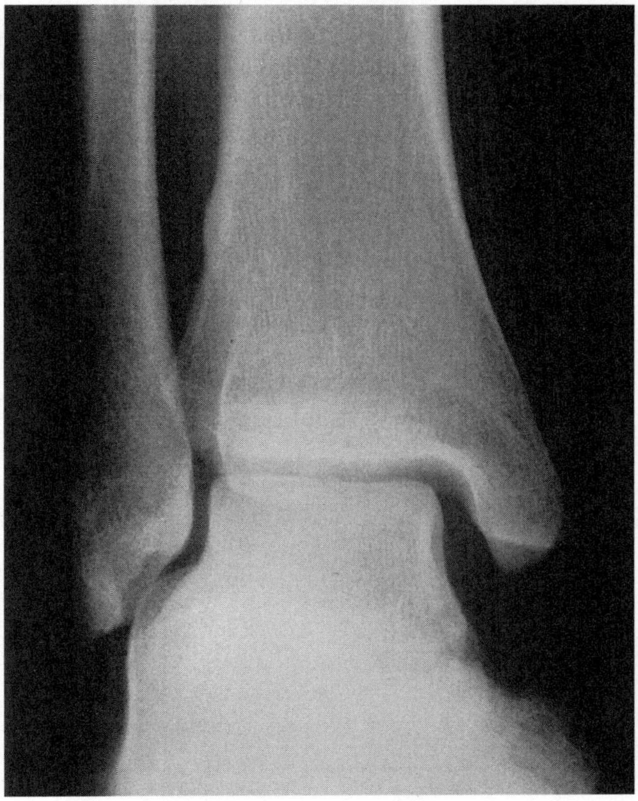

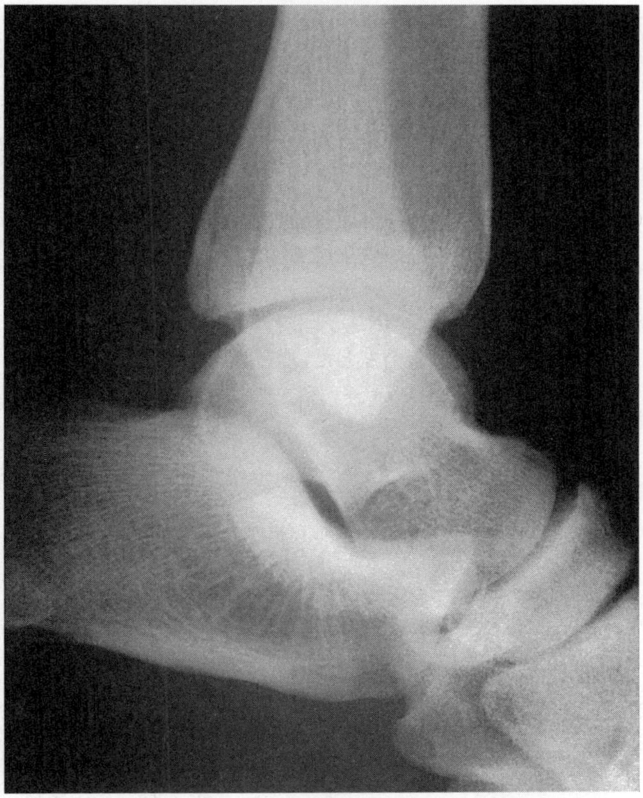

(A) closed reduction and cast immobilization
(B) a CT scan of the distal tibia and fibula
(C) plain radiographs of the proximal fibula
(D) open reduction and internal fixation
(E) application of a below-knee walking cast

688. A 23-year-old woman injured in a motor vehicle accident sustained the injuries shown. The most appropriate treatment is

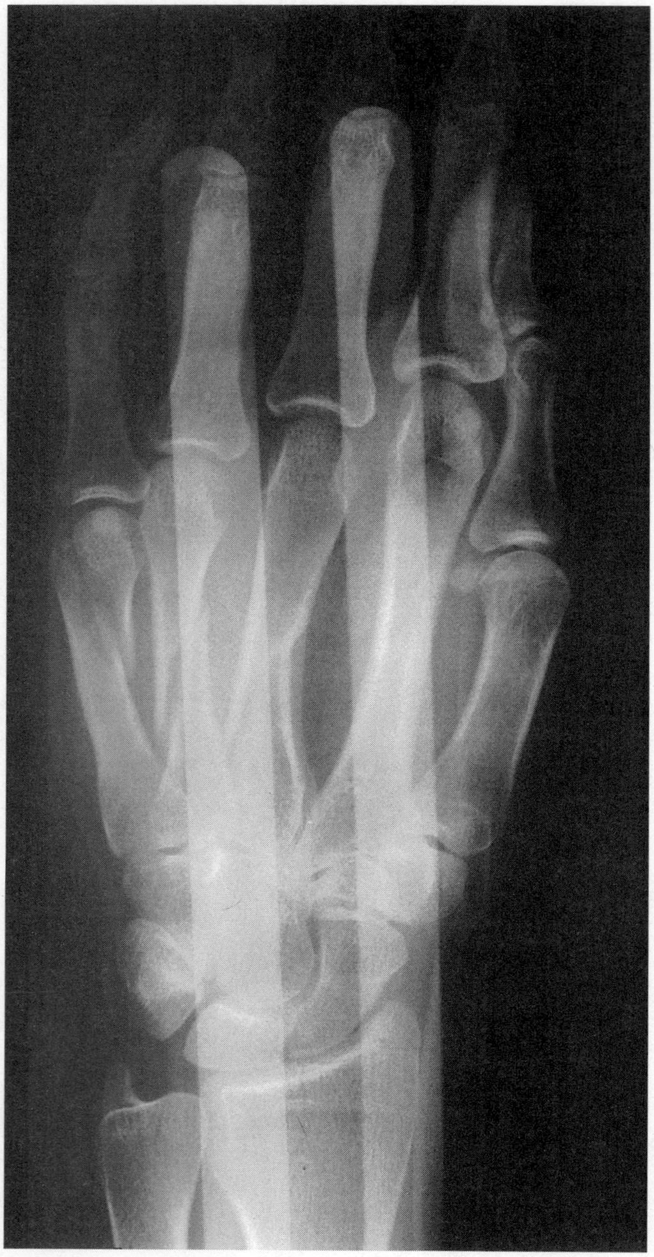

(A) application of a below-elbow cast with the metacarpophalangeal (MCP) joints in full extension
(B) application of a below-elbow cast with the MCP joints flexed 60°
(C) open reduction and internal fixation of the fifth metacarpal only
(D) open reduction and internal fixation of all fractured metacarpals
(E) external skeletal fixation

689. A 70-year-old man fell at home and sustained a displaced fracture of the surgical neck of the humerus. He was taken to the operating room where closed reduction under fluoroscopic guidance was attempted. The fracture was reducible, but redisplaced as soon as traction was released from the arm. The most appropriate management of this fracture is

(A) immobilization in a sling; early motion
(B) immobilization in a shoulder spica cast
(C) closed reduction and percutaneous pinning
(D) open reduction and internal fixation
(E) hemiarthroplasty of the shoulder

690. A 31-year-old woman sustained the injury shown below in a motor vehicle accident. The most appropriate treatment is

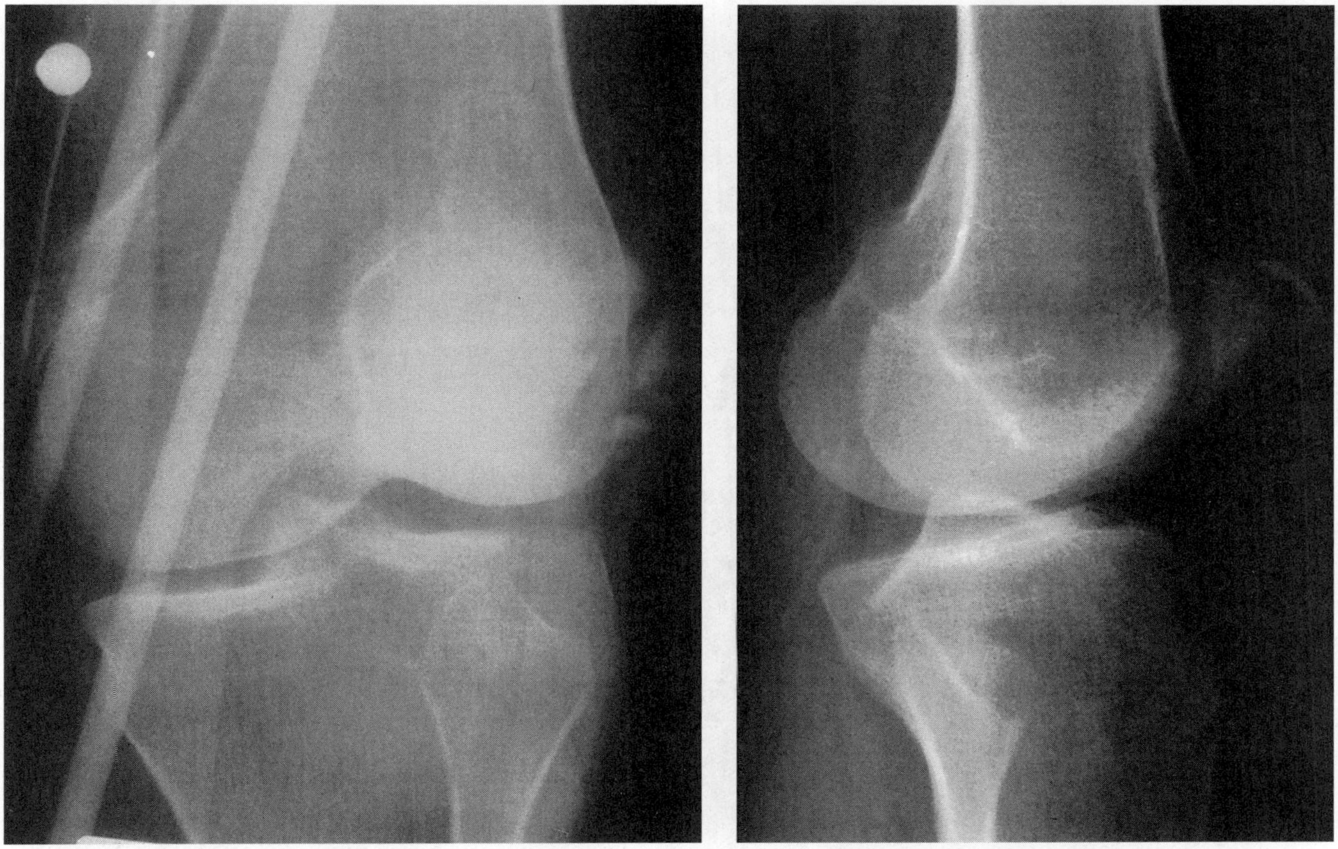

(A) open reduction and internal fixation
(B) excision of the fracture fragments
(C) immobilization in a cylinder cast
(D) application of a hinged knee brace
(E) patellectomy

691. A 35-year-old man involved in a pedestrian versus motor vehicle accident sustained a grade II open tibial shaft fracture and the injury in the figure. The most appropriate sequence for managing this patient's injuries is

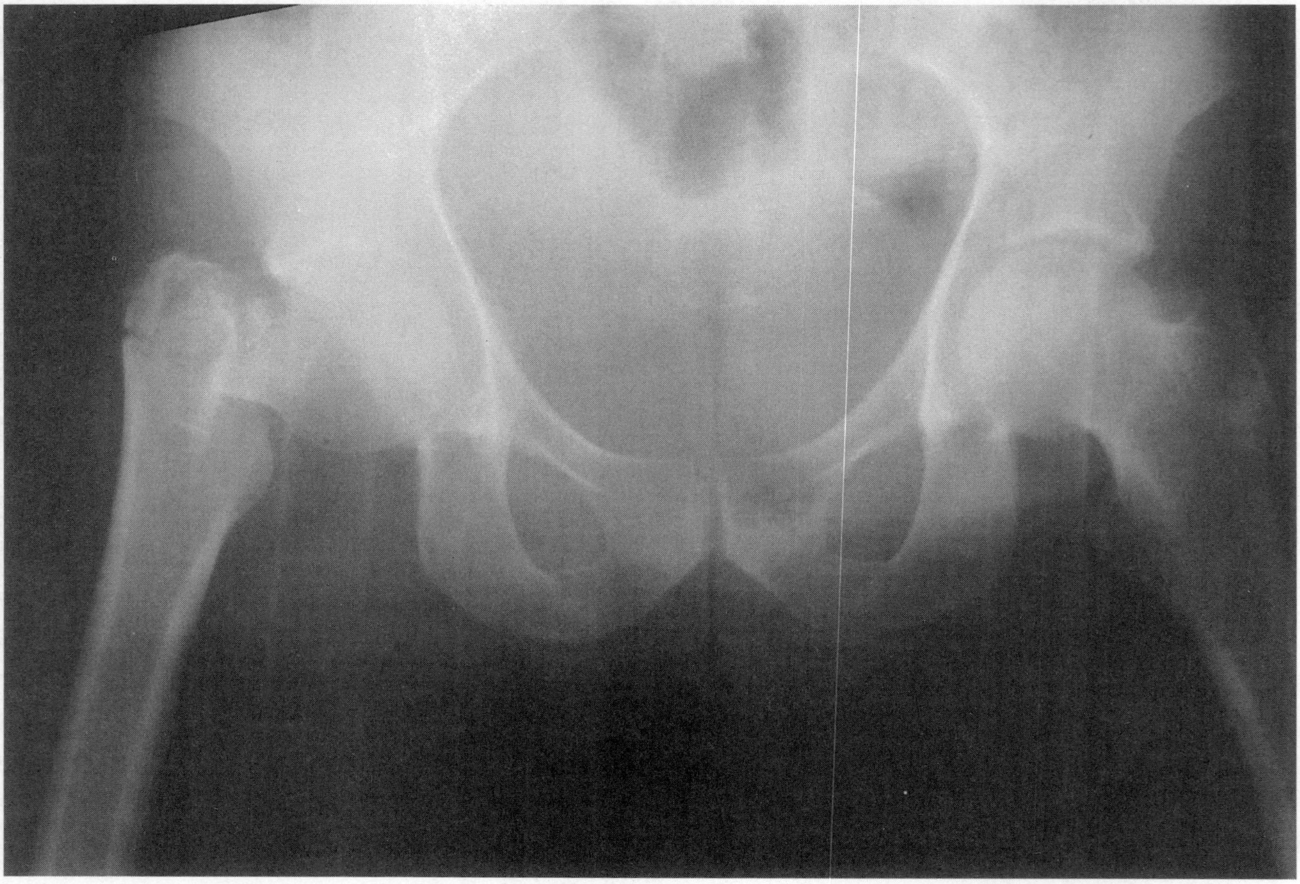

(A) reduction and stabilization of the femoral neck fracture; debridement and irrigation of the tibial fracture; stabilization of the tibial fracture
(B) debridement and irrigation of the tibial fracture; stabilization of the tibial fracture; reduction and stabilization of the femoral neck fracture
(C) debridement and irrigation of the tibial fracture; reduction and stabilization of the femoral neck fracture; stabilization of the tibial fracture
(D) debridement and irrigation of the tibial fracture; reduction and stabilization of the femoral neck fracture; casting of the tibial fracture
(E) debridement and irrigation of the tibial fracture; stabilization of the tibial fracture; bipolar hemiarthroplasty for the femoral neck fracture

692. A 35-year-old male pedestrian struck by a motor vehicle sustained a closed head injury, a splenic rupture, right femoral shaft and femoral neck fractures, and the injury in the figure. After insertion of an intracranial pressure monitor, splenectomy, and stabilization of the femoral neck and shaft fractures, the patient had received 10 units of packed red blood cells. His partial thromboplastin time (PTT) was 45 and his peak inspiratory pressures had slowly increased to 45 mmHg. The most appropriate management of the tibial fracture is

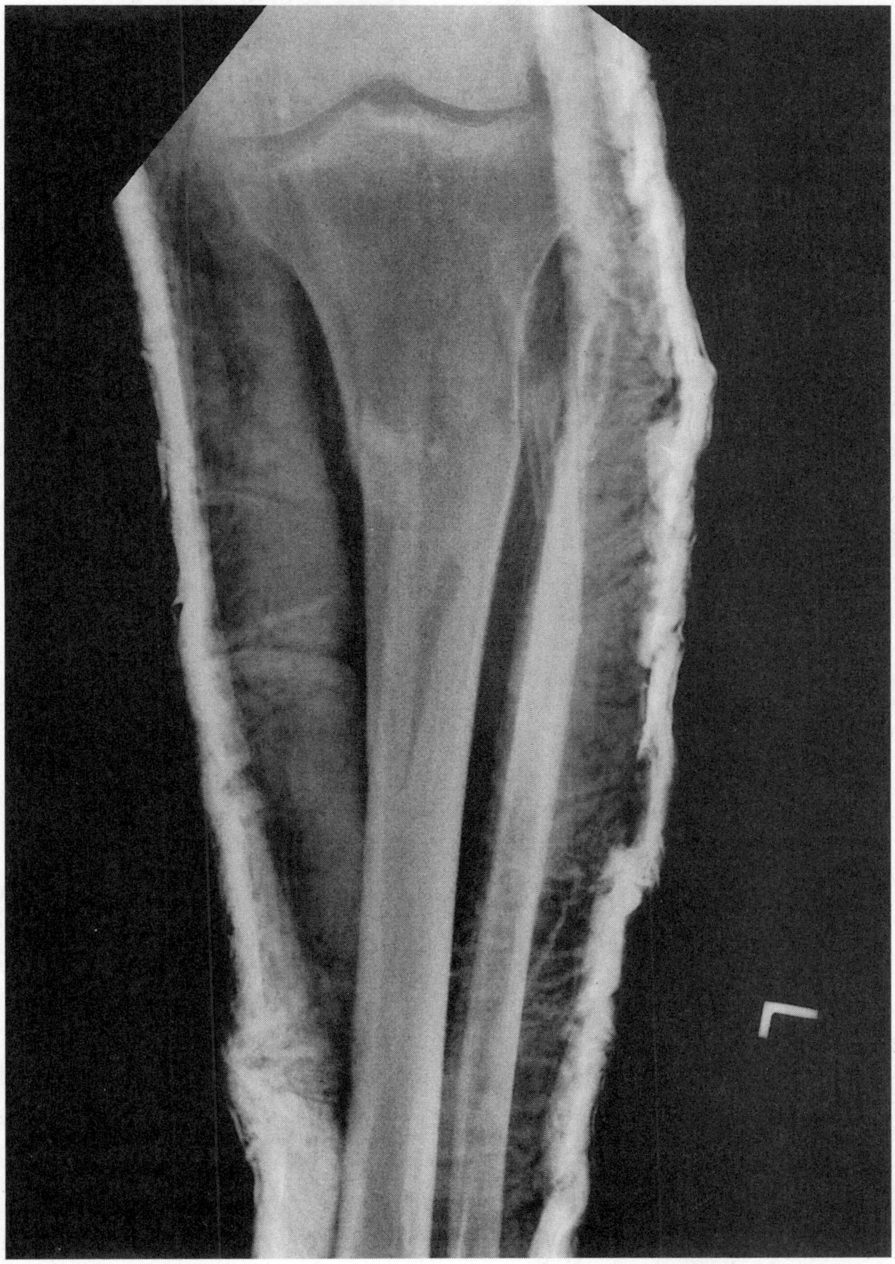

(A) application of an above-knee cast
(B) application of a knee immobilizer
(C) external skeletal fixation
(D) reamed intramedullary nailing
(E) open reduction and plate fixation

693. Twelve weeks following open reduction and internal fixation of a tibial plafond fracture, the radiograph below was obtained. The patient had been in a non-weight-bearing cast since the operation. The surgical incisions are clean and there is no edema or erythema. The optimal treatment is

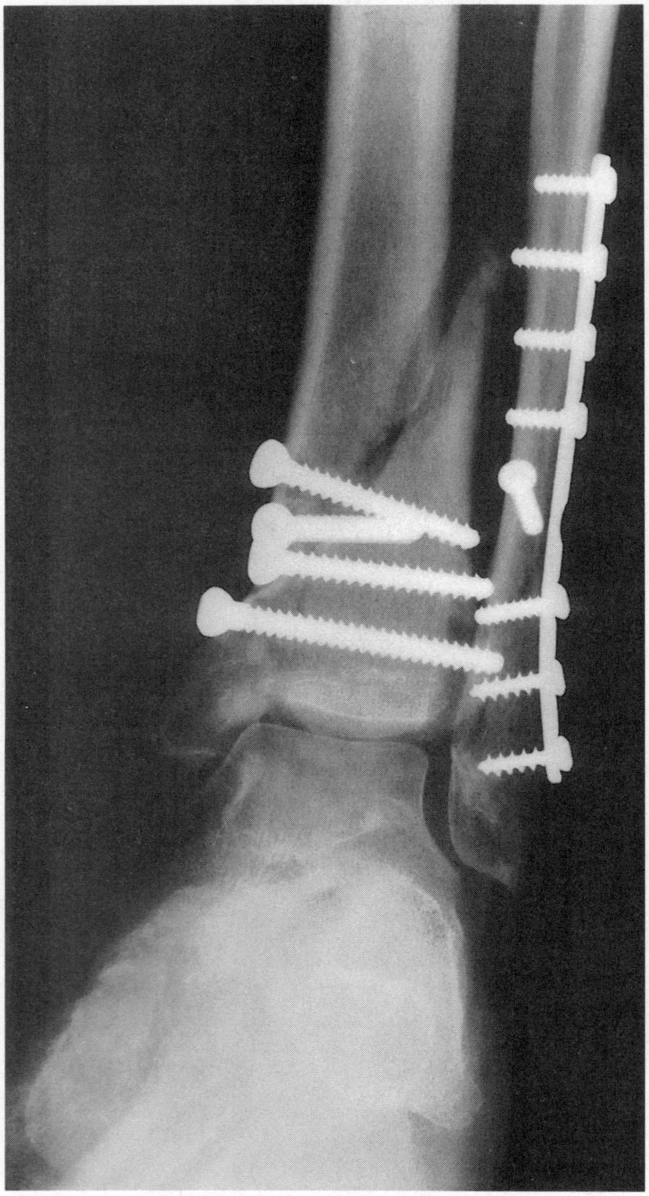

(A) continued immobilization in a non-weight-bearing cast
(B) application of a walking cast
(C) iliac crest bone grafting
(D) removal of hardware, bone grafting, and internal fixation
(E) arthrodesis of the ankle

694. A 45-year-old man sustained the injury in the figure. All the following statements about this patient are true EXCEPT

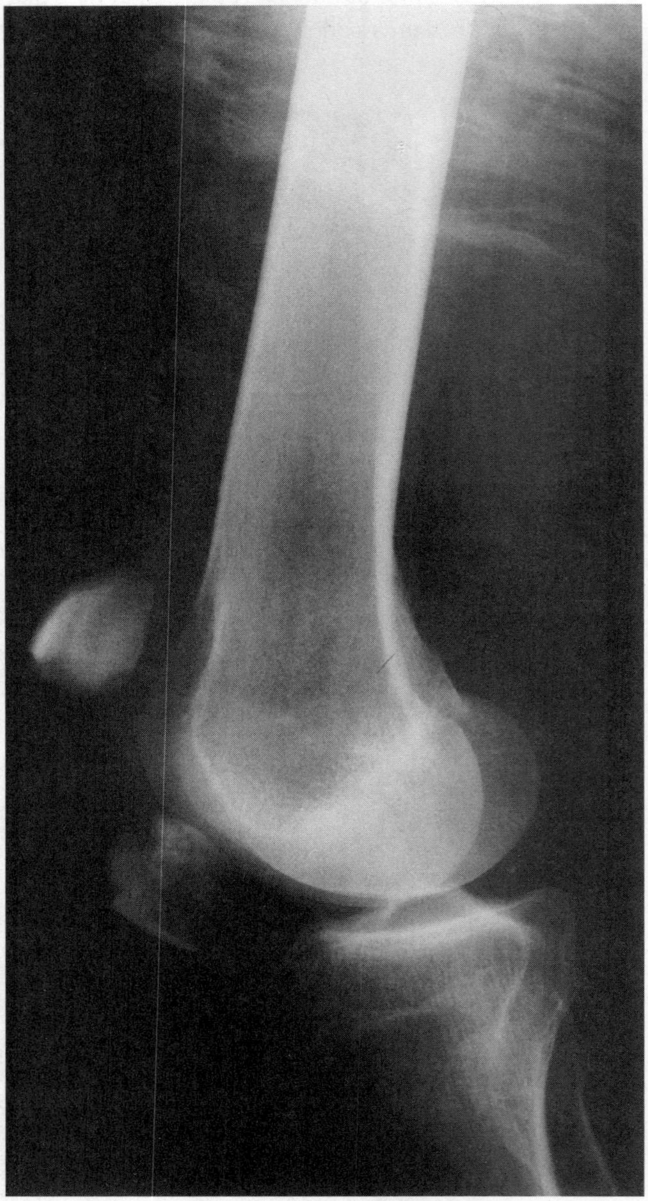

(A) the patella failed in tension
(B) a large hemarthrosis is present
(C) operative intervention is indicated
(D) passive knee extension will be limited
(E) the medial and lateral extensor retinacula are torn

695. An 82-year-old man fell at home and sustained the injury below. He lived alone and was an independent community ambulator with the aid of a cane. The most appropriate management is

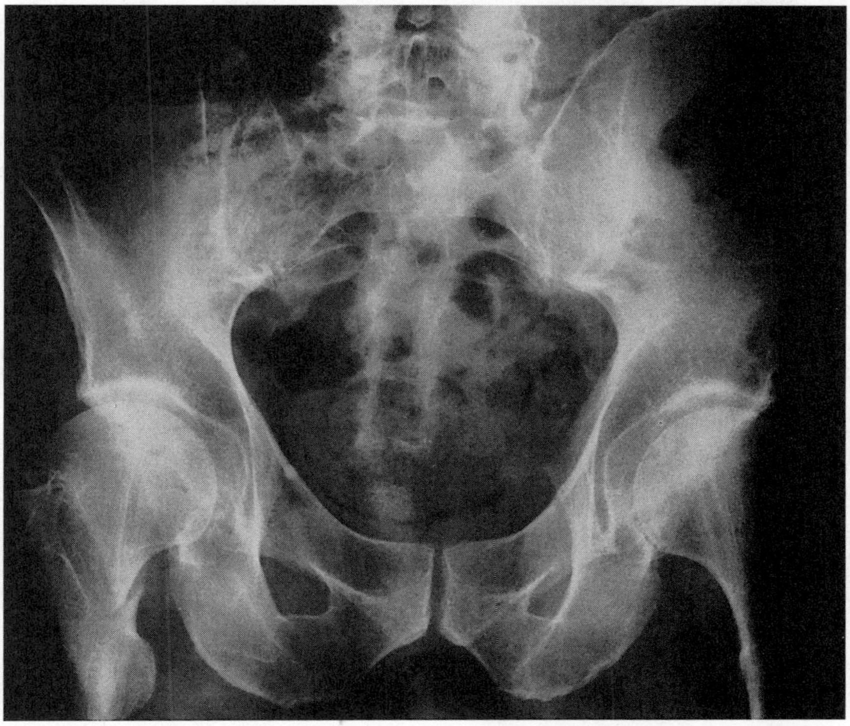

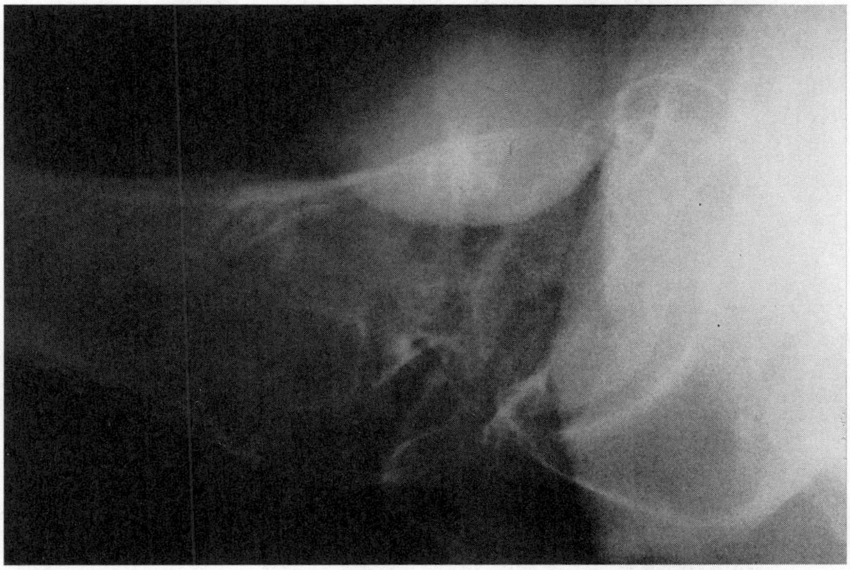

(A) nonoperative treatment
(B) percutaneous pin fixation in situ
(C) closed reduction and percutaneous pin fixation
(D) open reduction and internal fixation with a hip compression screw
(E) unipolar hemiarthroplasty

696. A 90-year-old female nursing home resident sustained the injury in the figure. She engaged in minimal household ambulation with the assistance of a walker. The most appropriate management is

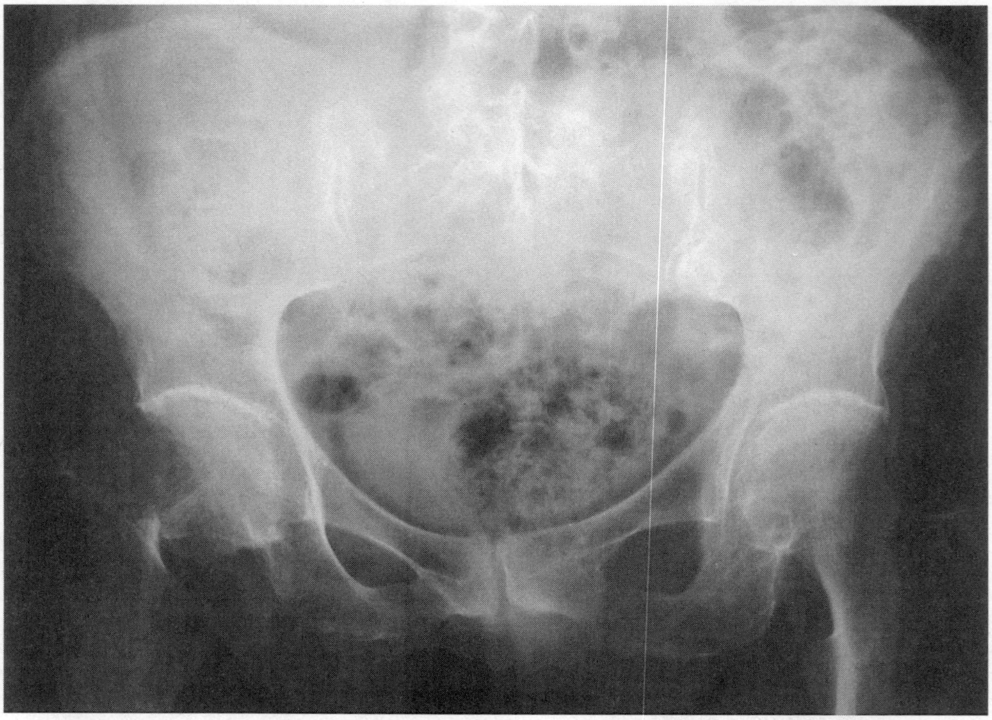

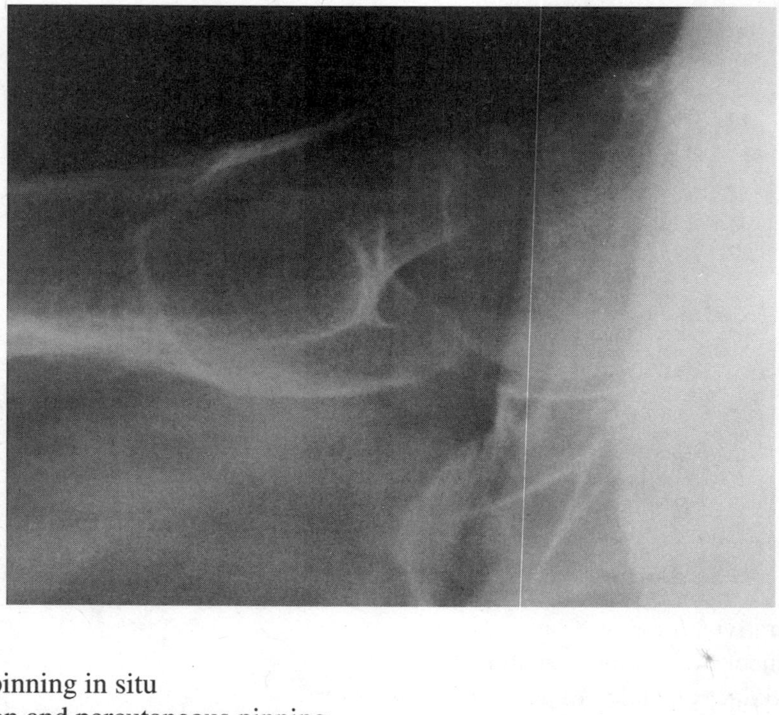

(A) nonoperative
(B) percutaneous pinning in situ
(C) closed reduction and percutaneous pinning
(D) unipolar hemiarthroplasty
(E) bipolar hemiarthroplasty

697. A 24-year-old man involved in a fist fight sustained the closed injury in the figure. The most appropriate treatment is

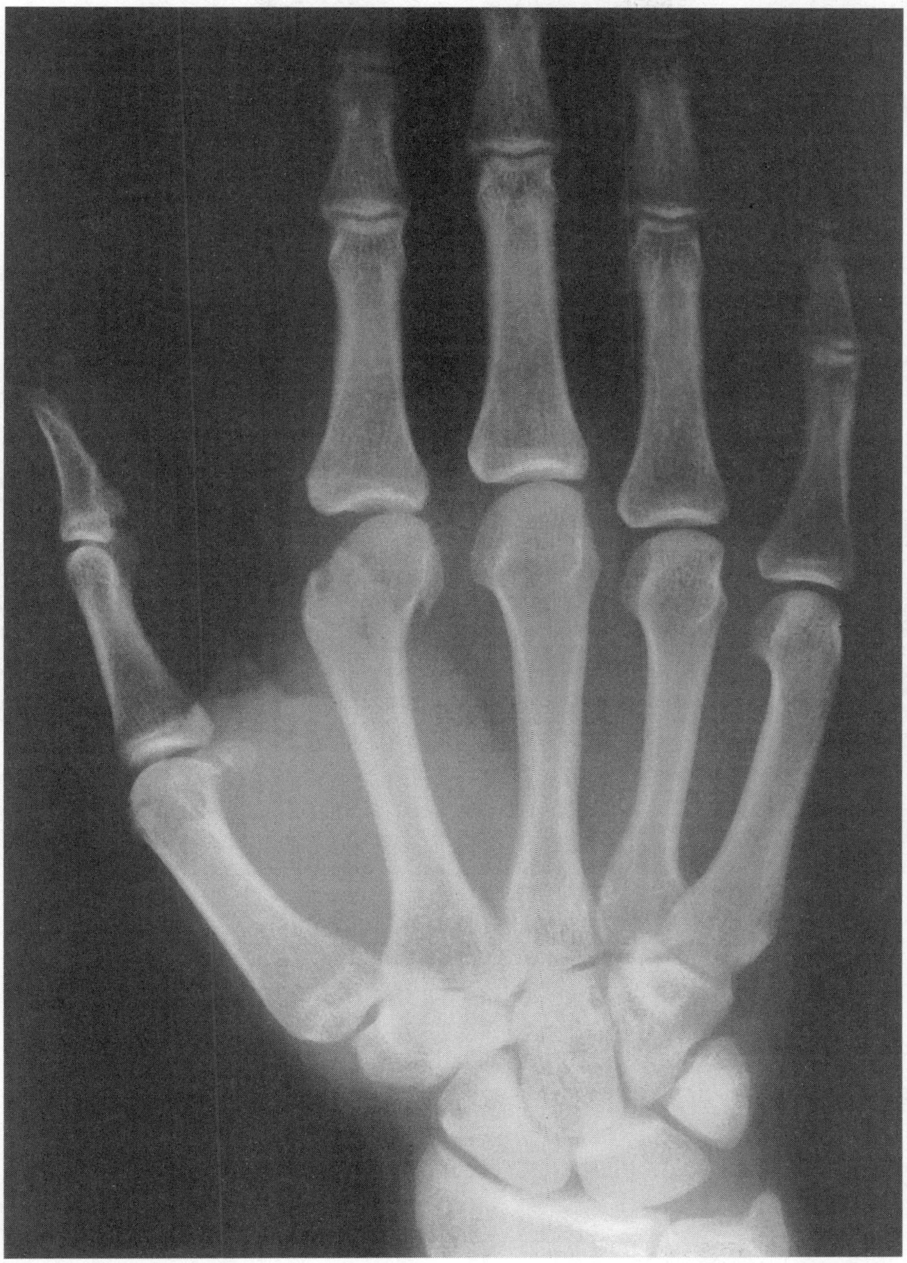

(A) splinting in situ
(B) "buddy-taping" to the adjacent finger
(C) closed reduction and cast immobilization
(D) open reduction and fixation with Kirschner wires
(E) open reduction and fixation with screws

698. A 29-year-old man fell and sustained the injury in the figure. All the following statements regarding this injury are true EXCEPT

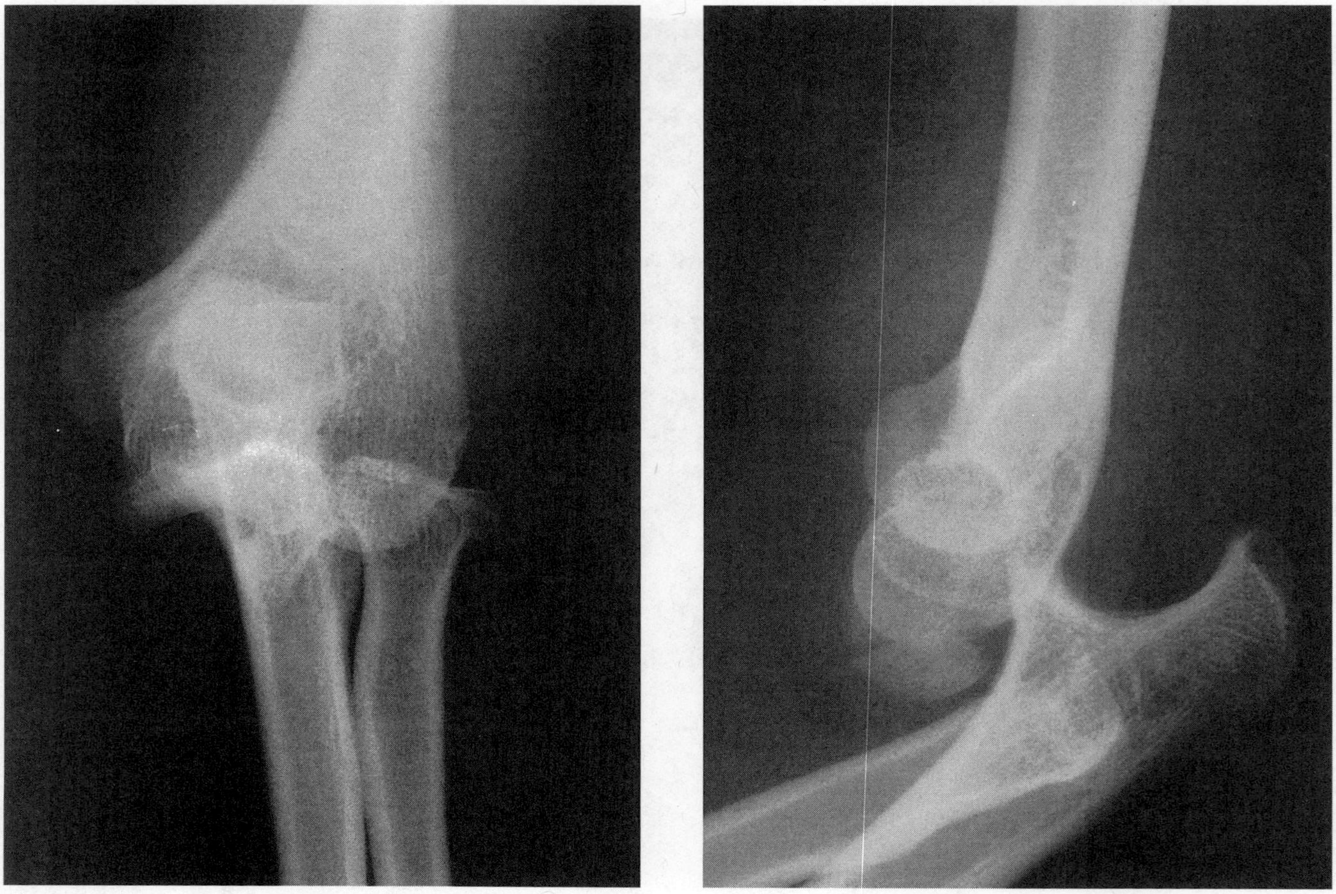

(A) open reduction of the dislocated elbow is likely to be required
(B) the medial collateral ligament is completely disrupted
(C) a favorable outcome is less common following this injury than following a simple dislocation of the elbow
(D) an effort should be made to preserve the radial head
(E) immobilization of the elbow for longer than 3 weeks is undesirable

699. A 38-year-old woman fell and sustained the fracture in the figure. All the following statements regarding this fracture are true EXCEPT that

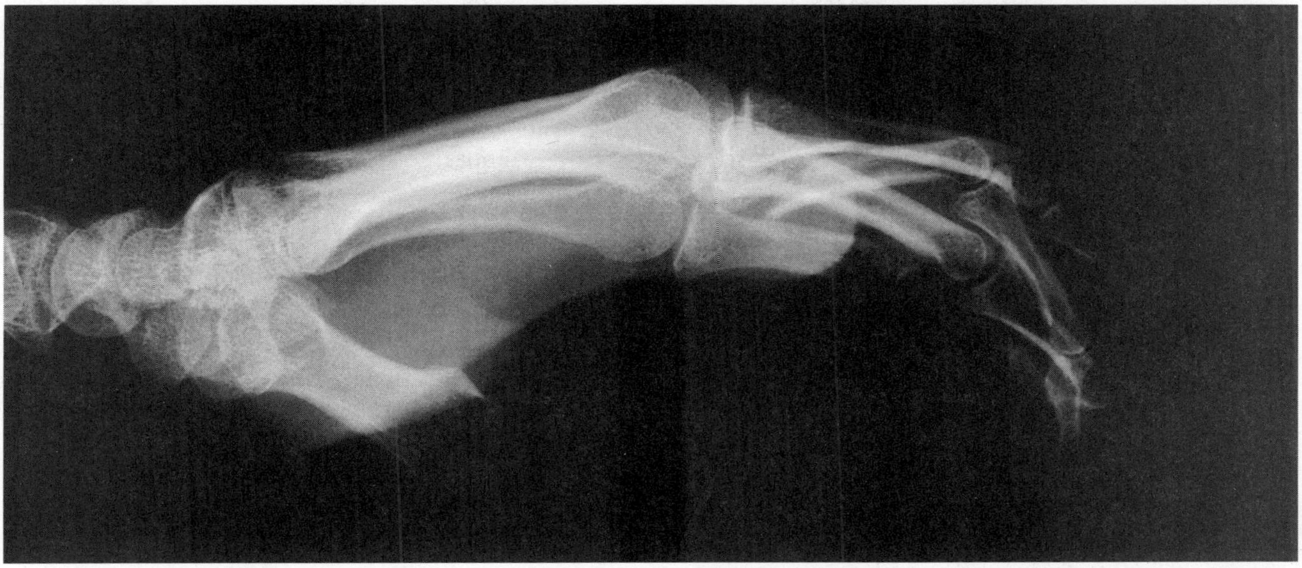

(A) the proximal portion of the phalanx is in flexion due to the pull of the superficialis tendon
(B) simple buddy-taping is inadequate treatment for this fracture
(C) if a stable closed reduction is achieved, casting to block extension is adequate immobilization
(D) if closed reduction is achieved but cannot be maintained, percutaneous Kirschner wire fixation is indicated
(E) clinical union will be achieved sooner than radiographic union

700. A 20-year-old woman involved in a motor vehicle accident sustained multiple injuries, including ipsilateral femoral neck and shaft fractures. The most appropriate treatment for this patient's orthopaedic injuries is

(A) skeletal traction until the patient is stable, then internal fixation of the femoral neck fracture and locked intramedullary nailing of the femoral shaft fracture
(B) skeletal traction until the patient is stable, then fixation of femoral neck and shaft fractures with a femoral reconstruction nail
(C) immediate fixation of femoral neck and shaft fractures with multiple screws and Enders' nails
(D) immediate fixation of the femoral neck and shaft fractures with multiple screws and retrograde intramedullary nailing
(E) immediate fixation of the femoral neck and shaft fracture with multiple screws and antegrade intramedullary nailing

701. A 28-year-old man involved in a motor vehicle accident sustained multiple injuries, including a closed head injury and a splenic rupture. His orthopaedic injuries included a displaced supratectal fracture of the right acetabulum and an ipsilateral fracture of the femoral shaft. The most appropriate management of this patient's orthopaedic injuries is

(A) skeletal traction for both the acetabular and femoral shaft fractures
(B) immediate intramedullary nailing of the femoral shaft fracture and ORIF of the acetabular fracture
(C) immediate intramedullary nailing of the femoral shaft fracture; delayed ORIF of the acetabular fracture
(D) delayed intramedullary nailing of the femoral shaft fracture and delayed ORIF of the acetabular fracture
(E) ORIF of the acetabular fracture; skeletal traction for the femoral shaft fracture

702. A 65-year-old woman involved in a motor vehicle accident sustained a grade II open fracture of the distal femur. She was taken immediately to the operating room where irrigation, debridement, and fracture stabilization were performed. Her postoperative radiograph is shown below. The most likely postoperative complication in this patient is

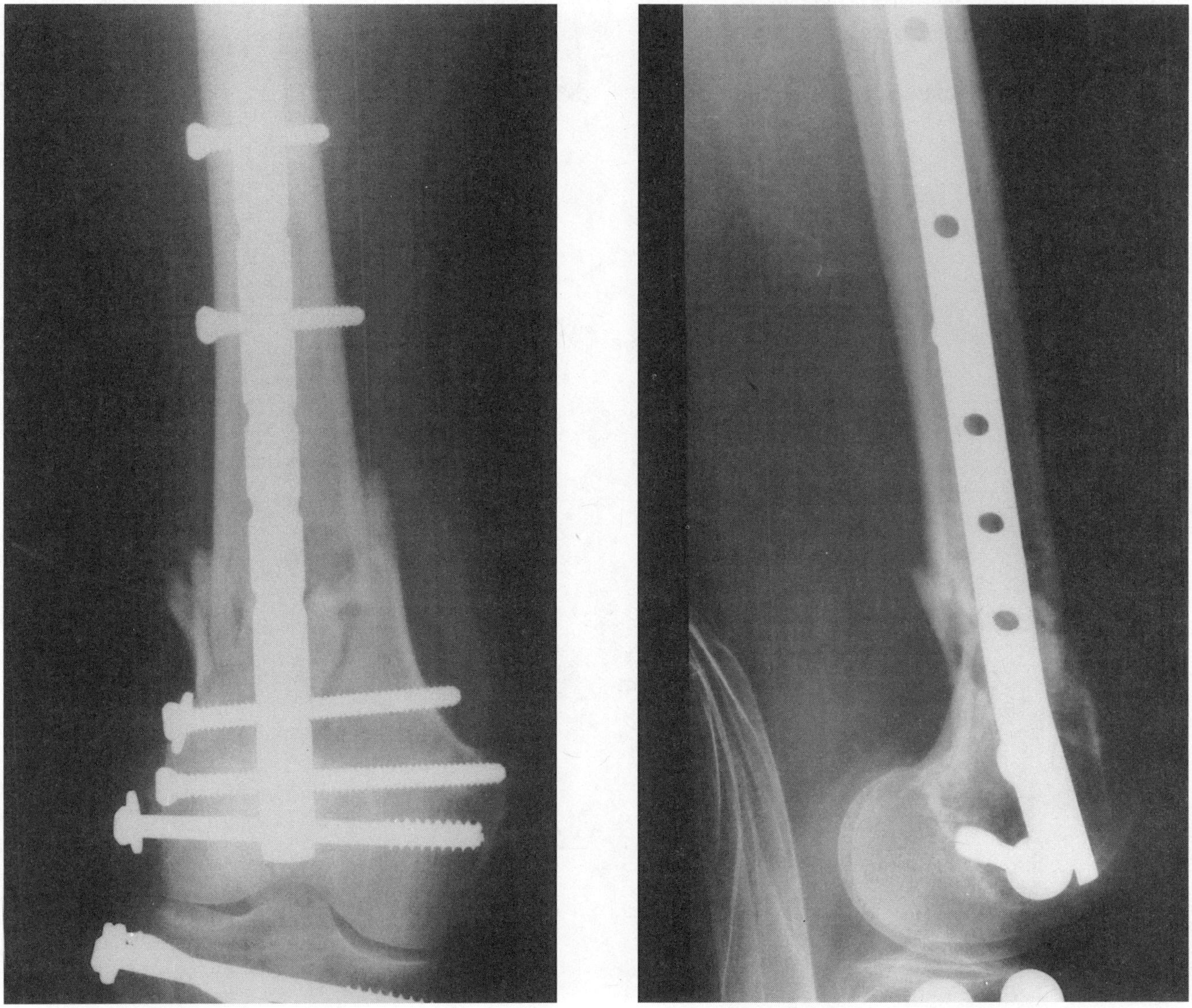

(A) infection
(B) nonunion
(C) malunion
(D) failure of the implant
(E) arthrofibrosis

703. Figures *A* and *B* show a transverse fracture of the patella in a 35-year-old man who fell 15 feet. Figures *C* and *D* show the postoperative reduction and stabilization. The most common complication after this treatment is

(A) loss of reduction
(B) avascular necrosis of the patella
(C) infection
(D) nonunion
(E) pain from retained hardware

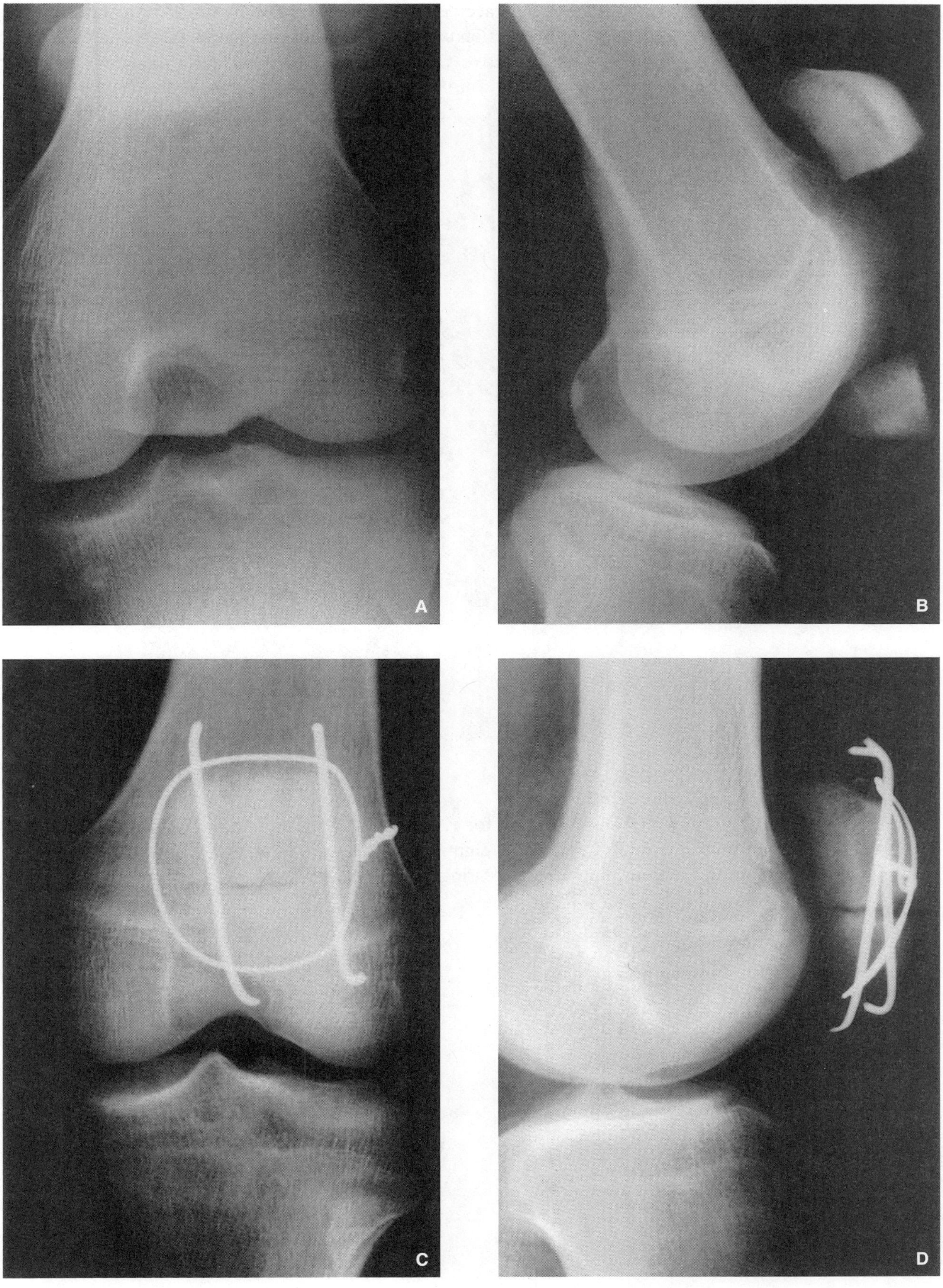
A
B
C
D

704. A 32-year-old man involved in a motor vehicle accident had the radiograph below. He was taken immediately to the operating room, where closed reduction was performed under general anesthesia. After reduction, the hip was clinically stable. A postoperative CT scan revealed a concentric reduction and no entrapped bodies within the hip joint. The most appropriate postoperative management of this patient is

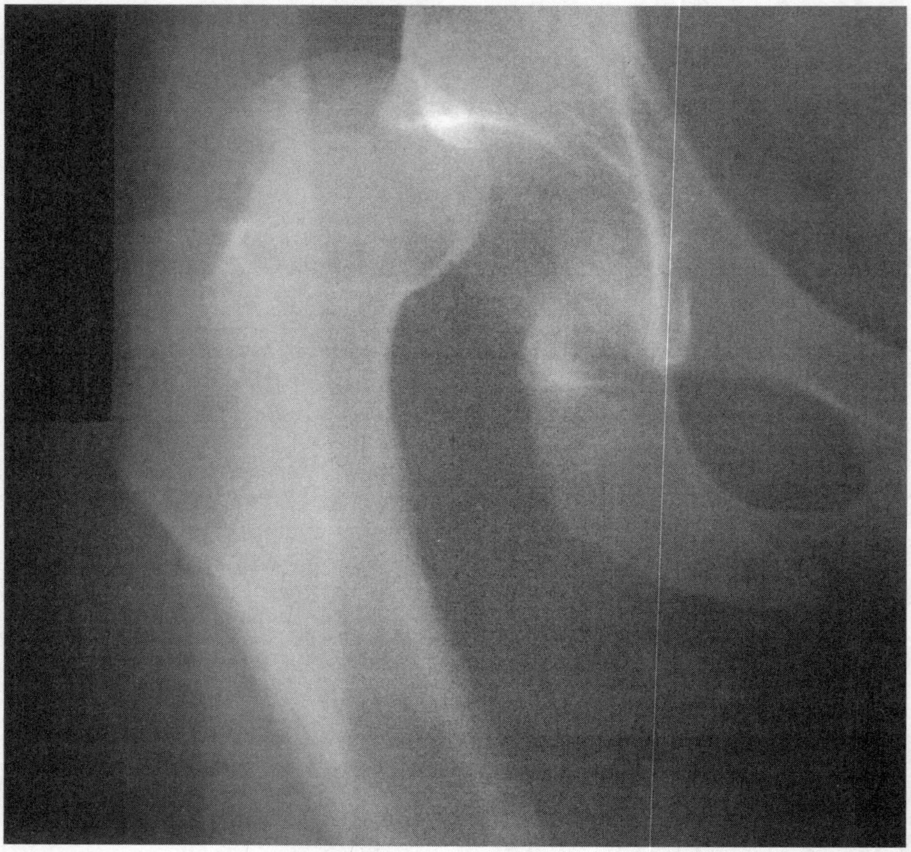

(A) immobilization in a hip spica cast
(B) use of an abduction orthosis for 6 weeks
(C) early motion of the hip; no weight-bearing for 12 weeks
(D) early motion of the hip; gradual return to weight-bearing over 2 to 4 weeks
(E) skeletal traction for 2 weeks; non-weight-bearing for 12 weeks

705. A 38-year-old man struck by a speeding car at 2 AM sustained the injury in the figure. The most appropriate treatment is

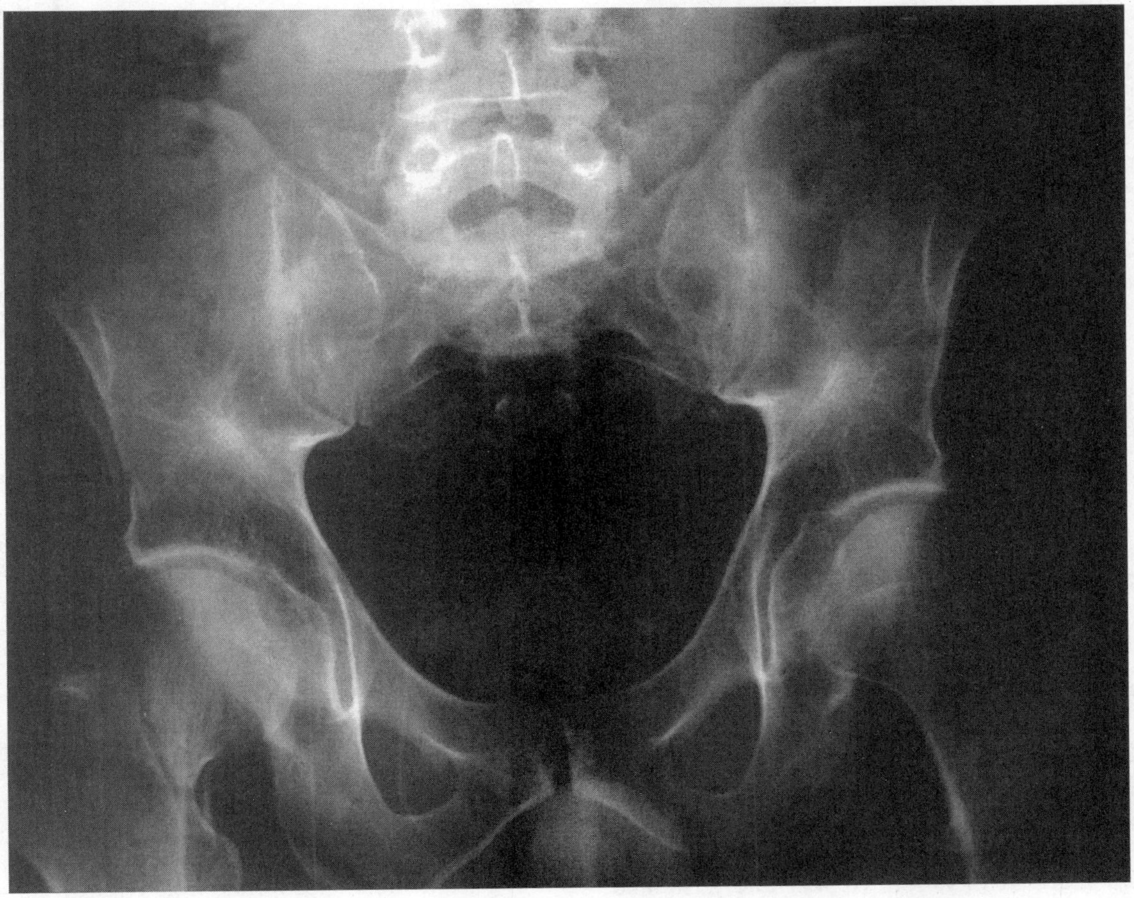

(A) immediate reduction and fixation with multiple screws
(B) immediate reduction and fixation with a compression hip screw
(C) reduction the next morning and fixation with multiple screws
(D) reduction the next morning and fixation with a compression hip screw
(E) bipolar hemiarthroplasty

Questions 706–707

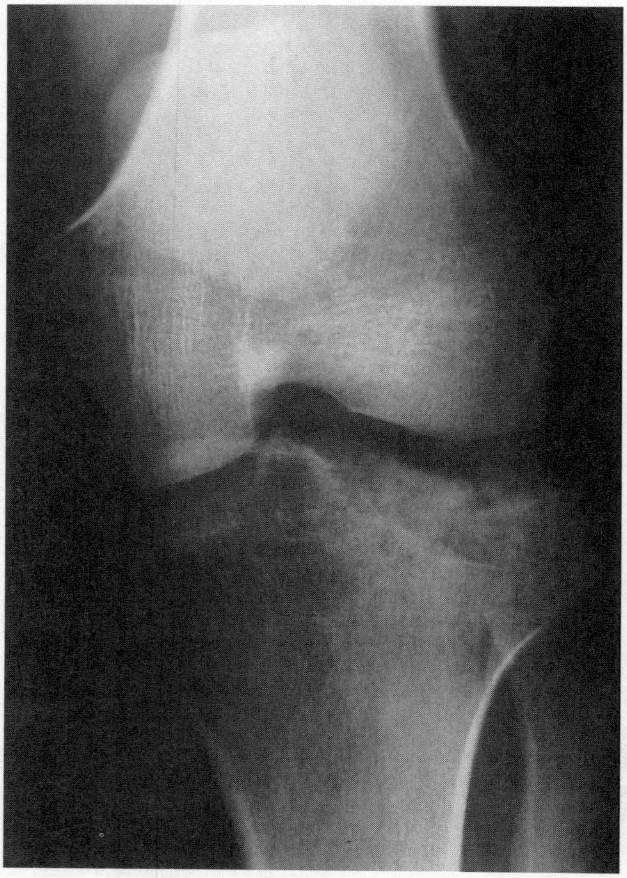

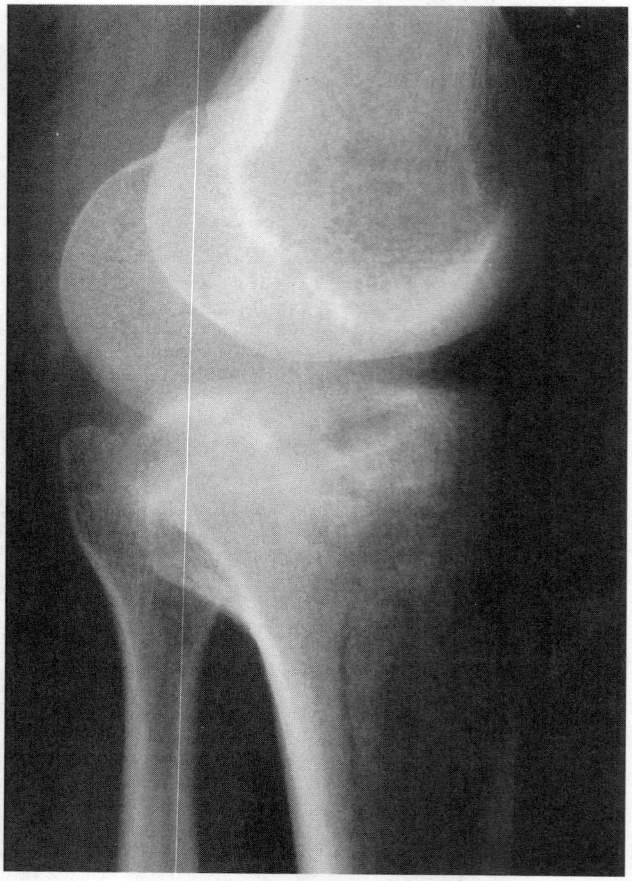

706. A 35-year-old man fell 10 feet and sustained the injury in the radiographs above. The most appropriate classification of this fracture is

(A) wedge
(B) depression
(C) wedge and depression
(D) bicondylar
(E) subcondylar

707. The most appropriate treatment of this injury is

(A) a bulky dressing and early motion
(B) a knee immobilizer for 6 weeks
(C) a cylinder cast for 6 weeks
(D) elevation of the depressed articular fragments, bone grafting, and a cylinder cast
(E) elevation of the depressed articular fragment, bone grafting, internal fixation, and early knee motion

708. A 42-year-old man sustained a gunshot wound to the leg, causing the injury shown below. The most appropriate treatment for this injury is irrigation and debridement of the gunshot wound and

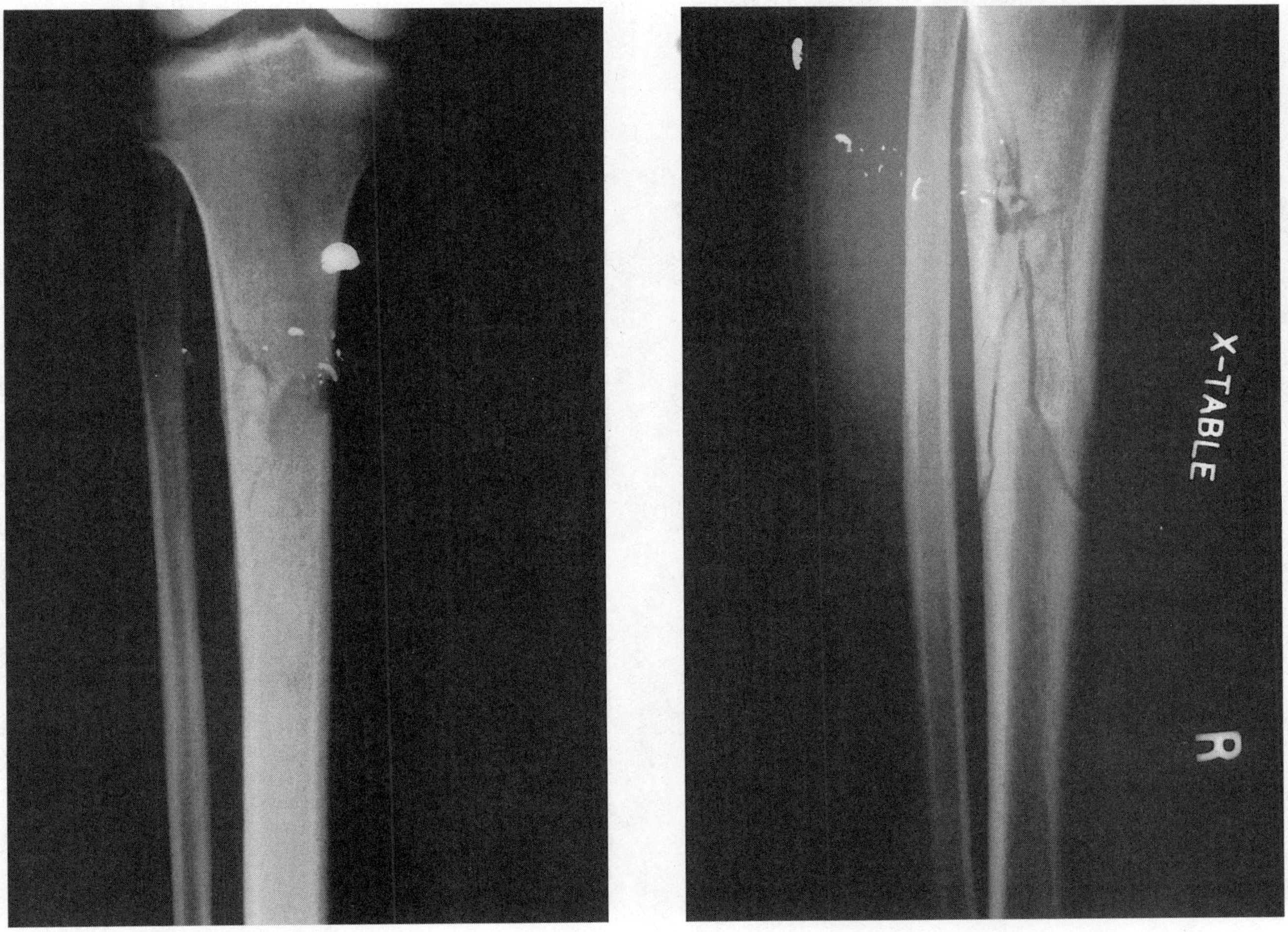

(A) immobilization in an above-knee cast
(B) external skeletal fixation
(C) removal of the metallic fragments; immobilization in an above-knee cast
(D) removal of the metallic fragments; external skeletal fixation
(E) removal of the metallic fragments; ORIF with a plate and screws

709. The radiographs below are of the tibia in a 70-year-old woman 6 months following a fracture treated by closed reduction and cast immobilization. The patient reported pain with attempted ambulation. There is no evidence of infection. The most appropriate treatment is

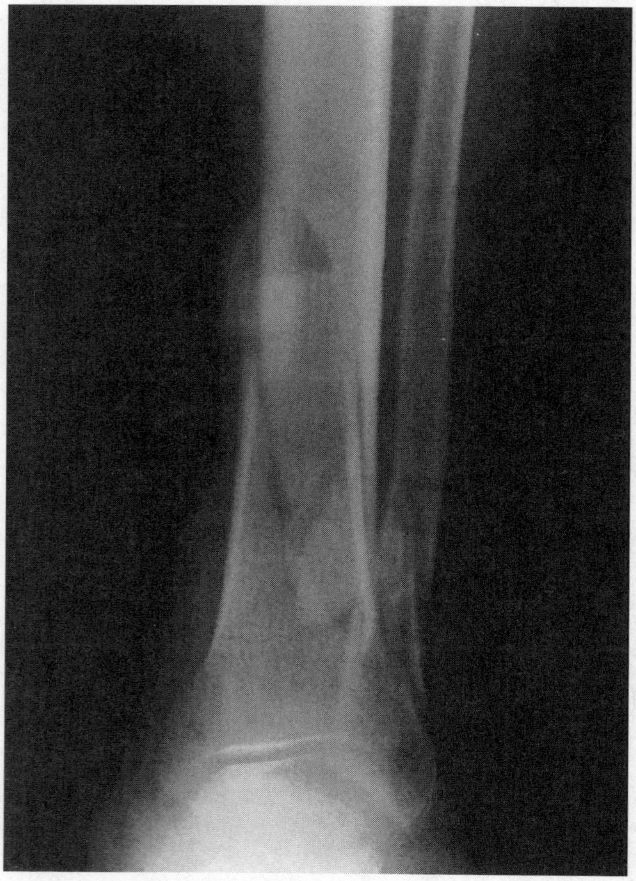

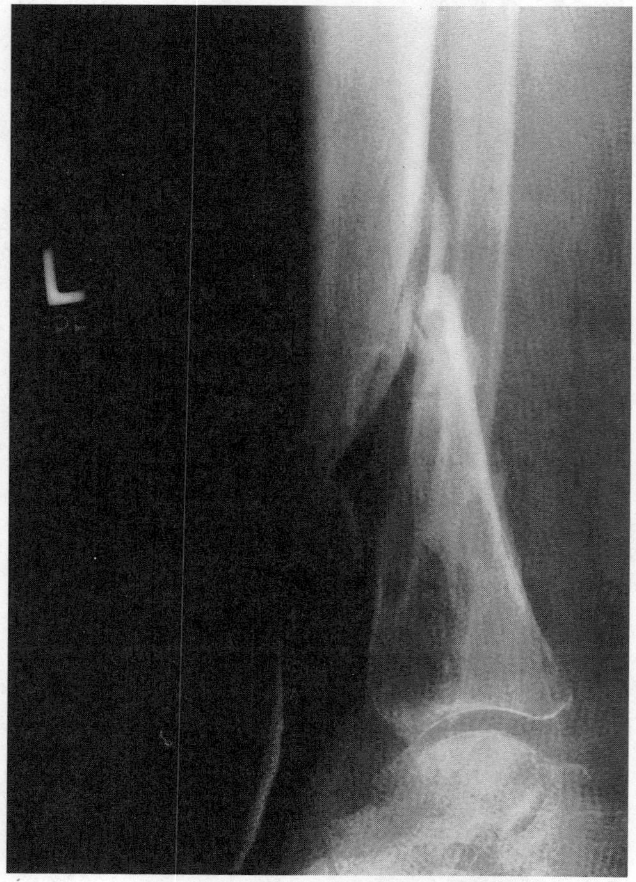

(A) posterolateral bone grafting
(B) fibulotomy and continued weight-bearing
(C) reamed intramedullary nailing
(D) open reduction, plate fixation, and bone grafting
(E) electrical stimulation

710. Six months following closed reduction and casting of a tibial shaft fracture, an 18-year-old man had pain when he ambulated more than 30 min at a time. Radiographs of his tibia are shown below. All the following forms of treatment could be justified in this patient EXCEPT

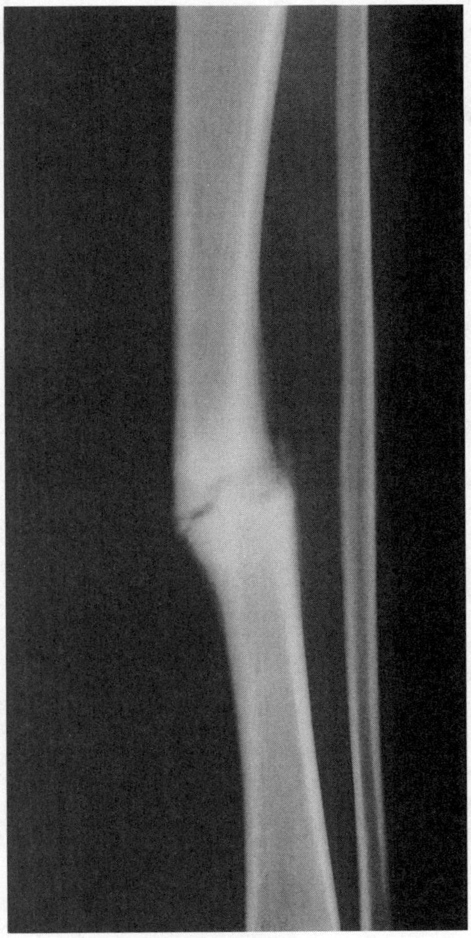
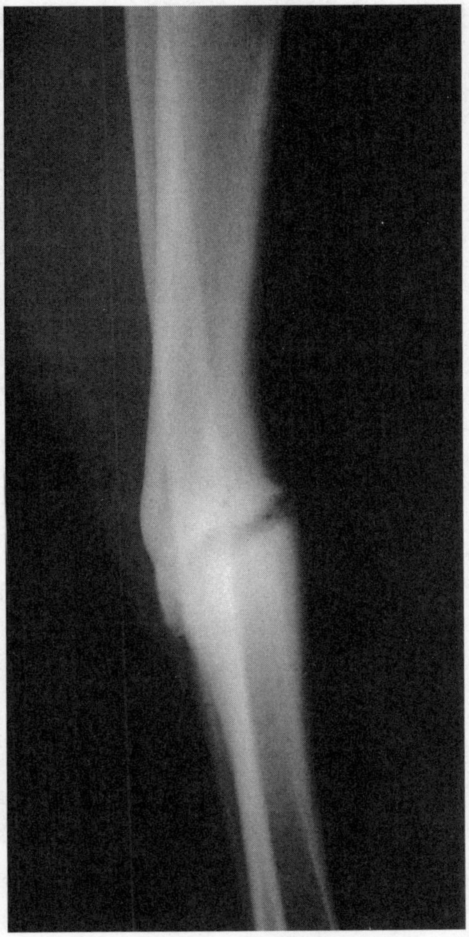

(A) resection of 2 cm of fibula
(B) posterolateral bone grafting
(C) pulsed electromagnetic field stimulation
(D) reamed intramedullary nailing
(E) take-down of the nonunion site, with plating and bone grafting

711. A 34-year-old man involved in a motor vehicle accident sustained the isolated, closed injury shown below. Closed reduction is achieved under general anesthesia. The most appropriate post-reduction management is

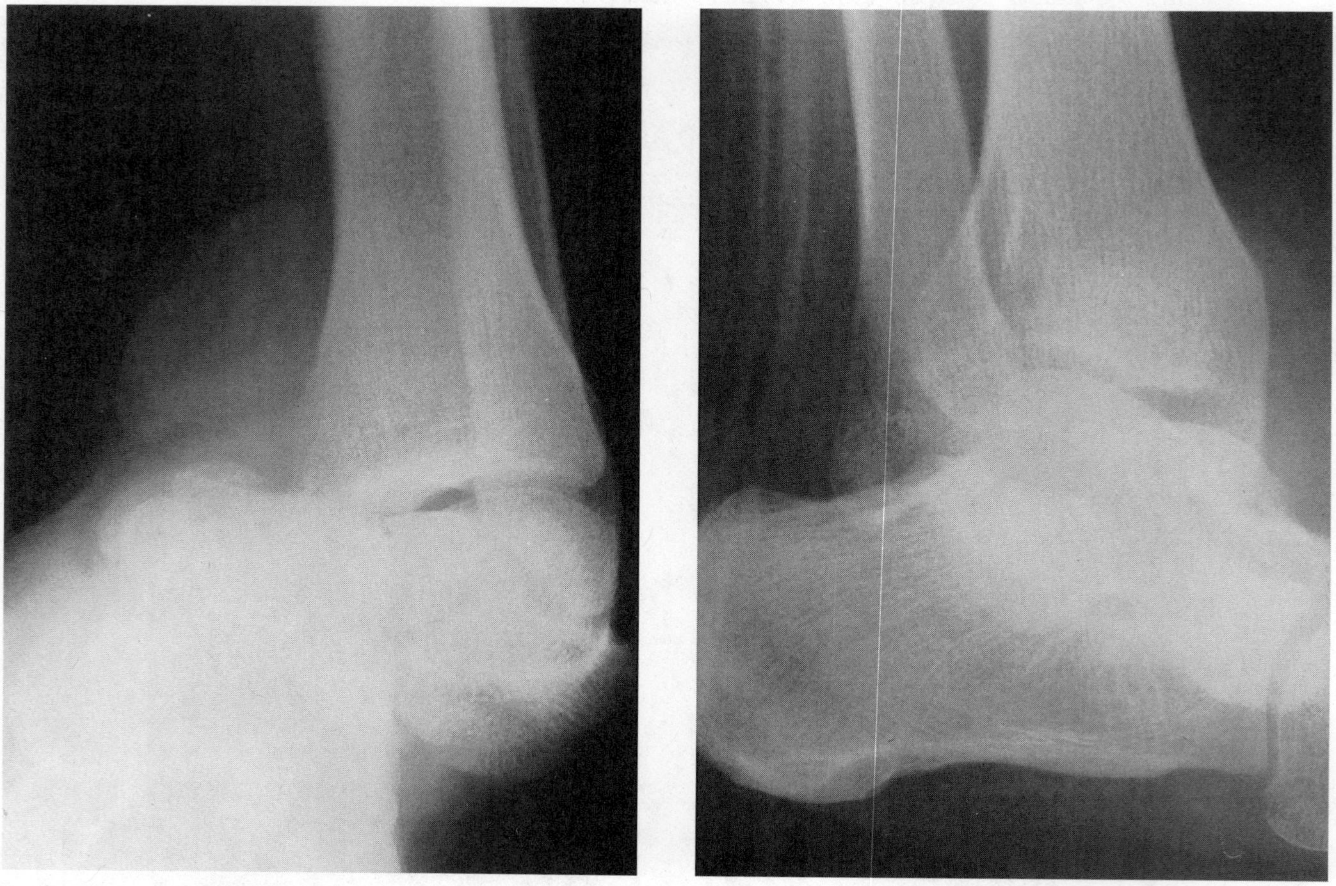

(A) fixation with percutaneous Kirschner wires; early ankle motion
(B) fixation with percutaneous Kirschner wires; immobilization for 4 weeks in a below-knee cast
(C) immobilization for 4 weeks in a below-knee cast
(D) immobilization for 4 weeks in an above-knee cast
(E) immobilization for 8 weeks in a below-knee cast

712. A 51-year-old patient fell while jogging and sustained the injury shown below. The most appropriate form of treatment is

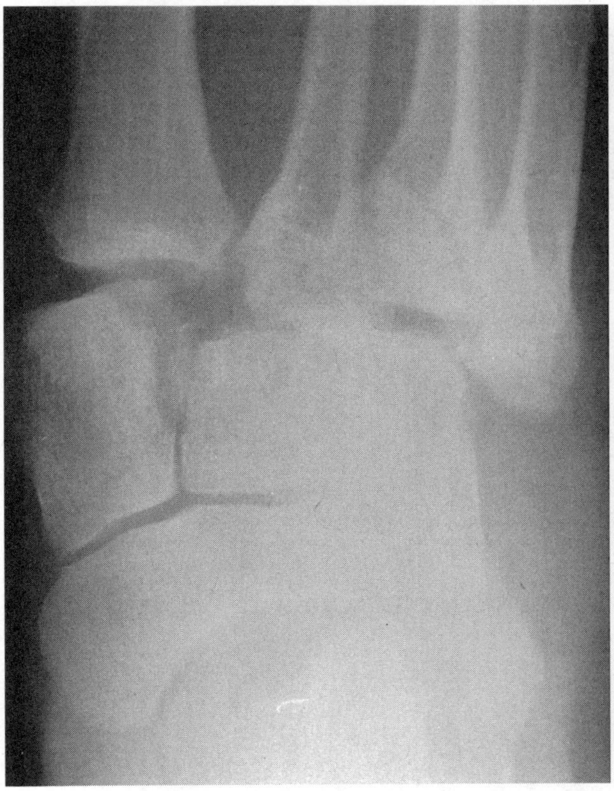

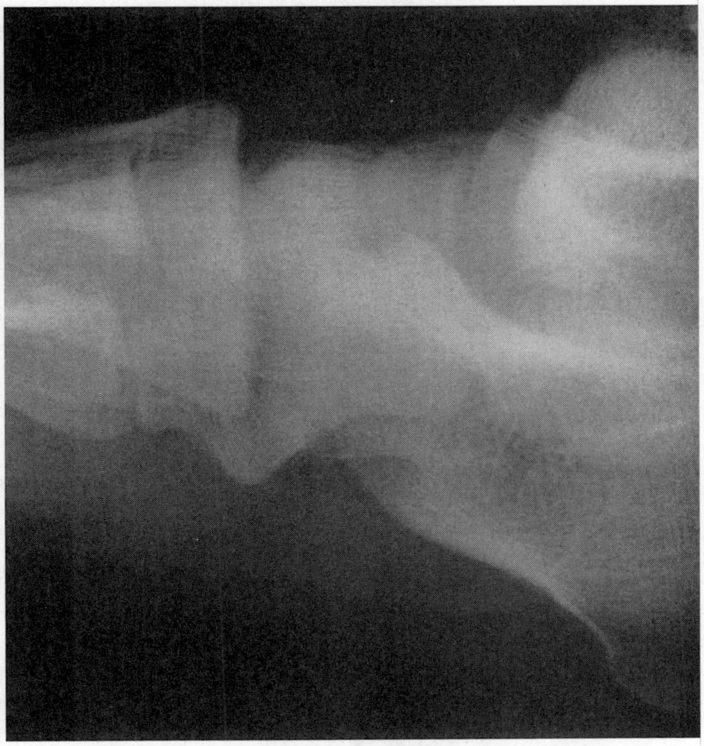

(A) immobilization in a below-knee cast
(B) closed reduction and immobilization in a below-knee cast
(C) closed reduction and percutaneous pin fixation
(D) open reduction and internal fixation
(E) arthrodesis of the first and second tarsometatarsal joints

713. A 21-year-old man sustained the injury in the figure in a fall onto his outstretched hand. The most appropriate management is

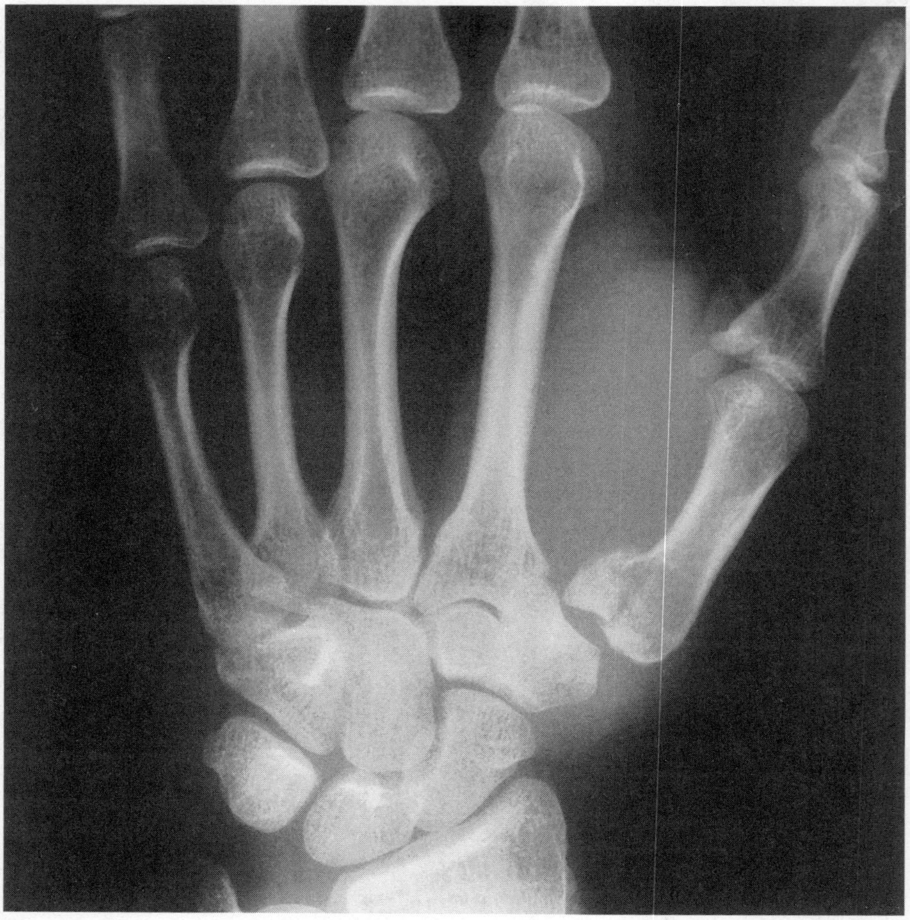

(A) immobilization in a thumb spica cast
(B) closed reduction; immobilization in a thumb spica cast
(C) closed reduction; percutaneous pin fixation; no immobilization
(D) closed reduction; percutaneous pin fixation; immobilization in a thumb spica cast
(E) ORIF with a minifragment plate and screws

714. The radiographs below show an abduction–external rotation injury of the ankle in a 38-year-old woman. At the time of surgery, structures requiring internal fixation are the

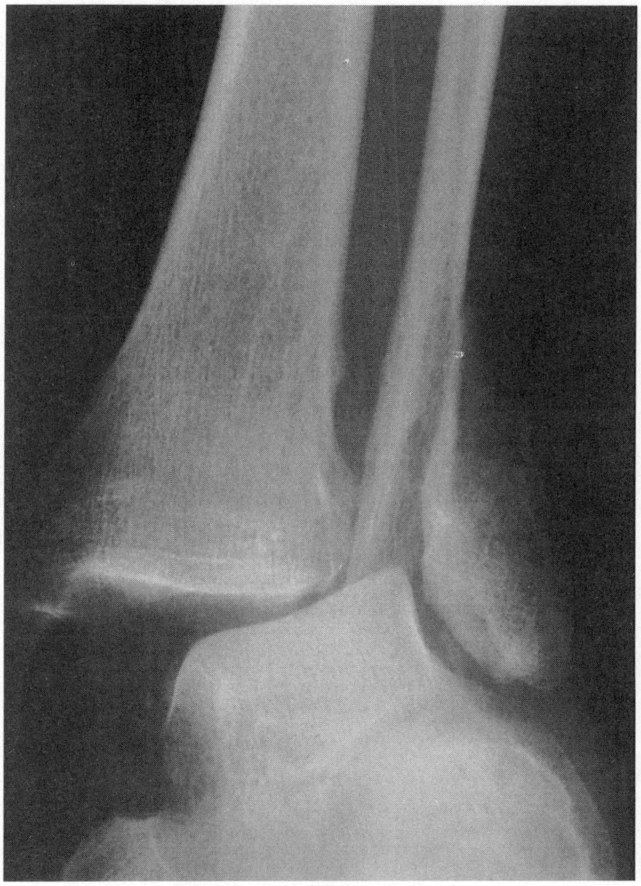

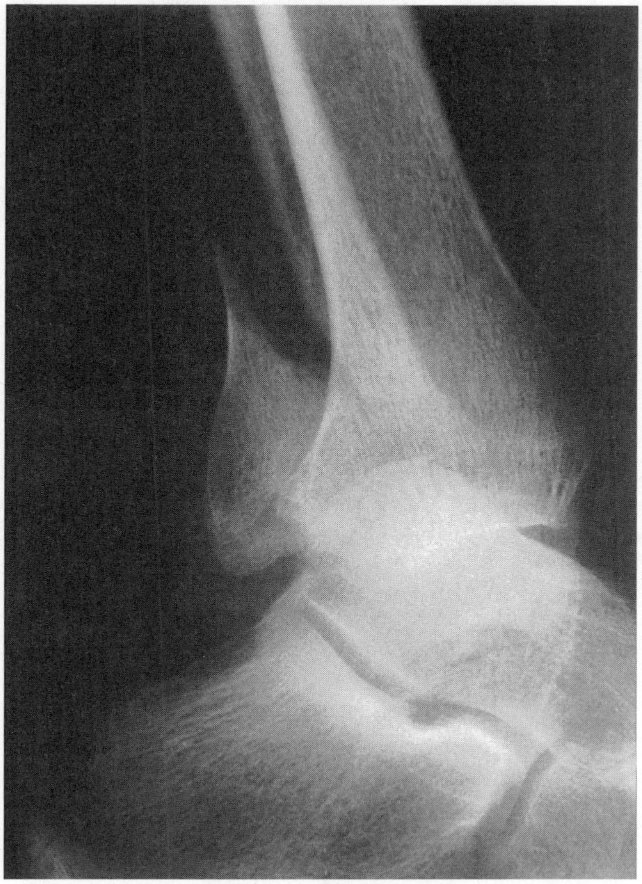

(A) lateral malleolus and tibiofibular syndesmosis
(B) medial and lateral malleoli
(C) medial, lateral, and posterior malleoli
(D) lateral and posterior malleoli
(E) medial and posterior malleoli

715. Figures *A* and *B* are radiographs of the forearm in a 28-year-old woman 8 months following a comminuted fracture of the radius and ulna treated with ORIF. The patient is pain-free, but the forearm is fixed in 5° of supination, and the patient wishes to achieve more forearm rotation. A bone scan of the forearm is shown in figure *C*. The recommended treatment is

(A) informing the patient that she will regain more forearm rotation with further time and observation
(B) informing the patient that she will regain no more forearm rotation and that surgery will not help
(C) administering indomethacin, 25 mg po tid for 6 weeks
(D) repeating the bone scan in 4 to 6 months
(E) performing resection of a synostosis; administering indomethacin, 25 mg po tid; beginning early motion

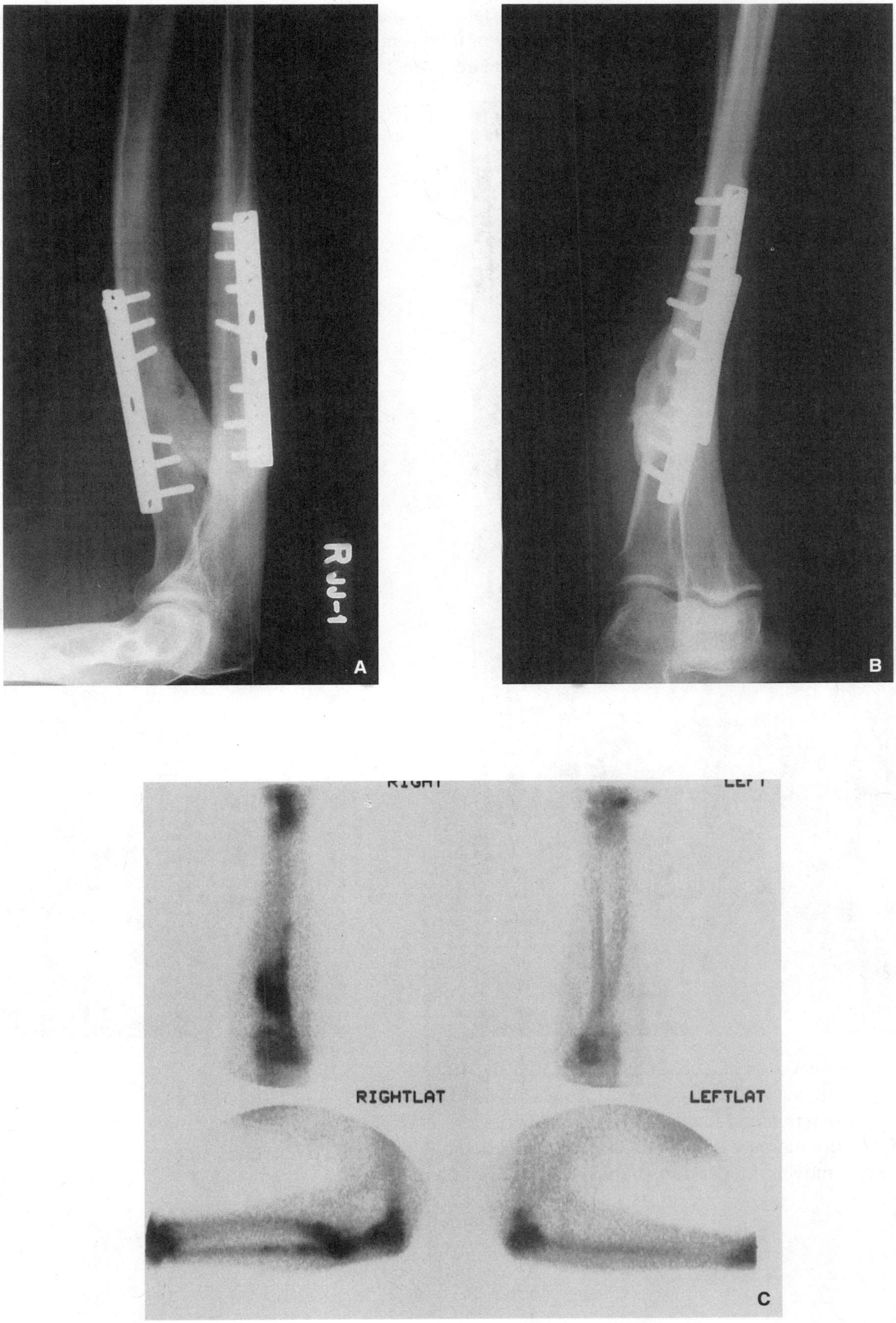
R JJ-1
A
B
RIGHTLAT
LEFTLAT
C

716. Four months following proximally and distally interlocked intramedullary nailing of a closed tibial fracture, a patient was fully weight-bearing but complained of mild pain at the fracture site with ambulation. Radiographs of the tibia are shown below. The most appropriate treatment is

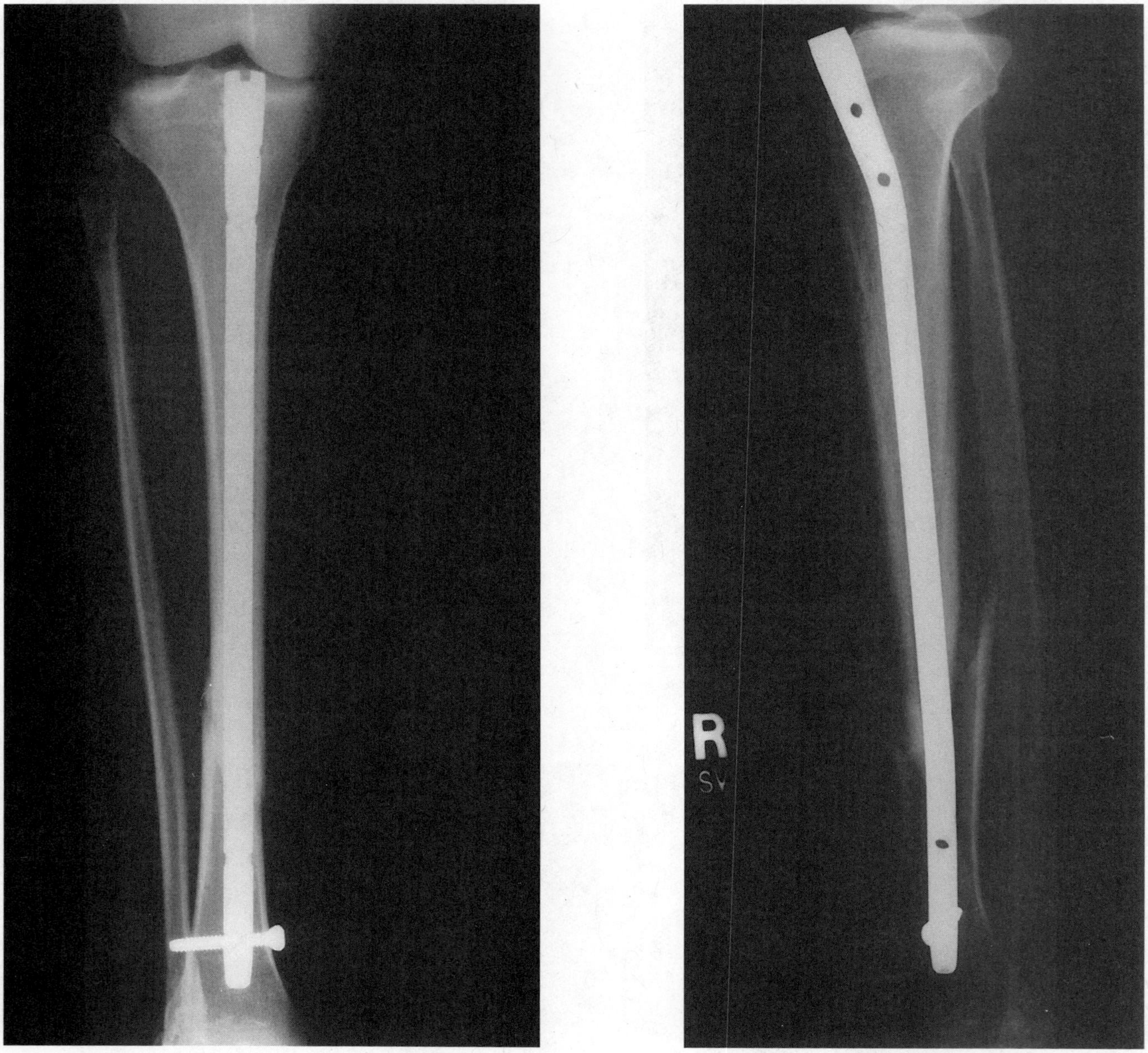

(A) observation and continued full weight-bearing
(B) removal of the distal interlocking screw and continued full weight-bearing
(C) posterolateral iliac crest bone grafting
(D) stimulation with a pulsed electromagnetic field
(E) removal of the intramedullary nail and replacement with a larger, reamed intramedullary nail

717. Radiographs of a 22-year-old man who injured his ankle are shown below. The mechanism of injury was most likely

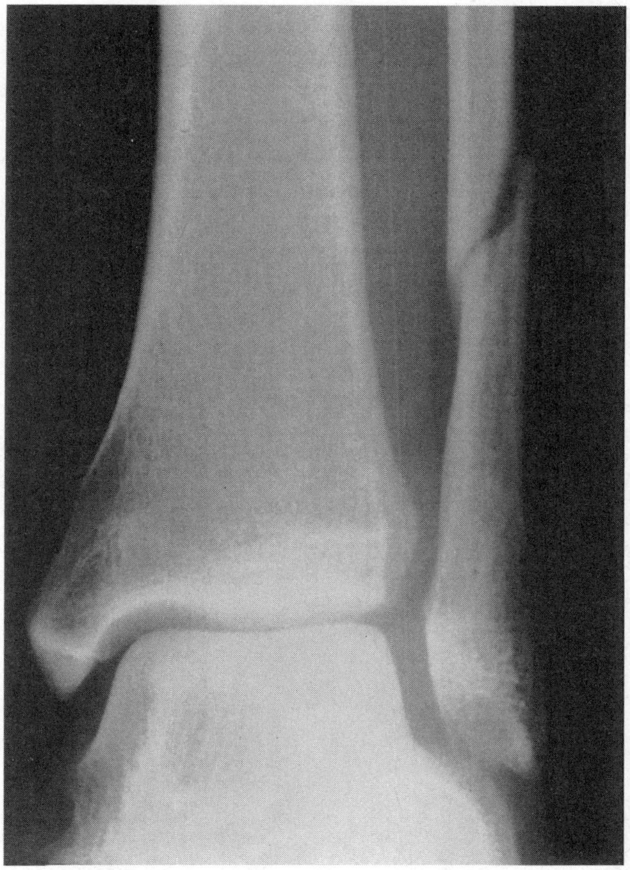

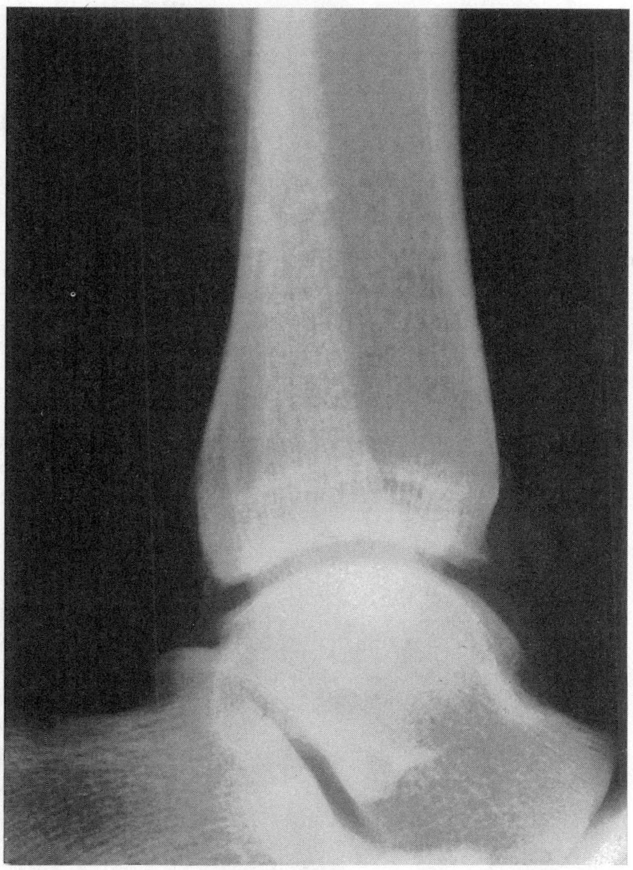

(A) adduction
(B) abduction
(C) external rotation
(D) direct trauma to the fibula
(E) adduction and external rotation

---

718. An inversion injury of the ankle may cause a fracture of all the following EXCEPT the

(A) tip of the lateral malleolus
(B) lateral process of the talus
(C) sustentaculum tali
(D) base of the fifth metatarsal
(E) anterior process of the calcaneus

719. All the following have been reported with severe inversion injuries to the ankle EXCEPT

(A) rupture of the calcaneofibular ligament
(B) rupture of the skin on the lateral aspect of the ankle
(C) injury to the peroneal nerve
(D) rupture of the peroneal tendons
(E) compartmental syndrome

720. All the following statements regarding ruptures of the Achilles' tendon are correct EXCEPT that they occur

(A) more commonly in males
(B) most commonly in middle age
(C) most commonly during high-demand sports
(D) in association with weakness of ankle plantar flexion
(E) in association with a positive Thomas test

721. Which of the following is the best indication for surgical treatment of a mallet-finger fracture?

(A) A widely displaced fracture
(B) A fracture involving more than 40 percent of the articular surface
(C) A fracture associated with volar subluxation of the distal phalanx
(D) A displaced fracture in the thumb
(E) A fracture in a growing child

---

722. All the following statements concerning the fracture in the radiographs below are correct EXCEPT that

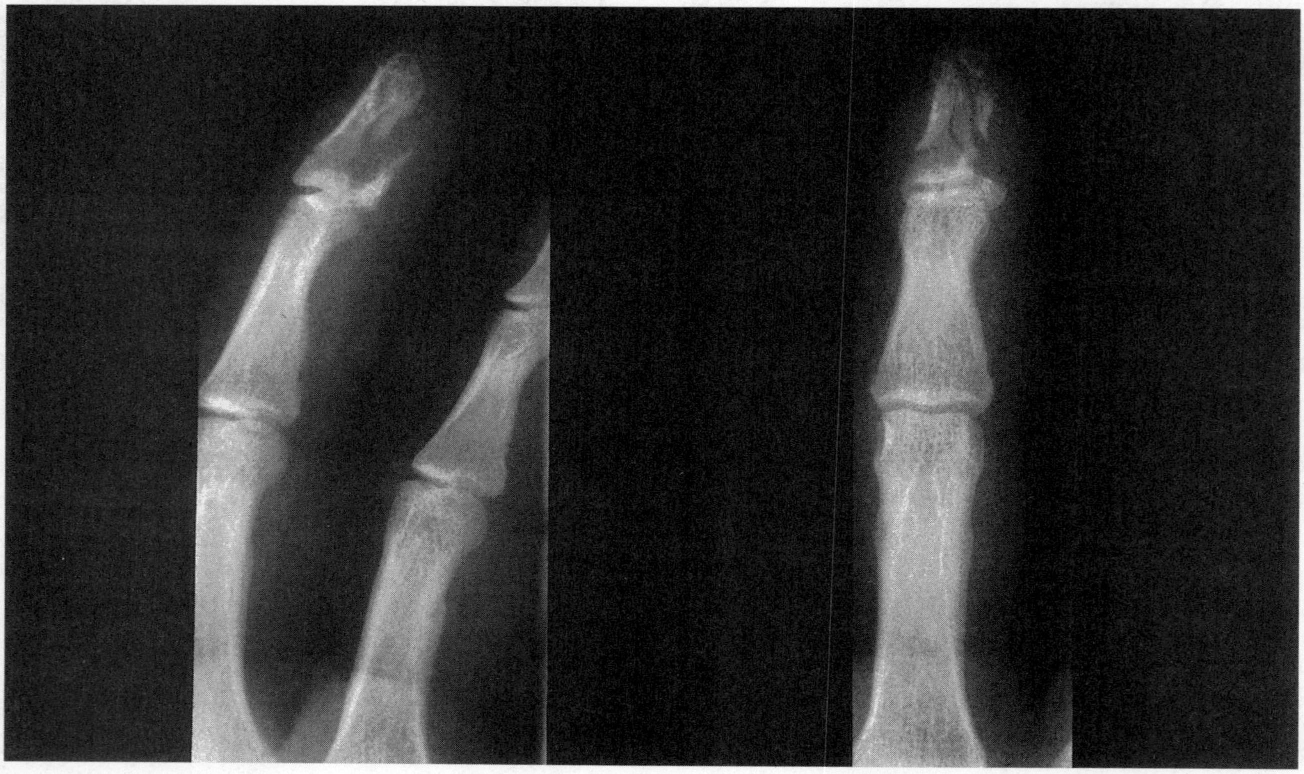

(A) drainage of a subungual hematoma may be required
(B) an open fracture may disrupt the nail bed
(C) treatment with a splint is usually adequate
(D) radiographic union will be present by 6 weeks
(E) the fingertip may be tender for months

723. Closed reduction of "complex" dorsal dislocations of the metacarpophalangeal joint are often unsuccessful because the

(A) spasm in the muscles crossing the joint cannot be overcome
(B) metacarpal head is trapped between the flexor tendon and lumbrical muscle
(C) palmar plate is wedged between the joint surfaces
(D) flexor tendon is trapped within the joint
(E) collateral ligament is trapped within the joint

724. In a patient with a complete tear of the ulnar collateral ligament of the thumb, the structure most likely to prevent ligamentous healing is the

(A) dorsal capsule of the metacarpophalangeal joint
(B) aponeurosis of the flexor pollicis brevis
(C) aponeurosis of the adductor pollicis
(D) the volar plate
(E) the extensor pollicis brevis

725. The most common mechanism by which a fracture of the scaphoid is produced is

(A) tension
(B) compression
(C) rotation
(D) tension on the palmar aspect of the bone and compression on the dorsal aspect
(E) compression on the palmar aspect of the bone and tension on the dorsal aspect

726. A 28-year-old man fell and sustained a minimally displaced fracture of the proximal pole of the scaphoid. The best treatment for this injury is

(A) a below-elbow cast
(B) an above-elbow thumb spica cast
(C) closed reduction and percutaneous pin fixation
(D) open reduction and internal fixation
(E) prosthetic replacement of the proximal pole of the scaphoid

727. The best treatment for an acute, complete rupture of the posterior tibial tendon in an otherwise healthy patient is

(A) below-knee casting for 6 weeks
(B) repair of the ruptured tendon
(C) repair of the ruptured tendon with augmentation from the adjacent toe flexor
(D) talocalcaneal arthrodesis
(E) triple arthrodesis

728. The LEAST appropriate method for internal fixation of a simple transverse closed fracture of the phalangeal shaft is

(A) crossed Kirschner wires
(B) intramedullary Kirschner wires
(C) intraosseous wires
(D) an interfragmentary compression screw
(E) external fixation

729. The optimal treatment for a minimally displaced Hawkins type I talar fracture is

(A) a below-knee cast in equinus
(B) a below-knee cast in neutral
(C) percutaneous Kirschner wire fixation
(D) percutaneous screw fixation
(E) open reduction and screw fixation

730. The change most likely to have resulted in a decrease in cervical spine injuries in football players is the

(A) improved construction of football helmets
(B) widespread use of neck rolls attached to shoulder pads
(C) improved strength training of football players
(D) improved endurance and conditioning of football players
(E) banning of the use of the helmet as the initial point of contact

731. Which of the following is the most common mechanism of cervical spine injury in football players?

(A) Hyperextension
(B) Hyperflexion
(C) Axial loading
(D) Distraction
(E) Rotation

732. Which of the following materials has been found experimentally to be associated with the highest rate of infection?

(A) Nylon
(B) High-density polyethylene
(C) Polymethyl methacrylate (PMMA)
(D) Surgical stainless steel
(E) Cobalt-chromium alloys

733. In a young, otherwise healthy patient involved in a motor vehicle accident, the best indicator of adequate fluid resuscitation is the

(A) pulse rate
(B) systolic blood pressure
(C) central venous pressure
(D) urine output
(E) hematocrit

734. The optimal tourniquet pressure for open reduction and internal fixation of an ankle fracture in a healthy 45-year-old patient is how many millimeters of mercury over systolic blood pressure?

(A) 50 mmHg
(B) 150 mmHG
(C) 250 mmHg
(D) 400 mmHg
(E) 500 mmHg

735. An 80-year-old woman with osteoporosis fell onto her right shoulder, sustaining a three-part fracture of the proximal humerus. There was 5 mm of superior displacement of the greater tuberosity, 10° varus tilting of the humeral head, and impaction of the anatomic neck into the humeral head. The most appropriate treatment is

(A) a sling and early physical therapy
(B) closed manipulation and a shoulder immobilizer for 6 weeks
(C) application of a shoulder spica cast and abduction for 6 weeks
(D) open reduction, internal fixation, and early physical therapy
(E) prosthetic replacement of the humeral head

736. Six months following reamed intramedullary nailing of an open femoral shaft fracture, a 30-year-old has continued thigh pain and drainage from a sinus located over the fracture site. Examination under fluoroscopy shows the fracture to be rigidly stabilized by the intramedullary device. The most appropriate management of this patient is now

(A) observation until the fracture unites and then removal of the intramedullary nail
(B) culture of the drainage, antibiotic treatment, observation until the fracture unites, and then removal of the nail
(C) debridement and culture of the infected tissues, antibiotic treatment, observation until the fracture unites, and then removal of the nail
(D) debridement and culture of the infected tissues, treatment with antibiotics, removal of the nail, and replacement with a larger, reamed nail
(E) debridement and culture of the infected tissues, treatment with antibiotics, removal of the nail, and stabilization with an external fixator

DIRECTIONS: The group of questions below consists of lettered headings followed by a set of numbered items. For each numbered item, select the **one** lettered heading with which it is **most** closely associated. Each lettered heading may be used **once, more than once, or not at all.**

Questions 737–742

For each numbered description below, select the neurologic syndrome with which it is most closely associated.

(A) Complete cord syndrome
(B) Central cord syndrome
(C) Anterior cord syndrome
(D) Posterior cord syndrome
(E) Brown-Séquard syndrome

737. The most common pattern of incomplete neurologic injury

738. The least common pattern of neurologic injury

739. The worst prognosis for return of function

740. Anatomically based on a unilateral cord injury

741. Quadriplegia with preservation of perianal sensation

742. Complete motor and sensory loss distal to the lesion but an intact bulbocavernosus reflex

Adult Trauma

Answers

596. The answer is E. *(Browner, pp 128–129.)* The role of EMTs in the field is very similar to that of the emergency department physician who is performing the primary survey. The establishment of an airway and ventilation is the first priority, followed by assessment of breathing, circulation, perfusion, and the need for hemorrhage control. The patient must be extricated prior to transport to an appropriate trauma center. Shock is controlled with intravenous fluids, control of exposure, application of antishock trousers as necessary, and stabilization of fractures. A trauma score is determined by the trauma team after arrival in the emergency department rather than by EMTs in the field.

597. The answer is C. *(Browner, pp 138–139.)* Pneumatic antishock garments are of value to help control hemorrhage in the face of significant pelvic fractures and in the setting of traumatic amputations of the lower limb. Inflation of the PASGs to greater than 30 mmHg may cause tissue anoxia, which can lead to a compartment syndrome. PASGs are not contraindicated in patients with spinal fractures. Lower limb fractures are a relative contraindication to the use of PASGs, but an absolute contraindication is the presence of a diaphragmatic rupture. Use of PASGs in this setting will force the abdominal contents into the thoracic cavity and make ventilation extremely difficult.

598. The answer is A. *(Browner, pp 133–134.)* Tension pneumothorax is caused by injury that produces a valvular mechanism in the chest wall or in the lung that results in an intrapleural collection of air that cannot escape. This leads to complete collapse of the ipsilateral lung and increasing pressure within the thoracic cavity. The mediastinum and trachea will deviate to the contralateral side, which interferes with venous return and ventilation of the contralateral lung. Physical findings include unilateral absence of breath sounds, tympany on percussion, distended neck veins, and hypotension. Paradoxical motion of the chest wall is indicative of a flail chest and not of a tension pneumothorax.

599. The answer is D. *(Browner, pp 137–138.)* The circulating blood volume is approximately 7 percent of body weight in adults or approximately 5 L in a 70-kg man. Class I hemorrhage is a loss of up to 15 percent of the circulating blood volume and results in no measurable change in the blood pressure or pulse. Class II hemorrhage is a loss of 15 to 30 percent of circulating blood volume and results in tachycardia and prolonged capillary refill, but no significant change in systolic blood pressure. A class III hemorrhage is a loss of 30 to 40 percent of circulating blood volume, or approximately 2000 mL in a 70-kg adult. This results in tachycardia, tachypnea, and systolic hypotension. A class IV hemorrhage involves greater than 40 percent loss of blood volume, which is life-threatening exsanguination; the patient will require immediate blood product replacement.

600. The answer is D. *(Browner, p 138.)* Initial resuscitation of the patient in traumatic shock entails administration of a large bolus of isotonic intravenous fluid. Although both normal saline and Ringer's lactate are relatively isotonic, Ringer's lactate contains a physiologic concentration of minor electrolytes and is the preferred resuscitation fluid in acutely traumatized patients. In adults, an initial bolus of 2 L should be given.

601. The answer is A. *(Browner, p 142.)* The most commonly injured intraabdominal organs following blunt trauma are the solid viscera. The hollow viscera, the small and large intestines, usually escape injury. The most commonly injured solid viscera are the liver and spleen, which are frequently the site of occult hemorrhage in the traumatized patient. Next, in descending order of frequency, are the kidney, pancreas, and small bowel. The prostate is rarely injured by blunt abdominal trauma.

602. The answer is B. *(Browner, pp 932–933.)* Radiographic criteria for acceptable alignment of middle third proximal phalangeal fractures include up to 10° of angulation in both sagittal and coronal planes. Up to 50 percent displacement at the fracture site is also acceptable. No rotational deformity, however, should be accepted. For metaphyseal fractures, up to 20° of angulation in the sagittal plane is acceptable.

603. The answer is D. *(Browner, pp 593–599.)* The anterior pin for a halo ring is best placed at a point just above the lateral third of the eyebrow. This is the area of thickest cranial bone and also lies just lateral to the supraorbital nerve. The supratrochlear nerve and frontal sinus lie almost in the midline above the bridge of the nose. Excessively lateral insertion of the pins puts the temporal artery and temporalis muscle at risk for injury. If the halo pins are too high on the convexity of the skull, slippage of the ring may occur when traction is applied.

604. The answer is B. *(Browner, pp 593–599.)* Recommendations for the initial tightening of halo pins are 6 to 8 inch-pounds in the older child and the adult. Recent studies of the complications of halo pins have revealed a lower rate of pin loosening and infection with an initial tightening torque of 8 inch-pounds. Pins should be retightened within 24 to 48 h and thereafter only if they are grossly loose.

605. The answer is C. *(Kretzler, Am J Sports Med 17:453–458, 1989.)* Rupture of the pectoralis major muscle most commonly occurs during weight-lifting activities, such as the bench press. Pain, deformity, and weakness are present, but pain is generally the patient's greatest concern. The muscle nearly always ruptures near its humeral insertion and deformity is obvious with muscle contraction. Early repairs are generally effective and, though retraction following muscle rupture can occur, late reattachment is possible with good functional results.

606. The answer is D. *(Rockwood, Matsen, pp 436–467.)* Controversy has surrounded the treatment of grade 3 acromioclavicular injuries. Many authors state that the best results can be obtained by operative treatment in those who do heavy labor and in young athletes. A review of the literature, however, shows that clinical results are similar following operative and nonoperative treatment. In one study, operatively treated patients had less abduction strength than did nonoperatively treated patients; however, other outcome parameters were comparable in the two groups. Complications with operative treatment have been reported in up to 50 percent of cases.

607. The answer is E. *(Poss, p 354.)* Disruption of the scapholunate ligament associated with angulated or displaced fractures of the carpal scaphoid should be suspected in patients with scaphoid fractures that do not reduce with the usual reduction maneuvers. The chance of an excellent functional outcome is decreased if a ruptured ligament is left unrepaired in the setting of an angulated or displaced scaphoid fracture.

608. The answer is A. *(Gelberman, J Bone Joint Surg 71-A:1560–1565, 1989.)* Although there are no studies specifically addressing late recognition of nondisplaced scaphoid fractures, nondisplaced fractures of the scaphoid can be effectively treated with cast immobilization up to 6 months after injury. Displaced or angulated fractures diagnosed late, however, require internal fixation and bone grafting after correction of the deformity. CT scanning is not indicated because the diagnosis can be made with plain radiographs.

609. The answer is B. *(Sandberg, J Bone Joint Surg 69-A:1120–1126, 1987.)* Studies indicate that isolated tears of the medial collateral ligament heal well when treated nonoperatively. Treatment is functional with the use of controlled flexion in a hinged brace to allow motion and prevent valgus stress. Patients treated in this manner regain strength and mobility more rapidly than patients treated with above-knee casting.

610. The answer is B. *(Josefsson, J Bone Joint Surg 69-A:605–608, 1987.)* Open reduction of simple elbow dislocations is rarely indicated. A recent prospective study showed no significant difference between the results of operative and nonoperative treatment of simple dislocations if no instability is present following reduction. Immobilization need be for only 7 to 10 days. If elbow instability is noted following concentric reduction, the elbow should be immobilized at 90° for 3 weeks. There were no redislocations or chronic instabilities in patients treated by this method. Immobilization beyond 3 weeks has significant adverse effects, including loss of motion and elbow flexion contracture.

611. The answer is D. *(Ovadia, J Bone Joint Surg 70-A:239–243, 1988.)* The most frequent complication with removal of Zickel nails is refracture of the proximal femur. This fracture nearly always occurs a few centimeters distal to the lesser trochanter, is often nondisplaced, and is occasionally not recognized intraoperatively.

612. The answer is C. *(Hougard, J Bone Joint Surg 69-A:679–683, 1987.)* A recent study indicated that a good result is obtained in only 31 percent of hip fracture/dislocations that are unstable after reduction. The age of the patient played a much smaller role in producing poor results. Open reduction, irrigation of the hip joint, and early weight-bearing or range of motion carried no negative implications.

613. The answer is E. *(Browner, pp 1350–1351.)* The management of all patients following closed reduction of a hip dislocation should include a CT scan of the hip and pelvis. Sections at 3-mm intervals through the entire acetabulum should be obtained and processed for bone and soft-tissue windows. The femoral head should be carefully analyzed for fractures or depressions, and the acetabulum should be examined for depression fractures. Finally, the presence of osteochondral fragments in the joint should be noted. Displaced fractures or incarcerated osteochondral fragments may require open reduction or removal.

614. The answer is E. *(Tencer, J Orthop Res 2:297–305, 1984.)* In a detailed evaluation of implant devices used for fixation of subtrochanteric fractures of the femur, a blade plate was found to have the highest resistance to torsional deformation. Blade plates were about 50 percent as stiff as the intact femur in torsion, while locked intramedullary nails were only 5 percent as stiff. Zickel nails and conventional femoral nails inserted without interlocks provided essentially no rotational resistance. In all modes of loading, Ender's nails were weaker in stabilizing subtrochanteric fractures than the other devices tested.

615. The answer is C. *(Sanders, J Bone Joint Surg 75-A:778–789, 1993.)* Although antibiotic prophylaxis, irrigation, skeletal stabilization, and soft-tissue coverage are all important aspects of the treatment of open tibial fractures, adequate, thorough, and complete debridement remains the single most important factor in attaining good results following these injuries. The common error made at the time of initial debridement is underestimation of the amount of muscle and soft-tissue damage. Failure to perform a thorough debridement places the patient at increased risk for infection, nonunion, and a poor clinical result.

616. The answer is C. *(Sanders, J Bone Joint Surg 75-A:778–789, 1993.)* Open fracture wounds are contaminated, and antibiotic treatment must be effective against gram-positive organisms, specifically *Staphylococcus aureus*, and gram-negative organisms. Most surgeons recommend a first- or second-generation cephalosporin with an aminoglycoside for grade III open fractures. If the injury is farm- or soil-related or has a severe crushing component, or if vascular compromise is present, penicillin G should be added as a third antibiotic.

617. The answer is D. *(Veitch, J Trauma 19:201–202, 1989.)* The organism most commonly associated with infections following cat bites is *Pasteurella multocida*. Aspiration at the site of infection is likely to reveal a thin, serous, cloudy fluid containing gram-negative rods. The drug of choice for treatment of this infection is penicillin.

618. The answer is E. *(Patzakis, Clin Orthop 220:237–240, 1987.)* Clenched fist injuries over the metacarpophalangeal joints usually penetrate the underlying joint or metacarpal. Trauma to the cartilage or bone and seeding of the metacarpophalangeal joint with bacteria are common. Surgical exploration and debridement of these deeper structures should be performed and intravenous antibiotics should be administered. Primary closure of the wound is contraindicated.

619. The answer is B. *(Bone, Instr Course Lect 37:557–563, 1986.)* Adult respiratory distress syndrome (ARDS) is a result of the complex sequelae of shock, systemic sepsis, trauma, or other insults. It affects approximately 150,000 persons annually and has a mortality of up to 50 percent. Clinically, it is characterized by declining arterial oxygen tension, decreased pulmonary compliance, and increased pulmonary vascular resistance. Analysis of serial blood gases is the most sensitive and earliest method of detecting ARDS. Bilateral diffuse alveolar infiltrates appear on chest radiographs only after ARDS is well established.

620. The answer is D. *(Fitzgerald, pp 71–82.)* *Staphylococcus epidermidis* is one of the most common organisms causing infection following implant surgery. Some microbiology laboratories report *S. epidermidis* as a skin contaminant and do not routinely perform sensitivity studies. An aspirate from deep in the tissues sent for culture and sensitivities can provide valuable information about the organisms involved in the infection. Increased uptake on a bone scan is not specific for infection only 6 weeks following fracture. An MRI scan would be difficult due to the implanted hardware, and operative debridement is not indicated until the diagnosis of deep infection is established.

621. The answer is A. *(Browner, pp 142–143.)* Rupture of the bladder or disruption of the membranous urethra is the most common genitourinary injury following displaced anterior pelvic fractures, occurring in 15 percent of cases. Evaluation of a suspected genitourinary injury should begin with a retrograde urethrogram prior to insertion of a Foley catheter. If the urethra is intact and hematuria is present, evaluation should proceed to a cystogram.

622. The answer is A. *(Poss, p 499.)* Optimal stability of femoral neck fractures against torsion and bending is achieved by fixation with multiple screws or pins. Sliding hip screw devices are generally reserved for intertrochanteric fractures or for fractures at the base of the femoral neck. Ender's nails are not indicated in the treatment of femoral neck fractures. A biomechanical study showed no justification for the use of more than three pins or screws, regardless of the type of implant chosen.

623. The answer is C. *(Browner, pp 869–872.)* The CT scan has revolutionized the assessment of injury to the posterior pelvic ring and is mandatory to determine the exact nature of injury. Inlet and outlet radiographs of the pelvis are important in assessing pelvic trauma, but are not as sensitive or as accurate as CT scanning. CT scanning with three-dimensional reconstruction can be helpful, but is time-consuming and often affords no advantage over standard CT scans. MRI scans currently play no role in the evaluation of pelvic trauma.

624. The answer is D. *(Smith, J Orthop Res 8:471–478, 1990.)* All internal fixation devices disturb diaphyseal circulation to some extent. The endosteal circulation of bone is much more important in supplying cortical blood flow than is the periosteal circulation. Thus, reamed intramedullary nailing produces the greatest injury to cortical circulation, resulting in the longest delay in revascularization. Unreamed intramedullary nailing is associated with more rapid revascularization because of the increased space between the implant and the endosteal surface. Plate and screw systems do not disturb the endosteal vascular supply. External fixation results in the least injury to cortical blood flow.

625. The answer is A. *(Epstein, J Bone Joint Surg 56-A:1103–1129, 1974.)* The length of time before reduction is a critical factor in the development of posttraumatic avascular necrosis of the femoral head following dislocations of the hip with and without associated fractures of the femoral head or acetabular lip. A dislocation of the hip requires closed or open reduction as soon as possible. A posterior surgical approach may jeopardize the vascular supply, but the length of time to reduction is a more critical factor. Other systemic injuries generally play no role in the development of osteonecrosis of the femoral head.

626. The answer is C. *(Sanders, J Bone Joint Surg 75-A:778–789, 1993.)* The location and severity of soft-tissue injury is the most important variable influencing the choice of skeletal stabilization following an open tibial fracture. Severe soft-tissue injuries require a method of stabilization that minimizes further injury to the vascular supply to the bone. Skeletal stabilization should also allow easy access for wound care or additional operative procedures. The fracture pattern may play a role in the form of stabilization used, but the severity of the soft-tissue injury is the more important variable. The age of the patient and the presence of other musculoskeletal injuries rarely determine the method of skeletal stabilization.

627. The answer is C. *(Gelberman, J Bone Joint Surg 75-A:1854–1878, 1993.)* Acute compression of the median nerve following fractures of the distal radius is being recognized with increasing frequency. The two factors most often associated with increased carpal canal pressure in this setting are the use of a circular cast and immobilization of the wrist in a position of flexion. When a patient complains of numbness in the distribution of the median nerve following reduction and immobilization of a distal radial fracture, the cast or splint should be immediately removed and the wrist extended to neutral. If symptoms do not improve within 2 to 4 h, measurement of carpal canal interstitial pressure, release of the transverse carpal ligament, or both are indicated.

628. The answer is B. *(Helal, Hand 14:41–47, 1982.)* Spontaneous rupture of the extensor pollicis longus tendon occurs following approximately 5 percent of distal radial fractures and can occur after minimally displaced fractures. Rupture most commonly occurs between 5 and 8 weeks following injury. Compression of the posterior interosseous nerve, compartment syndrome of the forearm, and displacement of the fracture are all unlikely to occur 5 weeks after fracture. Arthritis of the basilar joint of the thumb would not result in a sudden inability to extend the thumb.

629. The answer is D. *(Edwards, Clin Orthop 234:61–66, 1988.)* Disruption of the interosseous membrane and the distal radioulnar joint can occur in association with a fracture of the radial head. Radiographs of the entire forearm should be obtained in any patient with a radial head fracture. Although initial radiographic findings can be normal at the distal radioulnar joint, physical examination will reveal tenderness at this site. When recognized acutely, this may be an indication for open reduction and internal fixation or prosthetic replacement of the radial head.

630. The answer is C. *(Arntz, J Bone Joint Surg 70-A:173–181, 1988.)* Patients with fracture-dislocations of the tarsometatarsal joints do best with anatomic reduction and internal fixation. The fracture pattern, method of postoperative immobilization, and the method of stable internal fixation do not affect the functional outcome. The amount of damage to the articular surfaces has been shown to be directly related to the amount of pain and posttraumatic arthritis in patients treated with anatomic reduction and stable internal fixation.

631. The answer is D. *(Gelberman, J Bone Joint Surg 71-A:1560–1565, 1989.)* Follow-up studies of patients with nonunion of the scaphoid have revealed a high probability of the development of posttraumatic intercarpal arthritis. This natural history is unaffected by bracing of the wrist for strenuous activities. Radial styloidectomy may provide temporary relief of symptoms, but does not address the basic problem. Bone grafting and rigid internal fixation of the scaphoid provide optimal preservation of wrist function with the least risk of degenerative arthritis.

632. The answer is B. *(Browner, pp 1303–1305.)* Clavicular nonunions are uncommon; when they occur, they are usually in the central one-third of the bone and are hypertrophic nonunions. They have been associated with pain, functional limitation of the shoulder, and local compression of the subclavian vessels or brachial plexus. Surgery for cosmetic reasons alone is likely to be disappointing because the scar tissue generated at surgery may be as disfiguring as the prominence of the clavicular nonunion.

633. The answer is D. *(Browner, pp 1210–1213.)* Avulsion of the greater tuberosity occurs in 10 to 25 percent of anterior dislocations of the shoulder. If the greater tuberosity reduces to within 1 cm of its anatomic location following reduction of the shoulder dislocation, treatment with immobilization or gentle motion is indicated. Displacement of more than 1 cm is associated with a high incidence of late subacromial impingement, and open reduction, internal fixation, and rotator cuff repair are indicated.

634. The answer is D. *(Browner, pp 1181–1186.)* Closed, isolated fractures of the humeral shaft can be successfully treated by a variety of methods of supportive immobilization. Operative treatment is generally not indicated for these fractures. Although hanging arm casts, Velpeau dressings, and shoulder spica casts have been used successfully in the treatment of these fractures, all restrict shoulder and elbow motion. Functional bracing is the treatment of choice in these fractures; it provides adequate immobilization, but allows shoulder and elbow motion.

635. The answer is C. *(Browner, pp 1025–1027.)* Although any of these studies might confirm a suspected fracture of the scaphoid, three-phase bone scanning is the most reliable and sensitive. If the bone scan is negative, a fracture of the scaphoid has been ruled out. If the bone scan is positive, more specific studies such as tomography or CT scanning may be helpful. Arthroscopy of the wrist is unlikely to show a fracture not seen on plain radiographs but might be helpful in the diagnosis of a disruption of the scapholunate ligament.

636. The answer is E. *(Browner, pp 285–309.)* The earliest pathogenic factor in the production of an acute compartmental syndrome is increased tissue pressure, without which a compartmental syndrome cannot occur. Clinical manifestations of an acute compartmental syndrome include pain disproportionate to the injury, an alteration in sensation, a decrease in capillary refill, pain on passive stretch of the tendons traversing the compartment, and pulselessness. It must be remembered, however, that elevated tissue pressure, by definition, must precede the development of clinical signs and symptoms. The use of tissue pressure measurements allows the physician to diagnose acute compartment syndrome in the incipient rather than in the fulminant stage.

637. The answer is E. *(Browner, pp 285–309.)* If not treated promptly, a compartmental syndrome may progress to Volkmann's ischemic contracture. The only effective way of decompressing an acute compartmental syndrome is by surgical fasciotomy. Whatever surgical approach is used, it is mandatory that both the superficial and deep volar compartments be decompressed. There is some disagreement about the pressure beyond which fasciotomy is indicated, but pressures greater than 40 mmHg strongly indicate the need for fasciotomy.

638. The answer is C. *(Browner, pp 285–309.)* An incipient compartmental syndrome is defined as a compartmental syndrome that will develop if appropriate steps are not taken to prevent it. It is imperative to release tight dressings and casts; 40 percent less volume is required to raise intracompartmental pressures to equivalent levels in patients who are casted than in those who are not casted. Univalving a cast decreases intracompartmental pressures only 30 percent, while bivalving the cast and cast padding beneath results in a 55 percent decrease. Strict elevation of the limb in patients with incipient compartmental syndrome may result in reduced blood flow to the compartment and worsening of symptoms.

639. The answer is E. *(Bone, J Bone Joint Surg 68-A:945–949, 1986).* The polytraumatized patient has a much lower morbidity due to pulmonary problems and a better chance of recovery of function if treated by early stabilization of major long bone fractures. Overall nursing care and patient comfort, mobilization, and rehabilitation are also improved by early reduction and fixation of fractures. In this specific instance, fixation of the fractures of the upper limb would allow earlier elbow and wrist motion, return to self-care activities, and return to independent function.

640. The answer is C. *(Browner, pp 127–145.)* The history and physical examination of this patient indicate trauma to the head and face. Patients with blunt trauma to the head and maxillofacial region should be presumed to have an injury of the cervical spine until proved otherwise by radiographs. A pelvic radiograph will be obtained as part of the trauma evaluation, but, in this patient, the cervical spine radiograph has higher priority.

641. The answer is C. *(Browner, pp 134–135.)* The three traumatic conditions most often compromising ventilation in the hypoxemic patient whose condition does not improve with intubation and an increase in inspired oxygen are tension pneumothorax, open pneumothorax, and a large flail chest with pulmonary contusion. Decreased breath sounds in the right hemothorax suggest a tension pneumothorax, which is a clinical rather than a radiographic diagnosis. The initial management is insertion of a large-caliber needle in the second intercostal space at the midclavicular line. The definitive management is insertion of a chest tube.

642. The answer is C. *(Browner, pp 137–138.)* Initial resuscitation of a traumatized patient in shock consists of a 2000-mL bolus of Ringer's lactate solution. In this case, there is only a transient response to the fluid bolus, which indicates at least a class III hemorrhage. This patient requires continued administration of Ringer's lactate and immediate blood transfusion. Ringer's lactate is preferable to normal saline as a resuscitation fluid, and albumin is inferior to blood as colloid. No clinical indication for intubation exists. Hypotensive patients with collapsed veins should not have a central venous catheter inserted because of the risk of iatrogenic injury.

643. The answer is A. *(Maddox, p 115.)* The pH and P_{CO_2} of this patient indicate a metabolic acidosis partially corrected by hyperventilation. This, combined with the low bicarbonate level, indicates that the patient is inadequately resuscitated. The patient should receive more intravenous fluid to reduce hypovolemia. Administration of bicarbonate in a hypovolemic patient is contraindicated. There is no clinical indication for intubation, administration of more oxygen, or administration of dopamine.

644. The answer is D. *(Browner, pp 140–141.)* The radiograph in the figure shows a widened mediastinum. A traumatic injury of the aorta must be suspected in any patient with a history of a deceleration injury, such as that sustained in a head-on motor vehicle accident. Clues to the presence of an aortic injury include a widened mediastinum, fractures of the clavicle or upper two ribs, obliteration of the aortic knob, and deviation of the trachea and esophagus to the right. The diagnosis of aortic injury can be made definitively with an arch aortogram.

645. The answer is D. *(Browner, pp 1724–1729.)* The initial management of a posterior dislocation of the knee should be closed reduction. A complete neurologic and vascular examination should be performed prior to and following reduction. The necessity of arteriography following these injuries has been questioned recently. Open reduction is needed only if closed reduction fails. Application of a circular cast or constricting dressing is contraindicated for a dislocation of the knee. Immobilization with an external fixator may follow reduction but is not the *initial* management.

646. The answer is B. *(Browner, pp 133–134.)* In a patient with suspected cervical spine injury, it is critical that extension of the cervical spine be maintained during the management of the airway. Nasotracheal intubation is preferred for patients with an injury of the cervical spine who require intubation. Cricothyroidotomy is indicated in the apneic patient in whom nasotracheal intubation has been unsuccessful. Needle tracheostomy is not necessary in this situation, and open tracheostomy is reserved for the semielective setting.

647. The answer is C. *(Browner, pp 1799–1800.)* In a patient with a closed tibial fracture and acute compartmental syndrome requiring fasciotomies, the tibial fracture should be treated as though it were an open fracture. Although the fasciotomy dissection does not go down to bone, the vascular supply of the tibia is decreased because of the compartmental syndrome. Unreamed, locked, intramedullary nailing or external fixation is the preferred method of immobilization in this situation. Reamed intramedullary nailing and plate osteosynthesis may further disrupt the blood supply to the tibia. Above-knee casting and skeletal traction, though effectively immobilizing the fracture, do not allow close observation and easy care of the open fasciotomy wounds.

648. The answer is C. *(Bone, J Bone Joint Surg 68-A:945–949, 1986.)* An anteroposterior radiograph of the chest and pelvis and a lateral radiograph of the cervical spine are required for the evaluation of all multiply injured patients. After emergency laparotomy, the diagnosis of other injuries should proceed only after review of the chest, pelvic, and spinal radiographs.

649. The answer is A. *(Swiontkowski, Orthop Clin North Am 18:73–84, 1987.)* Ipsilateral fractures of the femoral neck occur in association with approximately 2.5 percent of fractures of the femoral shaft. The fracture of the femoral neck was missed on initial evaluation in 34 percent of published cases. Avascular necrosis of the femoral head followed less than 5 percent of these fractures.

650. The answer is A. *(Browner, pp 1632–1634.)* Successful treatment of an infected femoral shaft fracture requires fracture stability. If the intramedullary nail is providing stable fixation of the fracture, it should be left in place until union occurs. If the fracture is not stably fixed, the fixation device should be removed and stable fixation obtained. The primary goal is to achieve union of the fracture, followed by irradication of the infection. Neither skeletal traction, cast bracing, nor a combination of the two provides sufficient fracture stabilization to secure union.

651. The answer is D. *(Browner, pp 1625–1628.)* In most large series of femoral shaft fractures treated with closed, intramedullary nailing, the nonunion rate is less than 1 percent. In the absence of infection, treatment of a nonunion of the femoral shaft is straightforward. If an intramedullary nail is in place, simple exchange nailing with a nail 2 mm larger encourages fracture healing. Interlocking screws are usually unnecessary for simple nonunion patterns, and bone grafting is generally not required. There is virtually no place for the use of electrical stimulation in the treatment of nonunion or delayed union of a fracture of the femoral shaft.

652. The answer is B. *(Rockwood, pp 2093–2100.)* A subtalar dislocation is the simultaneous dislocation of the talocalcaneal and talonavicular joints. Medial dislocations are more common, are a result of inversion of the foot, and heal more rapidly than do lateral subtalar dislocations. Medial subtalar dislocations are generally stable following closed reduction, and avascular necrosis of the talus is rare, probably because the talus is not disrupted from the ankle mortise. The outcome of this injury is related to the mechanism, with low-energy injuries healing much more rapidly than high-energy, lateral subtalar dislocations.

653. The answer is D. *(Browner, pp 1578–1580.)* In the multiply injured patient, stabilization of a fracture of the femoral shaft in the first 24 h is critical for patient mobility, which allows better care of other injuries. Immediate stabilization decreases the incidence of pulmonary complications, such as fat embolism and ARDS. There is no increase in the rates of infection, nonunion, or shortening with delayed treatment of fractures of the femoral shaft.

654. The answer is D. *(Browner, p 1195.)* Radial nerve palsy occurs following up to 18 percent of closed fractures of the humeral shaft. More than 90 percent of palsies are neuropraxias in which radial nerve function will return spontaneously within 3 to 4 months of injury. In the absence of neurologic recovery, radial nerve dysfunction should be evaluated 6 weeks after injury by electromyography and nerve conduction studies. If fibrillation potentials are present, nonoperative management may be continued. However, if denervation is noted, operative treatment is indicated.

655. The answer is E. *(Sanders, J Bone Joint Surg 75-A:778–789, 1993.)* Initial antibiotic therapy in grade III open fractures of the tibia should include a cephalosporin and an aminoglycoside. Open fractures sustained in soil have the added potential for anaerobic infection, for which the addition of penicillin to the cephalosporin and aminoglycoside is strongly recommended.

656. The answer is C. *(Browner, pp 1402–1403.)* Stabilization of the fracture of the femoral neck must take precedence over that of the fracture of the femoral shaft because of the poor results of treatment of posttraumatic avascular necrosis. The neck fracture should be stabilized first, followed by treatment of the shaft fracture. With careful placement of the screws stabilizing the neck fracture, intramedullary nailing of the shaft fracture can be completed without the risk of further damage to the blood supply of the femoral head.

657. The answer is E. *(Browner, pp 140–142.)* Rib fractures constitute 40 percent of thoracic injuries from blunt trauma. Pulmonary and cardiac contusions occur less frequently and are often associated with multiple rib fractures. Pneumothoraces are also infrequent and are commonly associated with rib fractures. Aortic arch ruptures are very rare, but can be associated with fractures of the first or second ribs.

658. The answer is A. *(Browner, pp 337–366.)* Although early and complete debridement is the key to successful treatment of open fractures, obtaining prompt wound coverage with viable soft tissue is also of great importance. If possible, open fracture wounds should be covered within a week and before the wound is secondarily colonized with bacteria. Skin grafting is useful in areas covered with granulation tissue, but is not indicated to cover exposed bone. The medial gastrocnemius muscle flap is an excellent means of covering small defects on the medial side of the proximal third of the tibia. A free flap is indicated only if local muscle flaps are not adequate to cover the defect.

659. The answer is D. *(Browner, pp 1195–1197.)* Nonunion of humeral shaft fractures develops in 2 to 5 percent of nonoperatively managed injuries and in 25 percent of fractures managed by primary operation. Treatment of an established nonunion entails open reduction, bone grafting, and stable fixation. Plate osteosynthesis is preferred in patients with good bone stock, in midshaft fractures, and in hypertrophic nonunions with residual angulation. Intramedullary stabilization is preferred in patients with severe osteopenia, pathologic fractures, and fractures of the proximal third of the humerus.

660. The answer is D. *(Browner, pp 285–310.)* Compartmental syndromes may occur after closed, intramedullary nailing of the tibia and are probably caused by an expanding hematoma within a closed space, augmented by distraction of the limb and reaming. The diagnosis of acute compartmental syndrome is a clinical one, but the clinical findings are less reliable in a patient with a possible neurologic injury related to a fracture of the lumbar spine. The pressures should be measured in all four compartments and therapy based on intracompartmental pressures.

661. The answer is E. *(Browner, pp 1977–1982.)* The tarsometatarsal joints of the foot are very stable and are injured only by high-energy forces. The outcome following treatment of these injuries is related directly to the quality of reduction achieved; a 5-mm displacement at the first metatarsocuneiform joint is not adequate reduction. Open reduction and internal fixation with either screws or Kirschner wires should be performed.

662. The answer is D. *(Browner, pp 1878–1880.)* An inversion injury to the ankle would be expected to injure one or more of the lateral ankle ligaments. The anterior talofibular ligament is the primary support against inversion with the ankle in plantar flexion. The calcaneofibular ligament is brought into alignment with the fibula with dorsiflexion of the ankle. As the primary restraint to inversion in this position, it is the ligament most likely to be injured.

663. The answer is C. *(Browner, pp 1255–1257.)* Posterior dislocations of the shoulder are associated with fractures of the lesser tuberosity in 1.3 percent of cases. Sudden, marked internal rotation of the shoulder causes the lesser tuberosity to strike the glenoid, occasionally resulting in fracture. Anterior shoulder dislocations are commonly associated with greater tuberosity fractures.

664. The answer is A. *(Browner, pp 1251–1255.)* Fractures of the greater tuberosity constitute 14 percent of displaced proximal humeral fractures. Displacement is superior and posterior. Codman described this injury as one of the worst possible humeral fractures, since the supraspinatus is disrupted with fracture displacement. Displacement of the greater tuberosity of more than 5 to 10 mm is an indication for reduction and stabilization. A superiorly displaced greater tuberosity may heal to the articular surface of the humeral head and block forward elevation of the shoulder, resulting in stiffness, weakness, and pain. Early surgery is preferred to avoid this complication.

665. The answer is B. *(Pape, J Trauma 35:709–716, 1993.)* The advantages of immediate stabilization of long bone fractures in polytraumatized patients have been well established. Immediate stabilization results in lower morbidity, shorter ICU stays, and earlier mobilization. With the currently available intramedullary nails, adequate stabilization can be achieved either with reamed or unreamed techniques. Recent studies showed that in multiply injured patients, especially those with potential pulmonary contusions, reamed intramedullary nailing was associated with a deterioration of pulmonary function in the 48 h following surgery. Unreamed femoral nailing was not associated with changes in pulmonary function, thus reducing the risk of ARDS.

666. The answer is E. *(Browner, pp 358–359.)* In the distal third of the leg, coverage of soft-tissue defects with local muscle flaps is extremely difficult. Gastrocnemius and soleus muscle flaps will not reach the defect, and a flexor hallucis longus muscle flap is too small to cover a defect of this size. A free muscle transfer is the procedure of choice, with primary donor sites being the latissimus dorsi and the rectus abdominis muscles.

667. The answer is E. *(Browner, pp 1549–1553.)* Fractures of the femoral shaft in patients over 12 years of age should be treated as in adults. These patients are too large to be easily cared for in traction or a hip spica cast. Physiologically, bone development at this age is quite similar to that in an adult, with the exception of the open distal femoral physis. The greater trochanteric apophysis is well developed by age 12, and any injury to this area caused by intramedullary nailing will not result in significant disturbance of growth. Care should be taken not to penetrate the distal femoral physis.

668. The answer is E. *(Browner, pp 346–348.)* The workhorse for coverage of large soft-tissue defects on the dorsum of the hand and forearm is the groin flap. It almost always provides adequate tissue for coverage of defects on the dorsum of the hand, the wrist, and the distal forearm. Split thickness or full thickness skin grafting should not be performed over exposed extensor tendons or bone. The defect is too large for a rotation skin flap or a local muscle flap. A free muscle flap would provide coverage but is more difficult and less reliable than the pedicle groin flap. Free flaps should be reserved for larger and more complex defects in the hand and forearm.

669. The answer is D. *(Macy, J Am Acad Orthop Surg 2:36–43, 1994.)* Understanding the fracture pattern in acute calcaneal fractures is dependent on appropriate radiographic evaluation. Lateral and axial radiographs are essential for the preliminary investigation of the fracture. A Broden's view visualizes the posterior facet of the subtalar joint but is not as accurate as CT scanning for assessing the extent of comminution and congruity of the subtalar joint. MRI scanning is inferior to CT scanning in assessing the subtalar joint.

670. The answer is B. *(Browner, pp 849–899.)* Transiliac threaded bars may be used for internal fixation of posterior pelvic injuries, except when bilateral posterior pelvic disruption is present. Overtightening the nuts on transiliac bars can result in injury to a lumbosacral nerve root. Care must be taken not to compress the posterior fracture site when using this form of posterior pelvic stabilization.

671. The answer is C. *(Browner, pp 729–805.)* The figure shows a burst fracture of the L2 vertebra with approximately 15° of kyphosis and 60 percent compromise of the spinal canal caused by retropulsion of the posterior vertebral body fragment. The most critical factors determining the treatment of lumbar burst fractures are the amount of kyphosis, the neurologic condition of the patient, and the amount of spinal canal compromise. Kyphosis greater than 25° in the presence of an incomplete or progressive neurologic deficit is an indication for operative reduction and instrumentation. For the patient with intact neurologic function, the indications for operation are less clear, but many authors feel that greater than 25° of kyphosis or greater than 40 to 50 percent canal compromise warrants reduction and instrumentation. Laminectomy has no place in the treatment of burst fractures. Anterior decompression and instrumentation are indicated for burst fractures treated more than 1 to 2 weeks after injury and for fracture-dislocations with marked instability of the spine. Nonoperative treatment is a viable option for this patient, but would best consist of 1 to 2 weeks of bed rest, followed by mobilization in an extension orthosis.

672. The answer is C. *(Browner, pp 849–899.)* The figure shows a pubic symphysis diastasis and a vertical fracture through the sacrum. The patient is in hypovolemic shock as evidenced by the absence of a blood pressure response to fluid bolus. Although the patient may have other intraabdominal sources of hemorrhage, immediate external skeletal fixation of the anterior pelvis is indicated in this hemodynamically unstable patient. MAST trousers and a pelvic sling do not allow further examination or evaluation of the abdomen. Immediate internal fixation of anterior and posterior pelvic fractures is not appropriate for a hemodynamically unstable patient. Exploratory laparotomy to control intraabdominal sources of hemorrhage may be needed in this patient, but should be preceded by external fixation of the pelvis.

673. The answer is E. *(Browner, pp 849–899.)* The figure shows a vertical shear pelvic injury, with the posterior disruption occurring through the iliac wing. Nonoperative treatment would require lengthy immobilization of the patient and would likely result in an inequality of leg length. Late pain is common after nonoperative treatment of these injuries. Transilial bars and transilial sacral screws are not indicated because the fracture site is lateral to the insertion point of these fixation devices. The most appropriate treatment would be open reduction and internal fixation with plates and screws.

674. The answer is C. *(Browner, pp 1045–1053.)* The figure shows a transscaphoid perilunate fracture-dislocation. The mechanism of this injury, as in most carpal dislocations and fracture-dislocations, is axial loading of the hyperextended wrist. The most common carpal dislocations are the dorsal perilunate and volar lunate dislocations. The transscaphoid perilunate fracture-dislocation occurs by a mechanism similar to that of the dorsal perilunate dislocation except that the energy transmitted through the waist of the scaphoid causes it to fracture. Anatomic reduction of the scapholunate interval and of the scaphoid fracture is essential in the treatment of this injury.

675. The answer is E. *(Browner, pp 1096–1111.)* Displaced diaphyseal fractures of the forearm in adults are best treated by open reduction and internal fixation. Figure *C* shows formation of a radioulnar synostosis. An increased propensity for the formation of heterotopic bone in patients sustaining closed head injuries has been well documented, as have increased synostosis rates. Operative technique, delay to operation, and failure to bone graft have not been associated with a higher incidence of heterotopic bone formation in fractures of the forearm.

676. The answer is D. *(Browner, pp 1553–1555.)* All open fractures of the femoral shaft require immediate irrigation and debridement in the operating room. Immediate intramedullary nailing of grade II open femoral shaft fractures is the treatment of choice; recent series have noted infection rates from 1 to 5 percent. The infection rate after delayed intramedullary nailing is no lower than after immediate nailing.

677. The answer is B. *(Browner, pp 1793–1803.)* All open tibial fractures should be treated with immediate irrigation, debridement, and skeletal stabilization. Immediate skeletal stabilization is especially indicated in the polytraumatized patient and in the patient with ipsilateral tibial and femoral shaft fractures. Unreamed intramedullary nailing is the treatment of choice in this patient, as intramedullary reaming causes greater injury to the endosteal blood supply, increasing ischemia at the fracture site.

678. The answer is E. *(Browner, pp 1154–1162.)* The figure shows a displaced, intraarticular fracture of the distal humerus. Although nonoperative treatment is occasionally indicated in the elderly patient, the patient with multiple medical problems, and the patient with a severely comminuted fracture, operative treatment is generally felt to give better results. Reduction and stabilization of both medial and lateral columns is paramount for obtaining stable fixation of bicondylar distal humeral fractures. Percutaneous pin fixation may provide adequate alignment of the fragments but is insufficient fixation for early mobilization of the elbow.

679. The answer is B. *(Browner, pp 1944–1951.)* The figure shows a distal fibular fracture with rupture of the deltoid ligament and lateral translation of the talus in the ankle mortise. Closed reduction and cast immobilization of this fracture might be adequate treatment, but an above-knee cast would be necessary to maintain reduction. The distal tibiofibular syndesmosis is intact, so transsyndesmotic screw fixation is not indicated. Repair of the deltoid ligament is usually unnecessary because late insufficiency of the deltoid ligament is rare.

680. The answer is D. *(Browner, pp 1754–1757.)* The figure shows a depressed fracture of the lateral tibial plateau with displacement of the articular fragments. Among the goals of treatment for tibial plateau fractures are restoration of joint congruity and maintenance of the maximum area for articular contact. Although the amount of displacement seen in this patient might be accepted in an elderly patient, this patient is young, and accurate reduction and stable fixation of the intraarticular fragments is necessary for knee alignment, articular cartilage regeneration, and avoidance of osteoarthritic changes. The most appropriate treatment for this patient is open reduction, internal fixation, and bone grafting, with no weight-bearing until healing of the fracture.

681. The answer is D. *(Browner, pp 1931–1941.)* All the listed choices have been reported as complications associated with open reduction and plate fixation of tibial pilon fractures. The complication rate has approached 55 percent in some series, compared with 18 percent after external fixation. The most frequent complication is a wound slough or dehiscence, which occurs in up to 30 percent of patients treated with open reduction and plate fixation. Attention to detail and meticulous handling of soft tissues are necessary if plating is used for the treatment of pilon fractures.

682. The answer is D. *(Hawkins, J Bone Joint Surg 69-A:9–16, 1987.)* The importance of early diagnosis of posterior dislocations of the shoulder is well known, yet many are missed on the initial physical examination. Posterior dislocations of the shoulder more than 3 weeks old are rarely reducible by closed means, even under general anesthesia. An anterior surgical approach is generally preferred for these injuries, since it allows lengthening of the subscapularis tendon or transfer of the lesser tuberosity into the anterior humeral head defect. Following reduction of a posterior dislocation, the shoulder should be immobilized in slight external rotation to reduce tension on the attenuated posterior capsule.

683. The answer is C. *(Browner, pp 1113–1117.)* The figure shows a radial shaft fracture and a disruption of the distal radioulnar joint (DRUJ), a combination known as a *Galeazzi fracture*. Campbell, in 1941, termed this injury "a fracture of necessity," meaning that operative treatment is necessary for a satisfactory outcome. Stable internal fixation is most reliably achieved with a compression plate and screws. The DRUJ is then assessed; if it is unstable with forearm rotation, the patient is immobilized in supination for 4 to 6 weeks.

684. The answer is E. *(Browner, pp 1186–1192.)* The figure shows a fracture of the humeral shaft with unacceptable angular deformity in a patient with bilateral upper and lower limb fractures. Two indications for operative treatment of humeral shaft fractures are the failure to obtain or maintain reduction by closed techniques and a polytraumatized patient with multiple limb fractures. Plate osteosynthesis is the preferred method of internal fixation of humeral shaft fractures. External skeletal fixation is indicated primarily for extremely comminuted or open fractures with extensive soft-tissue injuries.

685. The answer is D. *(Browner, pp 1984–1986.)* The figure shows a fracture of the proximal metaphysis of the fifth metatarsal. The sclerotic bone edges confirm that the fracture is old, and the patient's increasing pain confirms that it is not healing. Although non-weight-bearing immobilization may be appropriate for an acute fracture, it is not the best treatment for delayed union. Although bone grafting alone may promote union, fracture stabilization will allow the patient normal ambulation. The best treatment would be intramedullary screw fixation and bone grafting of the delayed union.

686. The answer is E. *(Browner, pp 1088–1091.)* The figure shows loss of fixation of the distal radial fracture with volar displacement of the distal fragment. Significant deformity and disability would be anticipated if the fracture were allowed to heal in this position. Nineteen days following the fracture, it is unlikely that a closed reduction could be achieved. Open reduction is necessary to restore anatomic alignment.

687. The answer is C. *(Browner, pp 1908–1917.)* The figure shows no fracture, but there is widening of the distal tibiofibular syndesmosis. Syndesmotic widening coupled with an external rotation injury and tenderness over the distal tibiofibular syndesmosis should lead one to suspect a Maisonneuve fracture. Radiographs of the proximal fibula will show the fracture and confirm the need for operative stabilization of the syndesmosis.

688. The answer is D. *(Browner, pp 954–959).* Isolated fractures of the metacarpal shaft with little or no displacement are usually stable and readily treated by casting with the MCP joints in 60 to 70° of flexion. Multiple displaced fractures of the metacarpal shafts, especially when associated with soft-tissue trauma, are an indication for open reduction and internal fixation. Each fractured metacarpal should be anatomically reduced and rigidly stabilized. External skeletal fixation is generally reserved for fractures with extensive soft-tissue injuries.

689. The answer is C. *(Browner, pp 1244–1249.)* Most fractures of the surgical neck of the humerus are stable once reduced by longitudinal traction, flexion, and abduction while applying a posteriorly directed force to the upper humerus. Occasionally, these fractures redisplace as soon as the surgeon releases traction on the arm. Options for treatment include percutaneous pinning, external fixation, and open reduction and internal fixation. Closed reduction with percutaneous pinning is the treatment of choice in this elderly patient with poor bone stock.

690. The answer is B. *(Browner, pp 1690–1704.)* The figure shows a marginal fracture of the patella with marked comminution. The fracture is nondisplaced and does not disrupt the extensor mechanism of the knee. Neither total patellectomy nor open reduction and internal fixation is indicated for this injury. Nonoperative treatment is an option, but the likelihood of retropatellar pain from multiple displaced fracture fragments makes operative excision of the fracture fragments the treatment of choice.

691. The answer is C. *(Browner, pp 1397–1402.)* Because of the risk of avascular necrosis, reduction and stabilization of displaced femoral neck fractures in young persons are matters of great urgency. In the multiply injured patient, treatment of the femoral neck fracture should be preceded only by the debridement of contaminated open fractures and reduction of dislocations of the cervical spine. Bipolar hemiarthroplasty has no place in the treatment of femoral neck fractures in young persons.

692. The answer is C. *(Browner, pp 1792–1799.)* The ideal treatment for limb fractures in multiply injured patients is immediate stabilization to allow early mobilization of the patient. The patient is generally most stable during the initial operation, and stabilization of the fractures should proceed unless life-threatening hemodynamic instability occurs. Because of the increasing ventilatory pressures in this patient, the tibial fracture should be stabilized rapidly, and the method of choice is external skeletal fixation. Intramedullary nailing is also a possibility, but reaming may increase pulmonary complications in a patient with increasing peak inspiratory pressures.

693. The answer is C. *(Browner, pp 1931–1941.)* The radiograph shows delayed union of the fracture without loss of position. The fracture configuration is not such that weight-bearing should be permitted. Although the fracture may unite with continued treatment in a non-weight-bearing cast, iliac crest bone grafting is advisable to speed union. Arthrodesis of the ankle and revision of the internal fixation are not indicated at this time.

694. The answer is D. *(Browner, pp 1694–1699.)* A noncomminuted transverse fracture of the patella almost always results from failure of the bone in tension. More than 3 mm of separation between the fracture fragments indicates disruption of the extensor retinacula and is an indication for operative repair. A large hemarthrosis is present in all cases. Because of the disruption of the extensor mechanism, the patient will be unable to extend the knee actively; passive extension should be normal.

695. The answer is B. *(Browner, p 1399.)* Internal fixation is indicated for undisplaced fractures of the femoral neck. Nonoperative treatment is associated with a higher mortality than is internal fixation. The rate of displacement of the fracture with nonoperative treatment is 10 to 27 percent, and the rate of avascular necrosis doubles if displacement of the fracture occurs, so internal fixation with multiple pins is justified. Hemiarthroplasty has no place in the treatment of nondisplaced femoral neck fractures.

696. The answer is D. *(Browner, pp 1399–1402.)* The best method for treating displaced fractures of the femoral neck in the very elderly is controversial. In very elderly, low-demand patients, unipolar hemiarthroplasty is probably the treatment of choice. Bipolar hemiarthroplasty and total hip arthroplasty are best indicated for somewhat younger patients with moderate functional demands. Nonoperative treatment is rarely indicated.

697. The answer is E. *(Browner, pp 963–966.)* The primary goals of treatment of intraarticular fractures involving the head of the metacarpal are anatomic restoration of the joint surface and fixation stable enough to permit active mobilization. Immediate mobilization without internal fixation is indicated only for the most severely comminuted fractures. Kirschner wires, although effective in holding the fragments in place, do not provide sufficient stability for early mobilization, and the pins may irritate the surrounding soft tissues. For these reasons, minifragment screws or Herbert screws are the treatment of choice in minimally comminuted fractures of the metacarpal head.

698. The answer is A. *(Browner, pp 1143–1145.)* The outcome following fracture-dislocations of the radial head is considerably worse than after either injury alone. When faced with fracture-dislocations of the radial head, effort should be made to maintain the radiohumeral articulation, either through open reduction and internal fixation or by replacement with a silicone rubber prosthesis. The medial collateral ligament is completely disrupted in nearly all dislocations of the elbow, but open reduction is rarely necessary.

699. The answer is A. *(Browner, pp 982–985.)* Transverse fractures of the proximal phalanx angulate with the apex toward the palm because the intrinsics lie dorsal to the long axis of the phalanx. The superficialis tendon attaches at the base of the middle phalanx. Nondisplaced fractures may be treated with buddy-taping, but displaced fractures must be reduced prior to treatment. If a stable reduction is achieved, extension block casting is adequate immobilization; instability following closed reduction, however, is an indication for percutaneous K-wire fixation. Clinical union will occur in approximately 3 weeks, but radiographic union may take as long as 6 weeks.

700. The answer is E. *(Rockwood, Green, pp 1685–1688.)* Nonunion or avascular necrosis of the femoral head has been reported in 5 percent of combined femoral neck and shaft fractures. To avoid this complication, most surgeons advise immediate open reduction and internal fixation (ORIF) of the femoral neck fracture. Enders' nailing of the femoral neck fracture does not provide rigid enough stabilization to allow early mobilization of the patient. The preferred method of fixation is antegrade intramedullary nailing of the femoral shaft fracture combined with multiple-screw fixation of the femoral neck fracture. Retrograde intramedullary nailing of the femoral shaft fracture has been reported, but this method is exceedingly difficult.

701. The answer is C. *(Rockwood, Green, pp 1617–1625.)* In this young patient with ipsilateral acetabular and femoral shaft fractures, the best outcome will be achieved with internal fixation of both fractures. Early mobilization of this multiply injured patient may be critical to his survival, and immediate intramedullary nailing of the femoral shaft fracture is advisable. Immediate ORIF of the acetabular fracture, however, is not advisable, as severe hemorrhage could result in exsanguination of this multiply injured patient. The best management is immediate intramedullary nailing of the femoral shaft fracture, followed by delayed ORIF of the acetabular fracture.

702. The answer is A. *(Rockwood, Green, pp 1793–1794.)* The radiographs demonstrate a supracondylar/intercondylar fracture of the distal femur treated with percutaneous screw and retrograde intramedullary nail fixation. The main advantage of this mode of fracture stabilization is that it minimizes surgical dissection around the fracture fragments, optimizing blood supply to the fracture. Nonunion is infrequent following this method of treatment, provided rigid stabilization is achieved. Malunion and failure of the implant are also infrequent following this mode of stabilization, providing the patient is kept non-weight-bearing until consolidation of the fracture is seen. This method of fixation provides adequate stabilization for early motion of the knee. The major drawback to operative fixation of supracondylar fractures of the femur remains the risk of infection, especially in open fractures.

703. The answer is E. *(Rockwood, Green, pp 1775–1776.)* Pain from retained hardware is common following ORIF of displaced patellar fractures and is usually related to tendon or ligament irritation by Kirschner wires. Loss of reduction, avascular necrosis, and nonunion are infrequent, each having an incidence of less than 2 percent. Wound infections following ORIF of closed patellar fractures occur in less than 3 percent of cases.

704. The answer is D. *(Rockwood, Green, pp 1594–1605.)* The figure shows a posterior dislocation of the hip without associated fracture. The closed reduction was performed within 6 h and resulted in a concentrically reduced, stable hip. Immobilization of this patient is to be condemned because it prevents early joint motion that enhances healing of the damaged articular cartilage. The optimal time to begin weight-bearing after reduction is debated; however, in a patient with a stable, concentric reduction of an isolated posterior dislocation of the hip, weight-bearing in 2 to 4 weeks is appropriate.

705. The answer is A. *(Rockwood, Green, pp 1619–1622.)* There are three main criteria for successful treatment of femoral neck fractures in a young patient: (1) fixation within 12 h of injury, (2) anatomic reduction, and (3) stabilization with multiple screws. Immediate stabilization with multiple screws of femoral neck fractures in young patients has resulted in lower rates of nonunion and avascular necrosis than has immediate stabilization with compression hip screws.

706. The answer is B. *(Rockwood, Green, pp 1729–1731.)* The radiographs reveal a lateral tibial plateau fracture with an area of central depression. There is no fracture line exiting the lateral tibial metaphysis as seen in a wedge fracture; nor is there subcondylar or medial plateau involvement. The CT scan of this patient's proximal tibia confirmed a simple depression fracture with the articular fragment depressed 1 cm.

707. The answer is E. *(Rockwood, Green, pp 1735–1739.)* Elevation of the articular fragments and bone grafting of the underlying defect offer the best results following treatment of depression fractures of the tibial plateau. Cast or brace immobilization of the knee following this procedure does not provide the cartilage nutrition provided by early knee motion. Supporting the elevated articular fragments with one or two cancellous screws permits early knee motion. Fractures with less than 6 mm of depression of the articular surface may be treated with minimal external support, early knee motion, and delayed weight-bearing.

708. The answer is A. *(Rockwood, Green, pp 1756–1757.)* The patient has sustained a comminuted, nondisplaced fracture of the subcondylar region of the tibia. Although irrigation and debridement of the entrance wound is indicated, removal of the bullet fragments is not necessary to achieve a good result. Operative treatment with internal or external fixation is rarely needed. Isolated subcondylar fractures are usually managed nonoperatively with an above-knee cast that immobilizes the knee in extension.

709. The answer is D. *(Rockwood, Green, pp 1952–1954.)* The radiographs show a nonunion with angulation of a distal tibial fracture. Although fibulotomy with posterolateral bone grafting might lead to union, it would not correct the malalignment. Intramedullary nailing would be extremely difficult for this distal fracture. Electrical stimulation should probably not be used if there is a gap of 1 cm or more at the fracture site. Plate fixation with bone grafting is the treatment of choice.

710. The answer is E. *(Rockwood, Green, pp 1952–1954.)* The radiographs reveal a hypertrophic nonunion of the tibial shaft with good alignment. Increased compression of the fracture site, as would occur with resection of 2 cm of the fibula, posterolateral bone grafting, and closed, reamed intramedullary nailing would be expected to promote union of this fracture. Electrical stimulation could be considered, even though its success rate has been variable. Take-down of a hypertrophic nonunion is not indicated unless malalignment is present, as it may increase rather than decrease the time to union.

711. The answer is C. *(Rockwood, Green, pp 1751–1759.)* The radiographs show a medial subtalar dislocation without an associated fracture. Following closed reduction, this dislocation is stable and can be immobilized in a below-knee cast or splint, with the expectation of a good result. Above-knee casting or prolonged immobilization of simple dislocations may lead to joint stiffness and limited function.

712. The answer is D. *(Rockwood, Green, pp 2145–2149.)* The radiographs show a Lisfranc dislocation. The prognosis following this injury is directly related to obtaining and maintaining reduction of the tarsometatarsal joints during the healing period. Therefore, simple cast immobilization or closed reduction and cast immobilization are inadequate treatments. Although closed reduction is possible, it is the exception rather than the rule; ORIF is the best means of assuring anatomic reduction and rigid stabilization. Arthrodesis of the tarsometatarsal joints is a salvage procedure.

713. The answer is D. *(Rockwood, Green, pp 494–497.)* The radiographs reveal a displaced Bennett's fracture. Although many treatment methods have been used, the principle underlying all of them is reduction of the articular surface. It is extremely difficult to achieve and maintain this reduction without some form of skeletal fixation. The treatment of choice is closed reduction and percutaneous pin fixation with Kirschner wires, followed by immobilization in a thumb spica cast for 4 to 6 weeks. If closed reduction cannot be achieved, open reduction is indicated. Internal fixation may be attained with minifragment screws rather than Kirschner wires, but the fracture does not invite application of a plate.

714. The answer is B. *(Harper, J Bone Joint Surg 70-A:1348–1356, 1988.)* The radiographs show a trimalleolar fracture of the ankle with a small (less than 20 percent of the articular surface) posterior malleolar fracture. Because of the intact ligamentous attachments between the posterior malleolar and distal fibular fracture fragments, reduction and fixation of the fibular fracture will also stabilize the posterior malleolar fracture. Furthermore, reduction of a posterior malleolar fracture containing less than 25 percent of the articular surface is not necessary.

715. The answer is D. *(Browner, pp 1121–1122.)* Figures *A* and *B* show a synostosis between the proximal radius and ulna; figure *C* shows increased uptake of the radioisotope at this site. The synostosis is firmly established; therefore, continued observation or administration of indomethacin will not result in dissolution of the heterotopic bone. Although resection of a synostosis in the proximal third of the forearm carries a risk of neurologic and vascular injury, it can be performed and will improve forearm rotation. Excision, with or without interposition of muscle, fat, or silicone, may be considered when serial bone scans show maturity of the heterotopic bone.

716. The answer is B. *(Browner, pp 1846–1849.)* The radiographs show good alignment of the fracture with delayed union. The fibula is united, so malalignment following removal of the distal interlocking screws is unlikely. Although posterolateral bone grafting, electrical stimulation, or exchange intramedullary nailing might stimulate fracture healing, removal of the distal interlocking screw is the simplest way to promote union in this patient.

717. The answer is C. *(Browner, pp 1910–1915.)* A high fracture of the fibula associated with rupture of the tibiofibular syndesmosis results primarily from external rotation of the foot on the leg. A direct blow to the fibula could produce a similar fibular fracture, but the syndesmosis would have remained intact.

718. The answer is C. *(Browner, p 1944.)* It is vital to carefully inspect the radiographs of a patient with a presumed lateral ankle sprain. Osteochondral fractures may be present on either the lateral or medial talar dome. Avulsion of the base of the fifth metatarsal may occur as may avulsion of the tip of the lateral malleolus. Fracture of the anterior process of the calcaneus may simulate a lateral ankle sprain, as may a fracture of the lateral process of the talus. The sustentaculum tali is a medial structure and is not injured by inversion of the ankle.

719. The answer is D. *(Browner, p 1944.)* Forceful inversion of the ankle may result in injury of the peroneal nerve, rupture of the skin over the lateral malleolus, delayed compartmental syndrome, and tearing of the lateral ankle ligaments. Rupture of the peroneal tendons has not been reported with inversion injuries to the ankle.

720. The answer is E. *(Browner, pp 1947–1948.)* Ruptures of the Achilles' tendon are usually caused by forced dorsiflexion of the plantarflexed foot. Patients are usually middle-aged men, and ruptures commonly occur during high-demand sports such as basketball or tennis. Examination of a patient with an acute rupture of the Achilles' tendon usually demonstrates a defect in the heel cord, tenderness, and weakness in plantar flexion of the ankle. The *Thompson* test is performed by manually squeezing the calf, a maneuver that normally produces passive plantar flexion of the ankle. The *Thomas* test is a test for flexion contracture of the hip.

721. The answer is C. *(Browner, pp 1010–1014.)* Although most mallet-finger fractures may be treated successfully by nonoperative means, operation is indicated if the injury results in volar subluxation of the distal phalanx. Other less definite surgical indications include widely displaced fractures involving 50 percent or more of the articular surface, impaction injuries at the base of the distal phalanx, and displaced fractures of the thumb's interphalangeal joint. Physeal injuries in children are generally treated nonoperatively.

722. The answer is D. *(Browner, pp 1002–1004.)* Fractures of the distal phalangeal tuft are common and may be exceptionally painful, as there is little room for fracture hematoma within the pulp space. Release of the subungual hematoma and application of a protective splint are the only treatments needed for closed injuries. Open fractures may lacerate the nail bed or nail plate, which should be repaired. The fingertip is likely to be tender for months following injury. Radiographic union may take 6 months to a year.

723. The answer is C. *(Browner, p 1017.)* A dorsal dislocation of the metacarpophalangeal joint in which reduction is blocked by soft-tissue interposition is referred to as a "complex dislocation." Kaplan and others have suggested that the metacarpal head is trapped between the flexor tendon and the lumbrical muscle and therefore recommend a volar surgical approach. However, it is the palmar plate, still attached to the dorsally displaced proximal phalanx, that becomes wedged between the joint surfaces and prevents closed reduction, making a dorsal surgical approach safer and more straightforward.

724. The answer is C. *(Browner, pp 1017–1018.)* A completely torn ulnar collateral ligament is often displaced proximally, with the aponeurosis of the adductor muscle interposed between the ligament and its insertion. This interposition prevents anatomic reduction of the ligament by closed means and may impede healing, resulting in chronic instability of the thumb MCP joint. Surgical exploration is indicated if complete ligamentous disruption is suspected.

725. The answer is D. *(Browner, pp 1025–1027.)* Fractures of the scaphoid generally occur by an axial load applied to the radial half of the dorsiflexed wrist. It is surmised that the proximal pole of the scaphoid is fixed by the radius proximally, dorsally, and radially, and by the capitate and lunate ulnarly. At the same time, the distal pole is free to translate dorsally with the distal row of carpal bones, which results in fracture through the waist of the scaphoid. The palmar aspect of the bone fails in tension and the dorsal aspect in compression.

726. The answer is B. *(Browner, pp 1034–1036.)* Vascular studies have established that fractures through the proximal one-third of the scaphoid are likely to devascularize the proximal fragment because most of the blood supply enters the bone distal to this level. Nonetheless, if seen early, minimally displaced fractures of the proximal pole should be treated with a thumb spica cast until the outcome is obvious. The patient should also be cautioned that the fracture has a significant risk of nonunion. If nonunion or delayed union occurs, a cancellous bone graft with internal fixation is recommended.

727. The answer is C. *(Browner, pp 1948–1949.)* Acute ruptures of the posterior tibial tendon are difficult to diagnose and are frequently unrecognized for long periods of time. Complete ruptures that have been diagnosed early can be repaired with augmentation from the adjacent toe flexors. Cast immobilization does not result in functional healing of the ruptured tendon. Subtalar or triple arthrodesis should be reserved for patients with old, symptomatic posterior tibial tendon ruptures unresponsive to nonoperative measures.

728. The answer is D. *(Browner, pp 937–948.)* Crossed or intramedullary Kirschner wires and intraosseous wires have proved effective in the treatment of transverse phalangeal fractures. Although usually reserved for fractures with significant soft-tissue injuries, external skeletal fixation would provide good stabilization in a simple, closed transverse injury. Although lag screw fixation of phalangeal shaft fractures is effective for long oblique or spiral fractures, it is not applicable to simple transverse fractures of the phalangeal shaft. For fixation by screws alone, the length of the fracture line should be at least twice the diameter of the bone.

729. The answer is D. *(Browner, pp 1960–1964.)* A nondisplaced talar neck fracture requires rigid stabilization to prevent displacement and to lower the risk of avascular necrosis. In addition, early motion of the ankle and subtalar joints is beneficial to the articular cartilage and to the overall rehabilitation of the foot. Kirschner wires do not provide sufficient stabilization. Treatment of a nondisplaced talar neck fracture in a cast precludes early motion and should be considered only as a temporary measure. The ideal treatment for a nondisplaced or minimally displaced fracture is percutaneous screw fixation with one or two screws placed posteriorly to anteriorly.

730. The answer is E. *(Torg, Am J Sports Med 18:50–57, 1990.)* Analysis of injury films in high school and college football indicated that axial compression was the most common mechanism of cervical spine injury. In 1976, spearing was outlawed in high school and college football. The National Football Head and Neck Injury Registry then documented a marked decrease in the incidence of quadriplegia and cervical fractures from 1976 through 1984. Strength training, conditioning, and use of neck rolls are not effective in decreasing the risk of cervical spine injury; instruction in proper tackling technique remains the most effective means to decrease the rate of cervical spine injuries in football.

731. The answer is C. *(Torg, Am J Sports Med 18:50–57, 1990.)* Analysis in the early 1970s of cervical spine injuries in high school and college football revealed that the majority of these resulted from axial loading with the neck slightly flexed. This position straightens the normal lordotic curve of the cervical spine and allows it to be loaded as a column, producing an axial loading injury. Results of this investigation were used to outlaw use of the top of the helmet as the initial point of contact in high school and college football.

732. The answer is C. *(Petty, J Bone Joint Surg 67-A:1236–1244, 1985.)* Implantation of any foreign material lowers the host's resistance to infection. Microorganisms may exist in a relatively sheltered environment adjacent to the foreign body. In experimental studies, PMMA was found to be associated with a higher incidence of infection than other materials. This is thought to be related to the in vivo polymerization of the material and to heat-induced tissue necrosis.

733. The answer is D. *(Browner, pp 137–138.)* In an otherwise healthy individual, without preexisting cardiac or renal failure, the best indicator of adequate fluid resuscitation is a urine output of greater than 50 mL/h, which indicates adequate renal blood flow. The hematocrit indicates red cell mass only, takes time to equilibrate, and is not useful in the early resuscitation of the trauma patient. In the otherwise healthy patient with mild hypovolemia, pulse and blood pressure may be initially maintained, making them less useful as sensitive indicators of hypovolemia.

734. The answer is B. *(Chapman, pp 179–202.)* The optimal pressure for a tourniquet is the lowest possible pressure that will prevent arterial inflow to a limb. Higher pressures may result in an increased incidence of ischemic nerve injury and resultant tourniquet palsy. The optimal pressure for a lower limb tourniquet appears to be 100 to 150 mmHg above systolic blood pressure. Lower pressures may not stop arterial inflow, and higher pressures increase the chance of nerve injury.

735. The answer is A. *(Browner, pp 1257–1261.)* Three-part fractures of the proximal humerus constitute 3 to 29 percent of displaced proximal humeral fractures without a dislocation. In this case, the fracture is minimally displaced. Nonoperative management of these fractures with a sling and early physical therapy is the treatment of choice. Open reduction and internal fixation are indicated for displaced fractures unless osteoporosis or other bone conditions preclude secure fixation.

736. The answer is C. *(Rockwood, Green, pp 1708–1710.)* Most patients with infection develop drainage from a sinus tract or from the surgical incision. Most surgeons recommend the intramedullary device be retained if it provides rigid fracture stabilization. Debridement and culture of infected tissues is required to drain abscesses or remove sequestra and infected soft tissue. Culture of the drainage is not adequate, since contamination with skin flora commonly occurs. Most femoral fractures heal within 4 to 6 months, even in the presence of infection, so suppression of the infection with antibiotics is indicated until the fracture heals, at which time the intramedullary nail may be removed.

737–742. The answers are 737–B, 738–D, 739–C, 740–E, 741–B, 742–A. *(Browner, pp 589–591.)* Central cord syndrome is the most common pattern of injury and represents central gray matter destruction with preservation of only the peripheral spinal cord structures, most notably the spinothalamic and corticospinal tracts. The patient is usually quadriplegic, with intact perianal sensation, and has an early return of bowel and bladder control. The chance of functional motor recovery has been estimated to be 75 percent; return of motor function begins with the sacral elements and progresses upward.

Posterior cord syndrome is the rarest syndrome and consists of loss of deep pressure, deep pain, and proprioception, with otherwise normal spinal cord functions. The neurologic deficits are similar to those seen in tabes dorsalis; a patient with posterior cord syndrome will have a characteristic foot-slapping gait.

The patient with anterior cord syndrome has complete motor and sensory loss except for retained proprioception in the trunk and lower limbs, which is the opposite anatomically from the posterior cord syndrome. This syndrome has the worst prognosis for return of function with only a 10 percent chance of functional motor recovery.

The Brown-Séquard syndrome is based anatomically on a unilateral cord injury such as that produced by a bullet wound. It is characterized by an ipsilateral motor deficit in combination with contralateral pain and temperature hypesthesia. Almost all patients show partial recovery.

A complete cord syndrome is defined by the absence of neurologic function caudal to the spinal cord injury in the presence of an intact bulbocavernosus reflex. The bulbocavernosus reflex indicates that the S3–4 region of the conus medullaris is functional (i.e., spinal shock is not present). Ninety-nine percent of patients have return of the bulbocavernosus reflex within 24 h; the presence of a complete or incomplete neurologic deficit can be determined at this time.

Bibliography

Aisen ML (ed): *Orthotics in Neurologic Rehabilitation.* New York, Demos, 1992.

Albright JA, Brand RA (eds): *The Scientific Basis of Orthopaedics,* 2/e. East Norwalk, CT, Appleton & Lange, 1987.

Allison AE (ed): *Athletic Training and Sports Medicine.* Park Ridge, IL, American Academy of Orthopaedic Surgeons, 1986.

Anderson JE (ed): *Grant's Atlas of Anatomy,* 8/e. Baltimore, Williams & Wilkins, 1983.

Arntz CT, Beith CJ, Hansen ST: Fractures and fracture-dislocations of the tarsometatarsal joint. *J Bone Joint Surg* 70-A:173–181, 1988.

Baker AS, Dove J: Progressive scoliosis as the presenting sign of syringomyelia. *J Bone Joint Surg* 65-B: 472–473, 1983.

Barrow G, Sahos D: Menstrual irregularity and stress fractures in female distance runners. *Am J Sports Med* 16:209–216, 1988.

Bernick SM: Dental emergencies. *Clin Pediatr* 9:487–491, 1980.

Boden SD, Wiesel SW, Laws ER Jr, Rothman RH (eds): *The Aging Spine.* Philadelphia, Saunders, 1991.

Bone L, Bucholz R: The management of fractures in the patient with multiple trauma. *J Bone Joint Surg* 68-A:945–949, 1986.

Bone LB, Chapman MW: Initial management of the patient with multiple injuries. *Instr Course Lect* 37:557–563, 1986.

Bordelon L (ed): *Surgical and Conservative Foot Care.* Thorofare, NJ, Slack, 1988.

Bowker JH, Michael JW (eds): *Atlas of Limb Prosthetics: Surgical, Prosthetic, and Rehabilitation Principles,* 2/e. St. Louis, Mosby Yearbook, 1992.

Brandt KD (ed): *Cartilage Changes in Osteoarthritis.* Indianapolis, Indiana University School of Medicine, 1990.

Brighton CT: Longitudinal bone growth: The growth plate and its dysfunctions. *Instr Course Lect* 33:3–25, 1984.

Browner BD, Jupiter JB, Levine AM, Trafton PG (eds): *Skeletal Trauma.* Philadelphia, Saunders, 1992.

Bunch WH, et al (eds): *Atlas of Orthotics,* 2/e. St. Louis, Mosby, 1985.

Cantu R: Guidelines for return to sports after cerebral concussion. *Phys Sports Med* 14:76–80, 1986.

Caudle RJ, Crawford AH: Avulsion fracture of the lateral acetabular margin: A case report. *J Bone Joint Surg* 70-A:1568–1570, 1988.

Chan WP, Lang P, Genant HK (eds): *MRI of the Musculoskeletal System.* Philadelphia, Saunders, 1994.

Coleman SS, Chestnut WJ: A simple test for hindfoot flexibility in the cavovarus foot. *Clin Orthop* 123:60–68, 1977.

Cotran RS, Kumar V, Robbins SL (eds): *Pathologic Basis of Disease,* 5/e. Philadelphia, Saunders, 1994.

Cruess RL, Rennie WRJ (eds): *Adult Orthopaedics.* New York, Churchill Livingstone, 1984.

Dirschl DR: Acute hematogenous osteomyelitis in children. *Orthop Rev* 23:305–312, 1994.

Edwards G, Jupiter JB: The Essex-Lopresti lesion revisited. *Clin Orthop* 234:61–66, 1988.

Enzinger FM, Weiss SW (eds): *Soft Tissue Tumors,* 3/e. St. Louis, Mosby, 1995.

Epstein HC: Posterior fracture-dislocations of the hip: Long-term follow-up. *J Bone Joint Surg* 56-A:1103–1129, 1974.

Evarts CM (ed): *Surgery of the Musculoskeletal System*, 2/e. New York, Churchill Livingstone, 1990.

Favus MJ (ed): *Primer on the Metabolic Bone Diseases and Disorders of Mineral Metabolism*. Kelseyville, CA, American Society for Bone and Mineral Research, 1990.

Fitzgerald RH (ed): *Orthopaedic Knowledge Update 2*. Park Ridge, IL, American Academy of Orthopaedic Surgeons, 1987.

Friedlaender GE, Goldberg VM (eds): *Bone and Cartilage Allografts*. Park Ridge, IL, American Academy of Orthopaedic Surgeons, 1991.

Frymoyer JW (ed): *The Adult Spine: Principles and Practice*. Philadelphia, Saunders, 1992.

Frymoyer JW, Gordon SL (eds): *New Perspectives on Low Back Pain*. Rosemont, IL, American Academy of Orthopaedic Surgeons, 1988.

Gamble JG (ed): *The Musculoskeletal System: Physiological Basics*. New York, Raven, 1988.

Gelberman RH, Eaton R, Urbaniak JR: Peripheral nerve compression. *J Bone Joint Surg* 75-A:1854–1878, 1993.

Gelberman RH, Wolock BS, Siegel DB: Current concepts review: Fractures and non-unions of the carpal scaphoid. *J Bone Joint Surg* 71-A:1560–1565, 1989.

Gilman AG, Rall TW, Nies AS, Taylor P (eds): *The Pharmacologic Basis of Therapeutics*, 8/e. New York, Pergamon, 1990.

Gonzales P, Lomar SJ: Calcaneo-navicular coalition treated by resection and interposition of the extensor digitorum brevis muscle. *J Bone Joint Surg* 72-A:7179, 1990.

Green DP (ed): *Operative Hand Surgery*, 3/e. New York, Churchill Livingstone, 1993.

Greenspan A (ed): *Orthopaedic Radiology: A Practical Approach*. Philadelphia, Lippincott, 1988.

Harper MC, Harden G: Posterior malleolar fractures of the ankle associated with external rotation-abduction injuries. *J Bone Joint Surg* 70-A:1348–1356, 1988.

Hawkins RJ, Neer CS, Pianta RM, Mendosa FX: Locked posterior dislocation of the shoulder. *J Bone Joint Surg* 69-A:9–16, 1987.

Helal B, Chin SC, Lweybu G: Rupture of the extensor pollicis longus and undisplaced Colles' type of fracture. *Hand* 14:41–47, 1982.

Henry JH, Golutz TH: Lateral retinacular release in patellofemoral subluxation. *Am J Sports Med* 14:221, 1986.

Hershman EB, Asa JW, Bergfeld JA: Acute brachial neuropathy in athletes. *Am J Sports Med* 13:655–659, 1989.

Hollinshead WH, Rosse C (eds): *Textbook of Anatomy*, 4/e. Philadelphia, Harper & Row, 1985.

Hoppenfeld S: *Orthopaedic Neurology*. Philadelphia, Lippincott, 1977.

Hoppenfeld S, deBoer P: *Surgical Exposures in Orthopaedics*. Philadelphia, Lippincott, 1984.

Hotchkiss RN, Weiland AJ: Valgus stability of the elbow. *J Orthop Res* 5:372–377, 1987.

Hougard K, Thomsen PB: Coxarthrosis following traumatic posterior dislocation of the hip. *J Bone Joint Surg* 69-A:679–683, 1987.

Jenkins DB (ed): *Hollinshead's Functional Anatomy of the Limbs and Back*, 6/e. Philadelphia, Saunders, 1991.

Jokl P, Konstadt S: The effect of limb immobilization on muscle function and protein composition. *Clin Orthop* 174:222–229, 1983.

Josefsson PO, Gentz CF, Johnell O, et al: Surgical versus non-surgical treatment of ligamentous injuries following dislocation of the elbow joint. *J Bone Joint Surg* 69-A:605–608, 1987.

Kelley WN, Harris Jr ED, Ruddy S, Sledge CB (eds): *Textbook of Rheumatology*. Philadelphia, Saunders, 1989.

Kretzler HH, Richardson HB: Rupture of the pectoralis major muscle. *Am J Sports Med* 17:453–458, 1989.

Kuland, DW: *The Injured Athlete*. Philadelphia, Lippincott, 1982.

Lonstein JE, Carlson JM: Prediction of curve progression in untreated idiopathic scoliosis during growth. *J Bone Joint Surg* 66-A:1061–1071, 1984.

Lovell WW, Winter RB (eds): *Pediatric Orthopaedics*, 2/e. Philadelphia, Lippincott, 1986.

Macy LR, Benirschke SK, Sangeorzan BJ, Hansen ST: Acute calcaneal fractures: Treatment options and results. *J Am Acad Orthop Surg* 2:36–43, 1994.

Maddox K, Moore E, Feliciaro D, et al (eds): *Trauma*. East Norwalk, CT, Appelton & Lange, 1988.

Mann RA: Decision-making in bunion surgery. *Instr Course Lect* 39:3–13, 1990.

Miller MD: *Review of Orthopaedics*. Philadelphia, Saunders, 1992.

Mirra JM (ed): *Bone Tumors: Clinical, Radiologic, and*

Pathologic Correlations. Philadelphia, Lea & Febiger, 1989.

Morrissy RT (ed): *Lovell and Winter's Pediatric Orthopaedics*, 3/e. Philadelphia, Lippincott, 1990.

Mow VC, Hayes WC (eds): *Basic Orthopaedic Biomechanics*. New York, Raven, 1991.

Neer CS III, Watson KC, Stanton FJ: Recent experience in total shoulder replacement. *J Bone Joint Surg* 64-A:331–337, 1982.

Norkin CC, Levangie PK (eds): *Joint Structure and Function*. Philadelphia, Davis, 1992.

Oppenheim WL: Selective posterior rhizotomy in the treatment of spastic cerebral palsy. *Clin Orthop* 253:20–29, 1990.

Ovadia DN, Chess JL: Intraoperative and post-operative subtrochanteric fracture of the femur associated with removal of a Zickel nail. *J Bone Joint Surg* 70-A: 239–243, 1988.

Pape H, Regel F, Dwenger A, Crumm K, et al: Influences of different methods of intramedullary femoral nailing on lung function in patients with multiple trauma. *J Trauma* 35:709–716, 1993.

Pappas AN: Congenital posteromedial bowing of the tibia and fibula. *J Pediatr Orthop* 4:525–531, 1984.

Patzakis MJ, Wilins J: Surgical findings in clenched fist injuries. *Clin Orthop* 220:237–240, 1987.

Petty W, Spanier S, Shuster JJ, et al: The influence of skeletal implants on the incidence of infection: Experiments in a canine model. *J Bone Joint Surg* 67-A:1236–1244, 1985.

Pfeffer GB, Frey CC: *Current Practice in Foot and Ankle Surgery,* vol 1. New York, McGraw-Hill, 1993.

Phillips WA, Hensinger RN: The management of rotatory atlantoaxial subluxation in children. *J Bone Joint Surg* 71-A:664–668, 1989.

Pirone NA, Graham HK, Krajbick JE: Management of displaced extension type supracondylar fractures of the humerus in children. *J Bone Joint Surg* 70-A: 641–650, 1988.

Poss R, et al (eds): *Orthopaedic Knowledge Update 3*. Park Ridge, IL, American Academy of Orthopaedic Surgeons, 1990.

Rockwood CA, Green DP, Bucholz RW (eds): *Fractures in Adults*, 3/e. Philadelphia, Lippincott, 1991.

Rockwood CA, Matsen FA (eds): *The Shoulder*. Philadelphia, Saunders, 1990.

Rockwood CA, Wilkins KE, King RE (eds): *Fractures in Children*, 3/e. Philadelphia, Lippincott, 1991.

Roge JR, Simpson GP, McLone DG: Pediatric spinal injury in the very young. *J Neurosurg* 68:25–30, 1988.

Rothman RH, Simeone FA (eds): *The Spine,* 3/e. Philadelphia, Saunders, 1992.

Rubin E, Farber JL (eds): *Pathology,* 2/e. Philadelphia, Lippincott, 1994.

Samuelsson L, Skoog M: Ambulation in patients with myelomeningocele. *J Pediatr Orthop* 8:569–575, 1988.

Sandberg R, Dalkfers B, Nilsson B, et al: Operative versus non-operative treatment of recent injuries to the ligaments of the knee. *J Bone Joint Surg* 69-A:1120–1126, 1987.

Sanders R, Swiontkowski M, Nunley J, Spiegel P: The management of fractures with soft tissue disruptions. *J Bone Joint Surg* 75-A:778–789, 1993.

Schmalzried TP, Jasty M, Harris WH: Periprosthetic bone loss in total hip arthroplasty. *J Bone Joint Surg* 74-A:849–863, 1992.

Shapiro F, Specht L: The diagnosis and orthopaedic treatment of childhood spinal muscular atrophy, peripheral neuropathy, Friedreich ataxia, and arthrogryposis. *J Bone Joint Surg* 75-A:1699–1714, 1993.

Shapiro F, Specht L: The diagnosis and orthopaedic treatment of inherited muscular diseases of childhood. *J Bone Joint Surg* 75-A:439–454, 1993.

Sherk HH, Dunn EJ, Eismont FJ, et al (eds): *The Cervical Spine*, 2/e. Philadelphia, Lippincott, 1989.

Smith SR, Bronk JR, Kelly PJ: Effect of fracture fixation on cortical bone blood flow. *J Orthop Res* 8:471–478, 1990.

Sullivan JA, Grana WA (eds): *The Pediatric Athlete*. Park Ridge, IL, American Academy of Orthopaedic Surgeons, 1990.

Swiontkowski MF: Ipsilateral femoral shaft and hip fractures. *Orthop Clin North Am* 18:73–84, 1987.

Tachdjian MO (ed): *Pediatric Orthopaedics*, 2/e. Philadelphia, Saunders, 1990.

Tencer AF, Johnson KB, Johnston DWC, et al: A biomechanical comparison of various methods of stabilization of subtrochanteric fractures of the femur. *J Orthop Res* 2:297–305, 1984.

Tencer AF, Johnson KD, Kyle RF, Fu FH: Biomechanics of fractures and fracture fixation. *Instr Course Lect* 42:19–55, 1993.

Torg JS, Vagso JJ, O'Neill MJ, et al: The epidemiologic, pathologic, biomechanical, and cinematographic analysis of football-induced cervical spine trauma. *Am J Sports Med* 18:50–57, 1990.

Veitch JM, Omer GE: Treatment of cat bite injuries of the hand. *J Trauma* 19:201–202, 1989.

Vota S, Ewing J, Fleissner P, et al: Ankle arthroscopy: Neurovascular and arthroscopic anatomy of standard and trans-Achilles tendon portal placement. *Arthroscopy* 5:41–52, 1989.

Warren LF, Marshall, JL: The supporting structures and layers on the medial side of the knee. *J Bone Joint Surg* 61-A:56–62, 1979.

Wilson FC (ed): *The Musculoskeletal System*, 2/e. Philadelphia, Lippincott, 1983.

Wilson FC, Fay GF, LaMotte P, Williams JC: Triple arthrodesis. A study of the factors affecting fusion in 301 cases. *J Bone Joint Surg* 47-A:340–348, 1965.

Woodburne RT, et al (eds): *The Ciba Collection of Medical Illustrations,* vol 8. Summit, NJ, Ciba-Geigy Corporation, 1987.

Yates C, Grana WA: Patello-femoral pain. A prospective study. *Orthopaedics* 9:663, 1986.

NOTES

NOTES

NOTES

NOTES

NOTES

NOTES

NOTES

ISBN 0-07-052076-3
90000>
9 780070 520769